Mastering Health Data Science Using R

This book provides a practical, application-driven guide to using R for public health and health data science, accessible to both beginners and those with some coding experience. Each module starts with data as the driver of analysis before introducing and breaking down step-by-step the programming concepts needed to tackle the analysis. This book aims to equip readers with a practical and approachable programming guide tailored to those in health-related fields. Going beyond simple R examples, the programming principles and skills developed will give readers the ability to apply R skills to their own research needs. Practical case studies in public health are provided throughout to reinforce learning.

Topics include data structures in R, exploratory analysis, distributions, hypothesis testing, regression analysis, and larger scale programming with functions and control flows. The presentation focuses on implementation with R and assumes readers have had an introduction to probability, statistical inference, and regression analysis.

Key features:

- Includes practical case studies.
- Explains how to write larger programs.
- Contains additional information on Quarto.

Alice Paul is Assistant Professor of Biostatistics and Teaching Scholar, holding a Ph.D. in Operations Research from Cornell University. With 6 years of experience at the undergraduate, master's, and Ph.D. levels, she instructed students in diverse fields, including biostatistics, engineering, computer science, and data science at Brown University and Olin College of Engineering.

Mastering Health Data Science Using R

Alice Paul

CRC Press
Taylor & Francis Group
Boca Raton London New York

CRC Press is an imprint of the
Taylor & Francis Group, an **informa** business

A CHAPMAN & HALL BOOK

Designed cover image: Alice Paul

First edition published 2025
by CRC Press
2385 NW Executive Center Drive, Suite 320, Boca Raton FL 33431

and by CRC Press
4 Park Square, Milton Park, Abingdon, Oxon, OX14 4RN

CRC Press is an imprint of Taylor & Francis Group, LLC

ISBN: 978-1-032-72936-7 (hbk)
ISBN: 978-1-032-72993-0 (pbk)
ISBN: 978-1-003-42338-6 (ebk)

DOI: 10.1201/9781003423386

Typeset in Latin Modern font
by KnowledgeWorks Global Ltd.

Publisher's Note: This book has been prepared from camera-ready copy provided by the author.

To my students, who inspire me to grow and learn every day. And to my husband, whose endless support has made every endeavor possible.

Contents

Preface

This book serves as an interactive introduction to R for public health and health data science students. Topics include data structures in R, exploratory analysis, distributions, hypothesis testing, regression analysis, and larger scale programming with functions and control flows. The presentation assumes knowledge with the underlying methodology and focuses instead on how to use R to implement your analysis.

This book is written using Quarto Book. You can download the Quarto files used to generate this book or a corresponding Jupyter Notebook from the GitHub repository[1]. The GitHub repository also contains a few cheat sheets[2].

Acknowledgments

This book was written with the support of a Data Science Institute Seed Grant[3]. Thanks to students Thomas Arnold, Hannah Eglinton, Jialin Liu, Joanna Walsh, and Xinbei Yu for their help and feedback. Please contact Dr. Paul (alice_paul@brown.edu) with questions, suggested edits, or feedback.

---

[1]https://github.com/alicepaul/health-data-science-using-r
[2]https://github.com/alicepaul/health-data-science-using-r/tree/main/book/refs
[3]https://dsi.brown.edu/

Part I

Introduction to R

1

Getting Started with R

This chapter introduces you to R as a programming language and shows you how we can use this language in two different ways: directly through the R Console, and using the RStudio development environment. To start, you need to download R[1] and RStudio[2].

1.1 Why R?

What are some of the benefits of using R?

- R is built for statisticians and data analysts.

- R is open source.

- R has most of the latest statistical methods available.

- R is flexible.

Since R is designed for statisticians, it is built with data in mind. This comes in handy when we want to streamline how we process and analyze data. It also means that many statisticians working on new methods are publishing user-created packages in R, so R users have access to most methods of interest. R is also an interpreted language, which means that we do not have to compile our code into machine language first; this allows for simpler syntax and more flexibility when writing our code, which also makes it a great first programming language to learn.

Python is another interpreted language often used for data analysis. Both languages feature simple and flexible syntax, but while Python is more broadly developed for usage outside of data science and statistical analyses, R is a great programming language for those in health data science. I use both languages and find switching between them to be straightforward, but I do prefer R for anything related to data or statistical analysis.

---

[1] https://cran.rstudio.com/
[2] https://posit.co/download/rstudio-desktop/

1.1.1   Installation of R and RStudio

To run R on your computer, you need to download and install R[3]. This allows
you to open the R application and run R code interactively. However, to get
the most out of programming with R, you should install RStudio, which is
an integrated development environment (IDE) for R. RStudio offers a nice
environment for writing, editing, running, and debugging R code.

Each chapter in this book is written as a Quarto document and can also be
downloaded as a Jupyter notebook. You can open Quarto files in RStudio to
run the code as you read and complete the practice questions and exercises.

1.2   The R Console

The R Console provides our first intro to code in R. Figure 1.1 shows the
console's appearance when opened. You should see a blinking cursor; this is
where we can write our first line of code!

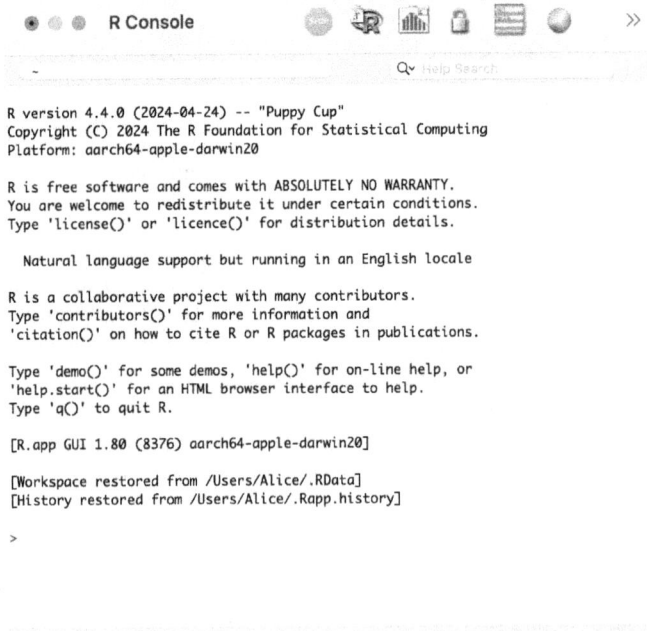

```
R version 4.4.0 (2024-04-24) -- "Puppy Cup"
Copyright (C) 2024 The R Foundation for Statistical Computing
Platform: aarch64-apple-darwin20

R is free software and comes with ABSOLUTELY NO WARRANTY.
You are welcome to redistribute it under certain conditions.
Type 'license()' or 'licence()' for distribution details.

  Natural language support but running in an English locale

R is a collaborative project with many contributors.
Type 'contributors()' for more information and
'citation()' on how to cite R or R packages in publications.

Type 'demo()' for some demos, 'help()' for on-line help, or
'help.start()' for an HTML browser interface to help.
Type 'q()' to quit R.

[R.app GUI 1.80 (8376) aarch64-apple-darwin20]

[Workspace restored from /Users/Alice/.RData]
[History restored from /Users/Alice/.Rapp.history]

>
```

Figure 1.1: The R Console.

---

[3]https://cran.rstudio.com/

To start, type 2+3 and press ENTER. You should see that 5 is printed below that code and that your cursor is moved to the next line.

1.2.1 Basic Computations and Objects

In the previous example, we coded a simple addition. Try out some other basic calculations using the following operators :

- Addition: 5+6

- Subtraction: 7-2

- Multiplication: 2*3

- Division: 6/3

- Exponentiation: 4^2

- Modulo: 100 %% 4

For example, use the modulo operator to find what 100 mod 4 is. It should return 0 since 100 is divisible by 4.

If we want to save the result of any computation, we need to create an object to store our value of interest. An **object** is simply a named data structure that allows us to reference that data structure. Objects are also commonly called **variables**. In the following code, we create an object x which stores the value 5 using the assignment operator <-. The assignment operator assigns whatever is on the right-hand side of the operator to the name on the left-hand side. We can now reference x by calling its name. Additionally, we can update its value by adding 1. In the second line of code, the computer first finds the value of the right-hand side by finding the current value of x before adding 1 and assigning it back to x.

```
x <- 2+3
x <- x+1
x
#> [1] 6
```

We can create and store multiple objects by using different names. The following code creates a new object y that is one more than the value of x. We can see that the value of x is still 5 after running this code.

```
x <- 2+3
y <- x
```

```
y <- y + 1
x
#> [1] 5
```

1.2.2   Naming Conventions

As we start creating objects, we want to make sure we use good object names. Here are a few tips for naming objects effectively:

- Stick to a single format. We use **snake_case**, which uses underscores between words (e.g., `my_var`, `class_year`).

- Make your names useful. Try to avoid using names that are too long (e.g., `which_day_of_the_week`) or that do not contain enough information (e.g., `x1`, `x2`, `x3`).

- Replace unexplained numeric values with named objects. For example, if you need to do some calculations using 100 as the number of participants, create an object `n_part` with value 100 rather than repeatedly using the number. This makes the code easy to update and helps the user avoid possible errors.

1.3   RStudio and Quarto

If we made a mistake in the code we typed in the console, we would have to re-enter everything from the beginning. However, when we write code, we often want to be able to run it multiple times and develop it in stages. R Scripts and R Markdown files allow us to save all of our R code in files that we can update and re-run, which allows us to create reproducible and easy-to-share analyses. We now move to RStudio as our development environment to demonstrate creating an R Script. When you open RStudio, there are multiple windows. Start by opening a new R file by going to File -> New File -> R Script. You should now see several windows as outlined in Figure 1.2.

1.3.1   Panes

There are four panes shown by default:

- **Source Pane** - used for editing code files such as R Scripts or Quarto documents.

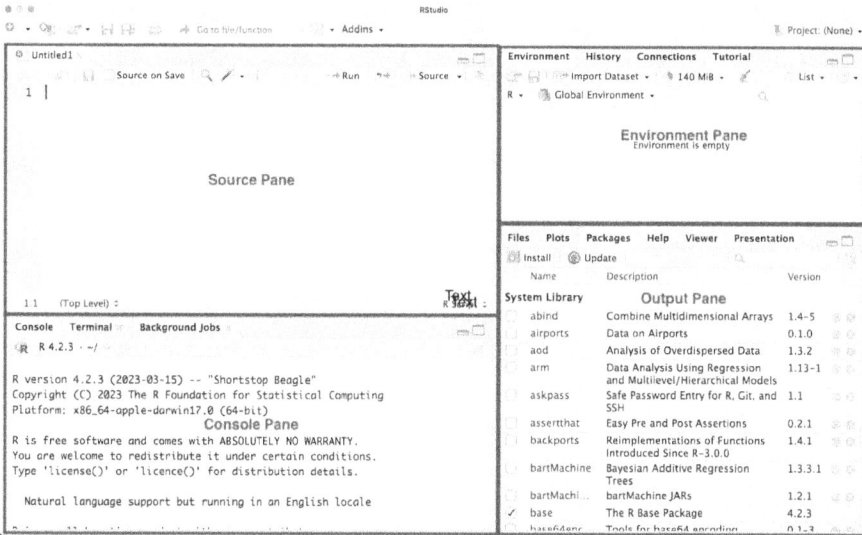

Figure 1.2: RStudio Layout and Panes.

- **Console Pane** - used to show the live R session.

- **Environment Pane** - contains the Environment and History tabs, used to keep track of the current state.

- **Output Pane** - contains the Plots and Packages tabs.

The source pane is the code editor window in the top left. This shows your currently blank R Script. Add the following code to your .R file and save the file as "test.R". Note that here we used snake_case to name our objects!

```
# Calculate primary care physician to specialist ratio
pcp_phys <- c(6300, 1080, 9297, 16433)
spec_phys <- c(6750, 837, 10517, 22984)
pcp_spec_ratio <- 1000 * pcp_phys / spec_phys
```

The first line starts with # and does not contain any code. This is a **comment** line, which allows us to add context, intent, or extra information to help the reader understand our code. A good rule of thumb is that we want to write enough comments so that we could open our code in 6 months and be able to understand what we were doing. As we develop longer chunks of code, this will become more important.

Unlike when we type code into the console, we can write multiple lines of code in our R Script without running them. In order to run the code in the script, we need to tell RStudio we are ready to run it. To run a single line of code,

we can either hit Ctrl+Enter when on that line or we can hit the Run button
⇢ Run ▾ at the top right of the source pane. This copies the code to the R
Console. Try this out to run the first line of code that defines `pcp_phys`. You
can see that the line of code has been run in the console pane. Now check your
environment pane. You should see that you have a new object representing
the one we just created. This pane keeps track of all current objects. Run the
second line of code and see how the environment updates. If you look at the
History tab within this pane, you see the history of R commands run.

If we want to run all lines of code in our script, we can use the Source button
⇥ Source . Before we do this, we will clear our environment. You can do this by

clicking the broom 🖌 in the environment pane, which deletes all objects in
the environment. Alternatively, you can go to Session -> Restart R in the main
menu, which restarts your whole R session. After clearing your environment,
click the Source button. You will see that in the R Console it shows that it
sourced this file. This means that it runs through all lines of code in this file.
You can see that our objects have been added back into our environment.

```
source("test.R")
```

Now suppose we want to update our script by adding a plot. Copy the code
in a subsequent code chunk, save your updated file, and then source your file.
You will see that the generated plot will appear in your output pane.

```
plot(spec_phys, pcp_phys)
```

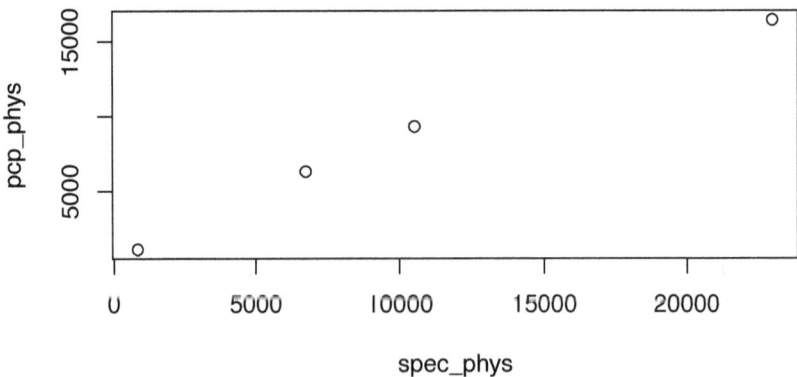

Unlike R Scripts which only contain R code, Quarto documents allow us to intersperse text and code. This breaks our code into chunks surrounded by text written in Markdown. Every chapter in this book is available as a Quarto document. Try opening the Quarto file for Chapter 2 of this book. You will see the first **code chunk** as in Figure 1.3. In order to run the code in a code chunk, we can again use Ctrl+Enter to run a single line or selected lines. Additionally,

we can use the Play button ▶ . This runs all the code within the chunk. We recommend using the available Quarto documents to follow along with the text. Writing your own Quarto documents is covered in Chapter 22.

```{r}
ex_num <- 4
```

Figure 1.3: Example Code Chunk.

1.3.2 Calling Functions

When we use R, we have access to all the functions available in base R. A **function** takes in one or more inputs and returns a single output object. Let's first use the simple function `exp()`. This exponential function takes in one (or more) numeric values and exponentiates them. The following code computes e^3.

```
exp(3)
#> [1] 20.1
```

Some other simple functions are shown that all convert a numeric input to an integer value. The `ceiling()` and `floor()` functions return the ceiling and floor of your input, and the `round()` function rounds your input to the closest integer. Note that the `round()` function rounds a number ending in 0.5 to the closest even integer.

```
ceiling(3.7)
#> [1] 4
```

```
floor(3.7)
#> [1] 3
```

```
round(2.5)
#> [1] 2
round(3.5)
#> [1] 4
```

If we want to learn about a function, we can use the help operator ? by typing it in front of the function we are interested in: this brings up the documentation for that particular function. This documentation often tells you the usage of the function, the **arguments** (the object inputs) and the **value** (information about the returned object), and it gives some examples of how to use the function. For example, if we want to understand the difference between `floor()` and `ceiling()`, we can call `?floor` and `?ceiling`. This should bring up the documentation in your help window. We can then read that the floor function rounds a numeric input down to the nearest integer, whereas the ceiling function rounds a numeric input up to the nearest integer.

1.3.3   Working Directories and Paths

Let's try using another example function: `read.csv()`. This function reads in a comma-delimited file and returns the information as a data frame (try typing `?read.csv` in the console to read more about this function). We learn more about data frames in Chapter 2. The first argument to this function is a file, which can be expressed as either a file name or a path to a file. First, download the file `fake_names.csv` from this book's github repository[4]. By default, R looks for the file in your current working directory To find the working directory, you can run `getwd()`. You can see in the following output that my current working directory is where the book content is on my computer.

```
getwd()
#> [1] "/Users/Alice/Dropbox/health-data-science-using-r/book"
```

You can either move the .csv file to your current working directory and load it in, or you can specify the path to the .csv file. Another option is to update your working directory by using the `setwd()` function.

```
setwd('/Users/Alice/Dropbox/health-data-science-using-r/book/data')
```

If you receive an error that a file cannot be found, you most likely have the wrong path to the file or the wrong file name. In the following code, I chose to

---

[4]https://github.com/alicepaul/health-data-science-using-r/tree/main/book/data

specify the path to the downloaded .csv file, saved this file to an object called df, and then printed that df object.

```
# update this with the path to your file
df <- read.csv("data/fake_names.csv")
df
#>                    Name Age     DOB            City State
#> 1             Ken Irwin  37 6/28/85      Providence    RI
#> 2 Delores Whittington    56 4/28/67      Smithfield    RI
#> 3         Daniel Hughes  41 5/22/82      Providence    RI
#> 4           Carlos Fain  83  2/2/40          Warren    RI
#> 5         James Alford   67 2/23/56 East Providence    RI
#> 6          Ruth Alvarez  34 9/22/88      Providence    RI
```

We can see that df contains the information from the .csv file, and that R has printed the first few observations of the data.

1.3.4 Installing and Loading Packages

When working with data frames, we often use the **tidyverse** package (Wickham 2023), which is actually a collection of R packages for data science applications. An R package is a collection of functions and/or sample data that allow us to expand on the functionality of R beyond the base functions. You can check whether you have the **tidyverse** package installed by going to the Package tab in the Output Pane in RStudio or by running the following command, which displays all your installed packages.

```
installed.packages()
```

If you don't already have a package installed, you can install it using the install.packages() function. Note that you have to include single or double quotes around the package name when using this function. You only have to install a package one time.

```
install.packages('tidyverse')
```

The function read_csv() is another function to read in comma-delimited files that is part of the **readr** package in the **tidyverse** (Wickham, Hester, and Bryan 2023). However, if we tried to use this function to load in our data, we would get an error that the function cannot be found. That is because we haven't loaded in this package. To do so, we use the library() function. Unlike the install.packages() function, we do not have to use quotes around the package name when calling this library() function. When we load in a package, we see some messages. For example, in the following output we see that this package contains the functions filter() and lag() that are also functions in base R. In future chapters, we suppress these messages to make the chapter presentation nicer. After loading the **tidyverse** package, we can now use the `read_csv()` function.

```
library(tidyverse)
```

```
df <- read_csv("data/fake_names.csv", show_col_types=FALSE)
df
#> # A tibble: 6 x 5
#>   Name                  Age DOB     City            State
#>   <chr>               <dbl> <chr>   <chr>           <chr>
#> 1 Ken Irwin              37 6/28/85 Providence      RI
#> 2 Delores Whittington    56 4/28/67 Smithfield      RI
#> 3 Daniel Hughes          41 5/22/82 Providence      RI
#> 4 Carlos Fain            83 2/2/40  Warren          RI
#> 5 James Alford           67 2/23/56 East Providence RI
#> 6 Ruth Alvarez           34 9/22/88 Providence      RI
```

Alternatively, we could have told R where to locate the function by adding `readr::` before the function. This tells it to find `read_csv()` function in the **readr** package. This can be helpful even if we have already loaded in the package, since sometimes multiple packages have functions with the same name.

```
df <- readr::read_csv("data/fake_names.csv", show_col_types = FALSE)
```

1.4 RStudio Projects and RStudio Global Options

You have now had a basic tour of RStudio. Once you close RStudio, you have the option of whether to store your current R environment. We highly recommend that you update your RStudio options to not save your workspace on exiting or load it on starting. This ensures that you have a fresh environment every time you open RStudio and helps you to create fully reproducible code and avoid possible errors or confusion (Figure 1.4).

Now when you re-open RStudio, it opens the files you had open previously and has your history of commands. This may become confusing when you are working on different files. RStudio projects allow us to create a folder that is associated with a single project. This means that when we open our project, it sets the appropriate work directory for us and only opens files related to

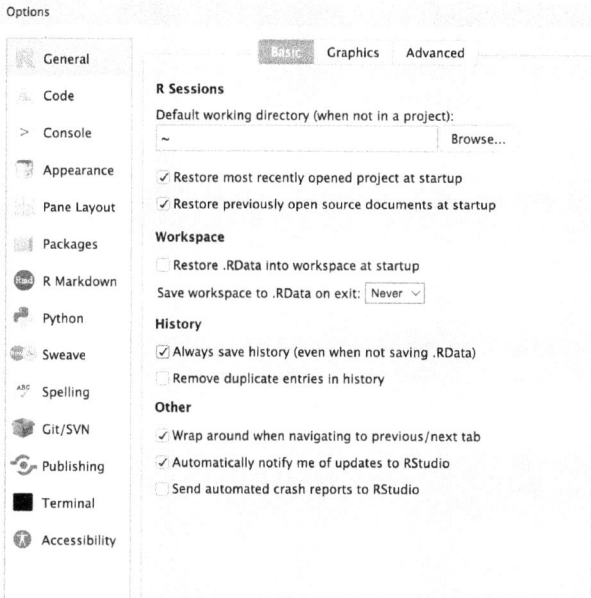

Figure 1.4: RStudio Global Options.

that project. In order to create a new R project, such as one associated with this book, you can go to File -> New Project. You can then choose whether to create a new directory or existing directory before selecting to create an empty project as in Figure 1.5. Within this directory you should see a .RProj file that allows you to re-open your project.

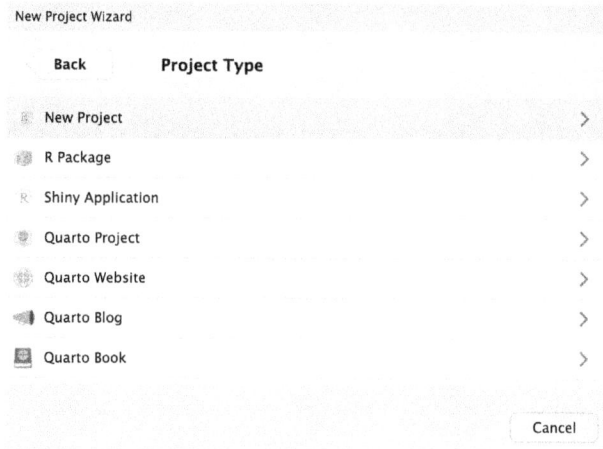

Figure 1.5: Creating a New RStudio Project.

1.5   Tips and Reminders

We end this chapter with some final tips and reminders.

- **Keyboard shortcuts**: RStudio has several useful keyboard shortcuts that make your programming experience more streamlined. It is worth getting familiar with some of the most common keyboard shortcuts using this book's cheat sheet[5].

- **Asking for help**: Within R, you can use the ? operator or the `help()` function to pull up documentation on a given function. This documentation is also available online[6].

- **Finding all objects**: You can use the environment pane or `ls()` function to find all current objects. If you have an error that an object you are calling does not exist, take a look to find where you defined it.

- **Checking packages**: If you get an error that a function does not exist, check to make sure you have loaded that package using the `library()` function. The list of packages used in this book is given on the GitHub repository homepage.

---

[5]https://github.com/alicepaul/health-data-science-using-r/blob/main/book/refs/r_stu dio_keyboard_shortcuts.pdf

[6]https://rdocumentation.org/

2

Data Structures in R

In this chapter, we demonstrate the key **data structures** in R. Data structures are how information is stored in R and refer to the types of objects we can create in R. The data structures that we use inform R how to interpret our code. Any **object** is a named instance of a data structure. For example, the object ex_num is a vector of numeric type.

```
ex_num <- 4
```

The main data structures in R are **vectors, factors, matrices, arrays, lists,** and **data frames**. These structures are distinguished by their dimensions and by the type of data they store. For example, we might have a one-dimensional vector that contains all numeric values, or we could have a two-dimensional data frame with rows and columns where we might have one numeric column and one character column. In Figure 2.1, there are two vectors with different types (character and numeric) on top, followed by a matrix and data frame below. In this chapter, we cover each data structure except for arrays. Arrays are an extension of matrices that allow for data that is more than two-dimensional and are not needed for the applications covered in this book.

2.1 Data Types

Each individual value in R has a type: **logical, integer, double,** or **character**. We can think of these as the building blocks of all data structures. We use the typeof() function to find the type of our vector ex_num, which shows that the value of ex_num is a **double**. A double is a numeric value with a stored decimal.

```
typeof(ex_num)
#> [1] "double"
```

On the other hand, an **integer** is a whole number that does not contain a

Vectors:

TRUE	FALSE	FALSE	FALSE

0	1	1	2	0	1	2	0

Matrix:

0	0	3	2
1	0	5	1
1	0	0	3
2	0	2	0
1	0	1	1

Data Frame:

name	visits	member
Alice	368	TRUE
Bob	47	FALSE
Carol	3	TRUE
Devon	65	FALSE
Eve	2	FALSE

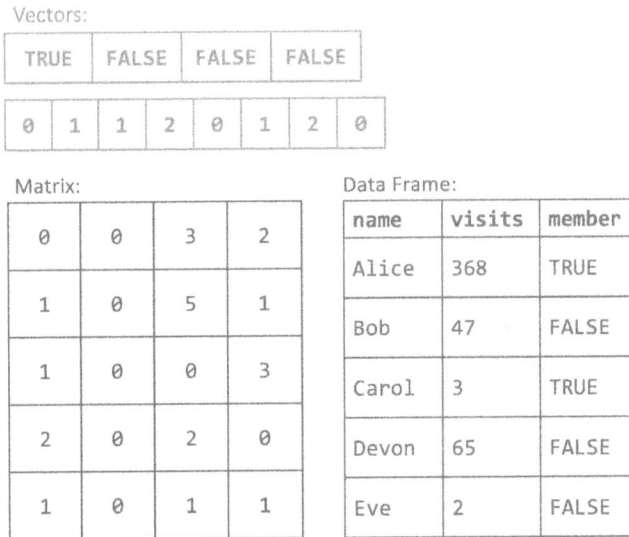

Figure 2.1: Data Structures.

decimal. We now create an integer object `ex_int`. To indicate to R that we want to restrict our values to integer values, we use an `L` after the number.

```
ex_int <- 4L
typeof(ex_int)
#> [1] "integer"
```

Both `ex_num` and `ex_int` are numeric objects, but we can also work with two other types of objects: **characters** (e.g., "php", "stats") and **Booleans** (e.g., TRUE, FALSE), also known as **logicals**.

```
ex_bool <- TRUE
ex_char <- "Alice"

typeof(ex_bool)
#> [1] "logical"
typeof(ex_char)
#> [1] "character"
```

One important characteristic of logical objects is that R also interprets them as 0/1. This means they can be added as in the following example: each TRUE has a value of 1, and each FALSE has a value of 0.

```
TRUE + FALSE + TRUE
#> [1] 2
```

To create all of these objects, we used the assignment operator <-, which we discussed in Chapter 1. You may see code elsewhere that uses an = instead. While = can also be used for assignment, it is more standard practice to use <-.

2.2 Vectors

In the previous examples, we created objects with a single value. R actually uses a vector of length 1 to store this information. **Vectors** are one-dimensional data structures that can store multiple data values of the same type (e.g., character, Boolean, or numeric). See Figure 2.2.

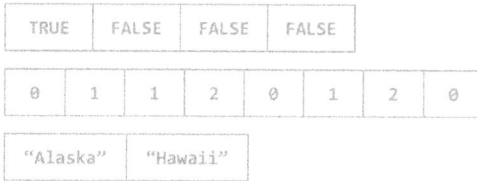

Figure 2.2: Vector Examples.

We can confirm this by using the is.vector() function, which returns whether or not the inputted argument is a vector.

```
is.vector(ex_bool)
#> [1] TRUE
```

One way to create a vector with multiple values is to use the combine function c(). In the following code, we create two vectors: one with the days of the week and one with the amount of rain on each day. The first vector has all character values, and the second one has all numeric values.

```
days <- c("Monday", "Tuesday", "Wednesday", "Thursday", "Friday")
rain <- c(5, 0.1, 0, 0, 0.4)
```

Remember, a vector can only store values of the same type. Because of this, in the following code, R automatically converts the numeric value to be a character in order to store these values in a vector together.

```
c("Monday", 5)
#> [1] "Monday" "5"
```

The class() function returns the data structure of an object. If we check the classes of these two objects using the class() function, we see that R tells us that the first is a character vector, and the second is a numeric vector. This matches the data type in this case.

```
class(days)
#> [1] "character"
class(rain)
#> [1] "numeric"
```

What happens when we create an empty vector? What is the class?

```
ex_empty <- c()
class(ex_empty)
#> [1] "NULL"
```

In this case, there is no specified type yet. If we wanted to specify the type, we could make an empty vector using the vector() function.

```
ex_empty <- vector(mode = "numeric")
class(ex_empty)
#> [1] "numeric"
```

Another way to create a vector is with the rep() or seq() functions. The first function rep(x, times) takes in a vector x and a number of times and outputs x repeated that many times. Let's try this with a single value. The second function seq(from, to, step) takes in a numeric starting value from, end value to, and step size step and returns a sequence starting at from in increments of step until a maximum value of to is reached.

```
rep(0, 5)
#> [1] 0 0 0 0 0
rep("Monday", 4)
#> [1] "Monday" "Monday" "Monday" "Monday"
```

```
seq(1, 5, 1)
#> [1] 1 2 3 4 5
seq(0, -10, -2)
#> [1]    0  -2  -4  -6  -8 -10
```

2.2.1 Indexing a Vector

Once we have a vector, we may want to access certain values stored in that vector. To do so, we index the vector using the position of each value: the first value in the vector has index 1, the second value has index 2, etc. When we say a vector is one-dimensional, we mean that we can define the position of each value by a single index. To index the vector, we then use square brackets [] after the vector name and provide the position. We use these indices to find the value at index 1 and the value at index 4.

```
days[1]
#> [1] "Monday"
days[4]
#> [1] "Thursday"
```

We can either access a single value or a subset of values using a vector of indices. Let's see what happens when we use a vector of indices `c(1,4)` and then try using `-c(1,4)` and see what happens. In the first case, we get the values at index 1 *and* at index 4. In the second case, we get all values *except* at those indices. The - indicates that we want to remove rather than select these indices.

```
days[c(1, 4)]
#> [1] "Monday"    "Thursday"
days[-c(1, 4)]
#> [1] "Tuesday"   "Wednesday" "Friday"
```

However, always indexing by the index value can sometimes be difficult or inefficient. One extra feature of vectors is that we can associate a name with each value. In the subsequent code, we update the names of the vector `rain` to be the days of the week and then find Friday's rain count by indexing with the name.

```
names(rain) <- days
print(rain)
#>    Monday   Tuesday Wednesday  Thursday    Friday
```

```
#>       5.0        0.1        0.0        0.0        0.4
rain["Friday"]
#> Friday
#>    0.4
```

The last way to index a vector is to use TRUE and FALSE values. If we
have a vector of Booleans that is the same length as our original vector, then
this returns all the values that correspond to a TRUE value. For example,
indexing the days vector by the logical vector ind_bools returns its first and
fourth values. We will see more about using logic to access certain values later
on.

```
ind_bools <- c(TRUE, FALSE, FALSE, TRUE, FALSE)
days[ind_bools]
#> [1] "Monday"    "Thursday"
```

2.2.2   Modifying a Vector and Calculations

The mathematical operators we saw in the last chapter (+, -, *, /, ^, %%) can
all be applied to numeric vectors and are applied element-wise. That is, in the
code examples, the two vectors are added together by index. This holds true
for some of the built-in math functions as well:

- exp() - exponential
- log() - log
- sqrt() - square root
- abs() - absolute value
- round() - round to nearest integer value
- ceiling() - round up to the nearest integer value
- floor() - round down to the nearest integer value
- signif(, dig) - round to dig number of significant digits

```
c(1, 2, 3) + c(1, 1, 1)
#> [1] 2 3 4
c(1, 2, 3) + 1 # equivalent to the code above
#> [1] 2 3 4
sqrt(c(1, 4, 16))
#> [1] 1 2 4
signif(c(0.23, 0.19), dig = 1)
#> [1] 0.2 0.2
```

After we create a vector, we may need to update its values. For example, we may want to change a specific value. We can do so using indexing. We then update the rain value for Friday using the assignment operator.

```
rain["Friday"] <- 0.5
rain
#>    Monday   Tuesday Wednesday  Thursday    Friday
#>       5.0       0.1       0.0       0.0       0.5
```

Further, we may need to add extra entries. We can do so using the c() function again but this time passing in the vector days as our first argument. This creates a single vector with all previous and new values. In the following code, we add two days to both vectors and then check the length of the updated vector rain. The length() function returns the length of a vector.

```
length(rain)
#> [1] 5
days <- c(days, "Saturday", "Sunday") # add the weekend with no rain
rain <- c(rain,0,0)
length(rain)
#> [1] 7
```

We can also call some useful functions on vectors. For example, the sum(), max(), and min() functions returns the sum, maximum value, and minimum value of a vector, respectively.

2.2.3 Practice Question

Create a vector of the odd numbers from 1 to 11 using the seq() function. Then, find the third value in the vector using indexing, which should have value 5.

```
# Insert your solution here:
```

2.2.4 Common Vector Functions

The following list contains some of the most common vector functions that are available in base R. All of these functions assume that the vector is numeric. If we pass the function a logical vector, R converts the vector to 0/1 first, and if we pass the function a character vector, R gives us an error message.

- sum() - summation
- median() - median value

- `mean()` - mean
- `sd()` - standard deviation
- `var()` - variance
- `max()` - maximum value
- `which.max()` - index of the first element with the maximum value
- `min()` - minimum value
- `which.min()` - index of the first element with the minimum value

Try these out using the vector `rain`. Note that R is case sensitive - `Mean()` is considered different from `mean()`, so if we type `Mean(rain)`, R tells us that it cannot find this function.

```
mean(rain)
#> [1] 0.8
min(rain)
#> [1] 0
which.min(rain)
#> Wednesday
#>         3
```

We may also be interested in the order of the values. The `sort()` function sorts the values of a vector, whereas the `order()` function returns the permutation of the elements to be in sorted order. The last line of the following code sorts the days of the week from smallest to largest rain value.

```
rain
#>    Monday   Tuesday Wednesday  Thursday    Friday
#>       5.0       0.1       0.0       0.0       0.5       0.0       0.0
order(rain)
#> [1] 3 4 6 7 2 5 1
days[order(rain)]
#> [1] "Wednesday" "Thursday"  "Saturday"  "Sunday"    "Tuesday"
#> [6] "Friday"    "Monday"
```

Both of these functions have an extra possible argument `decreasing`, which has a default value of FALSE. We can specify this to be TRUE to find the days of the week sorted from largest to smallest rainfall. Note that in the case of ties, the first occurrence gets the higher rank.

```
days[order(rain, decreasing=TRUE)]
#> [1] "Monday"    "Friday"    "Tuesday"   "Wednesday" "Thursday"
#> [6] "Saturday"  "Sunday"
```

2.3 Factors

A **factor** is a special kind of vector that behaves like a regular vector except that it represents values from a category. In particular, a factor keeps track of all possible values of that category, which are called the **levels** of the factor. Factors are especially helpful when we start getting into data analysis and have categorical columns. The `as.factor()` function converts a vector to a factor.

```
days <- c("Monday", "Tuesday", "Wednesday", "Monday",
          "Thursday", "Wednesday")
days_fct <- as.factor(days)

class(days_fct)
#> [1] "factor"
levels(days_fct)
#> [1] "Monday"    "Thursday"  "Tuesday"   "Wednesday"
```

In the previous example, we did not specify the possible levels for our column. Instead, R found all values in the vector `days` and set these equal to the levels of the factor. Because of this, if we try to change one of the levels to 'Friday', we get an error. Uncomment the following line to see the error message.

```
#days_fct[2] <- "Friday"
```

We can avoid this error by specifying the levels using the `factor()` function instead of the `as.factor()` function.

```
days <- c("Monday", "Tuesday", "Wednesday", "Monday", "Thursday",
          "Wednesday")
days_fct <- factor(days,
            levels = c("Monday", "Tuesday", "Wednesday",
                       "Thursday", "Friday", "Saturday", "Sunday"))

class(days_fct)
#> [1] "factor"
levels(days_fct)
#> [1] "Monday"    "Tuesday"    "Wednesday" "Thursday"  "Friday"
#> [6] "Saturday"  "Sunday"
days_fct[2] <- "Friday"
```

Factors can also be used for numeric vectors. For example, we might have a vector that is 0/1 that represents whether or not a day is a weekend. This can also only take on certain values (0 or 1).

```
weekend <- as.factor(c(1, 0, 0, 0, 1, 1))
levels(weekend)
#> [1] "0" "1"
```

2.4 Matrices

Matrices are similar to vectors in that they store data of the same type. However, matrices are two-dimensional consisting of both rows and columns (see Figure 2.3), as opposed to one-dimensional vectors.

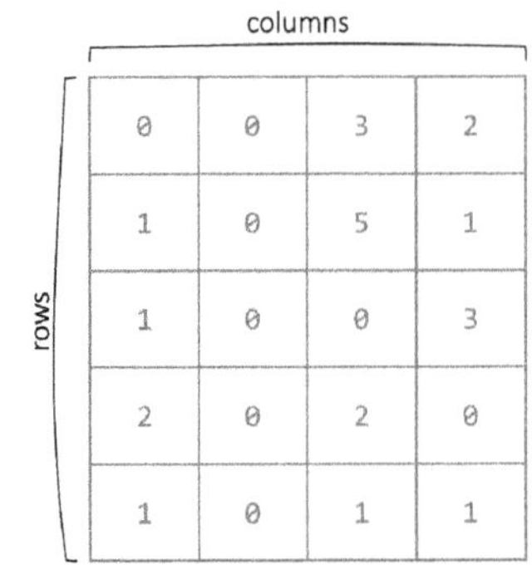

Figure 2.3: Matrix Example.

In the following code, we create a matrix reporting the daily rainfall over multiple weeks. We can create a matrix using the `matrix(data, nrow, ncol, byrow)` function. This creates a `nrow` by `ncol` matrix from the vector `data` values filling in by row if `byrow` is TRUE and by column otherwise. Run the code. Then, change the last argument to `byrow=FALSE` and see what happens to the values.

```
rainfall <- matrix(c(5, 6, 0.1, 3, 0, 1, 0, 1, 0.4, 0.2,
                     0.5, 0.3, 0, 0),
                 ncol=7, nrow=2, byrow=TRUE)
rainfall
#>      [,1] [,2] [,3] [,4] [,5] [,6] [,7]
```

```
#> [1,]    5 6.0  0.1  3.0  0.0    1    0
#> [2,]    1 0.4  0.2  0.5  0.3    0    0
```

We can find the dimensions of a matrix using the `nrow()`, `ncol()`, or `dim()` functions, which return the number of rows, the number of columns, and both the number of rows and columns, respectively.

```
nrow(rainfall)
#> [1] 2
ncol(rainfall)
#> [1] 7
dim(rainfall)
#> [1] 2 7
```

2.4.1 Indexing a Matrix

Since matrices are two-dimensional, a single value is indexed by both its row number and its column number. This means that to access a subset of values in a matrix, we need to provide row and column indices. In the subsequent code, we access a single value in the first row and the fourth column. The first value is always the row index and the second value is always the column index.

```
rainfall[1, 4]
#> [1] 3
```

As before, we can also provide multiple indices to get multiple values. In the subsequent example, we choose multiple columns, but we can also choose multiple rows (or multiple rows and multiple columns).

```
rainfall[1, c(4, 5, 7)]
#> [1] 3 0 0
```

As with vectors, we can also use Booleans to index a matrix by providing Boolean values for the rows and/or columns. Note that in the following example we give a vector for the row indices and no values for the columns. Since we did not specify any column indices, this selects all of them.

```
rainfall[c(FALSE, TRUE), ]
#> [1] 1.0 0.4 0.2 0.5 0.3 0.0 0.0
```

Let's do the opposite and select some columns and all rows.

```
rainfall[ ,c(TRUE, TRUE, FALSE, FALSE, FALSE, FALSE, FALSE)]
#>       [,1] [,2]
#> [1,]    5  6.0
#> [2,]    1  0.4
```

As with vectors, we can specify row names and column names to access entries instead of using indices. The `colnames()` and `rownames()` functions allow us to specify the column and row names, respectively.

```
colnames(rainfall) <- c("Monday", "Tuesday", "Wednesday", "Thursday",
                        "Friday", "Saturday", "Sunday")
rownames(rainfall) <- c("Week1", "Week2")
rainfall["Week1", c("Friday","Saturday")]
#>   Friday Saturday
#>        0        1
```

2.4.2 Modifying a Matrix

If we want to change the values in a matrix, we need to first index those values and then assign them the new value(s). In the subsequent code chunks, we change a single entry to be 3 and then update several values to all be 0. Note that we do not provide multiple 0's on the right-hand side, as R infers that all values should be set to 0.

```
rainfall["Week1", "Friday"] <- 3
```

```
rainfall["Week1", c("Monday", "Tuesday")] <- 0
print(rainfall)
#>       Monday Tuesday Wednesday Thursday Friday Saturday Sunday
#> Week1      0     0.0       0.1      3.0    3.0        1      0
#> Week2      1     0.4       0.2      0.5    0.3        0      0
```

Further, we can append values to our matrix by adding rows or columns through the `rbind()` and `cbind()` functions. The first function appends a row (or multiple rows) to a matrix and the second appends a column (or multiple columns). Note that in the following example I provide a row and column name when passing in the additional data. If I hadn't specified these names, then those rows and columns would not be named.

```
rainfall <- rbind(rainfall, "Week3" = c(0.4, 0.0, 0.0, 0.0, 1.2, 2.2,
                                         0.0))
rainfall <- cbind(rainfall, "Total" = c(7.1, 2.4, 3.8))
print(rainfall)
#>        Monday Tuesday Wednesday Thursday Friday Saturday Sunday Total
#> Week1     0.0     0.0       0.1      3.0    3.0      1.0      0   7.1
#> Week2     1.0     0.4       0.2      0.5    0.3      0.0      0   2.4
#> Week3     0.4     0.0       0.0      0.0    1.2      2.2      0   3.8
```

Here is an example where we bind two matrices by column. Note that whenever we bind two matrices together, we have to be sure that their dimensions are compatible and that they are of the same type.

```
A <- matrix(c(1, 2, 3, 4), nrow=2)
B <- matrix(c(5, 6, 7, 8), nrow=2)
C <- cbind(A, B)
C
#>      [,1] [,2] [,3] [,4]
#> [1,]    1    3    5    7
#> [2,]    2    4    6    8
```

As with vectors, most mathematical operators (+, -, *, /, etc.) are applied element-wise in R.

```
A+B
#>      [,1] [,2]
#> [1,]    6   10
#> [2,]    8   12
```

```
exp(C)
#>      [,1] [,2] [,3] [,4]
#> [1,] 2.72 20.1  148 1097
#> [2,] 7.39 54.6  403 2981
```

2.4.3 Practice Question

Create a 3×4 matrix of all 1's using the `rep()` and `matrix()` functions. Then select the first and third columns using indexing which returns a 3×2 matrix of all 1's.

```
# Insert your solution here:
```

2.5 Data Frames

Matrices can store data like the rainfall data, where everything is of the same type. However, if we want to capture more complex data records, we also want to allow for different measurement types: this is where data frames come in. A data frame is like a matrix in that data frames are two-dimensional, but unlike matrices, data frames allow for each column to be a different type (see Figure 2.4). In this case, each row corresponds to a single data entry (or observation) and each column corresponds to a different variable.

name	visits	member
Alice	368	TRUE
Bob	47	FALSE
Carol	3	TRUE
Devon	65	FALSE
Eve	2	FALSE

Figure 2.4: Data Frame Example.

For example, suppose that, for every day in a study, we want to record the temperature, rainfall, and day of the week. Temperature and rainfall can be numeric values, but day of the week is character type. We create a data frame using the data.frame() function. Note that I am providing column names for each vector (column).

The head() function prints the first six rows of a data frame (to avoid printing very large datasets). In our case, all the data is shown because we only created four rows. The column names are displayed as well as their type. By contrast, the tail() function prints the last six rows of a data frame.

```
weather_data <- data.frame(day_of_week = c("Monday", "Tuesday",
                                           "Wednesday", "Monday"),
                           temp = c(70, 62, 75, 50),
```

```
                            rain = c(5, 0.1, 0.0, 0.5))
head(weather_data)
#>    day_of_week temp rain
#> 1       Monday   70  5.0
#> 2      Tuesday   62  0.1
#> 3    Wednesday   75  0.0
#> 4       Monday   50  0.5
```

The `dim()`, `nrow()`, and `ncol()` functions return the dimensions, number of rows, and number of columns of a data frame, respectively.

```
dim(weather_data)
#> [1] 4 3
nrow(weather_data)
#> [1] 4
ncol(weather_data)
#> [1] 3
```

The column names can be found (or assigned) using the `colnames()` or `names()` function. These were specified when I created the data. On the other hand, the row names are currently the indices.

```
colnames(weather_data)
#> [1] "day_of_week" "temp"        "rain"
rownames(weather_data)
#> [1] "1" "2" "3" "4"
names(weather_data)
#> [1] "day_of_week" "temp"        "rain"
```

We update the row names to be more informative as with a matrix using the `rownames()` function.

```
rownames(weather_data) <- c("6/1", "6/2", "6/3", "6/8")
head(weather_data)
#>     day_of_week temp rain
#> 6/1      Monday   70  5.0
#> 6/2     Tuesday   62  0.1
#> 6/3   Wednesday   75  0.0
#> 6/8      Monday   50  0.5
```

2.5.1 Indexing a Data Frame

We can select elements of the data frame using its indices in the same way as we did with matrices. In the subsequent code, we access a single value and then a subset of our data frame. The subset returned is itself a data frame. Note that the second line returns a data frame.

```
weather_data[1, 2]
#> [1] 70
weather_data[1, c("day_of_week", "temp")]
#>      day_of_week temp
#> 6/1       Monday   70
```

Another useful way to access the columns of a data frame is by using the $ accessor and the column name.

```
weather_data$day_of_week
#> [1] "Monday"    "Tuesday"   "Wednesday" "Monday"
weather_data$temp
#> [1] 70 62 75 50
```

The column `day_of_week` is a categorical column, but it can only take on a limited number of values. For this kind of column, it is often useful to convert that column to a factor as we did before.

```
weather_data$day_of_week <- factor(weather_data$day_of_week)
levels(weather_data$day_of_week)
#> [1] "Monday"    "Tuesday"   "Wednesday"
```

2.5.2 Modifying a Data Frame

As with matrices, we can change values in a data frame by indexing those entries.

```
weather_data[1, "rain"] <- 2.2
weather_data
#>      day_of_week temp rain
#> 6/1       Monday   70  2.2
#> 6/2      Tuesday   62  0.1
#> 6/3    Wednesday   75  0.0
#> 6/8       Monday   50  0.5
```

The rbind() functions and cbind() functions also work for data frames in the same way as for matrices. However, another way to add a column is to directly use the $ accessor. We add a categorical column called aq_warning, indicating whether there was an air quality warning that day.

```
weather_data$aq_warning <- as.factor(c(1, 0, 0, 0))
weather_data
#>      day_of_week temp rain aq_warning
#> 6/1      Monday   70  2.2          1
#> 6/2     Tuesday   62  0.1          0
#> 6/3   Wednesday   75  0.0          0
#> 6/8      Monday   50  0.5          0
```

2.5.3 Practice Question

Add a column to weather_data called air_quality_index using the rep() function so that all values are NA (the missing value in R). Then, index the second value of this column and set the value to be 57. The result should look like Figure 2.5.

A data.frame: 4 × 5

	day_of_week	temp	rain	aq_warning	air_quality_index
	<fct>	<dbl>	<dbl>	<fct>	<dbl>
6/1	Monday	70	2.2	1	NA
6/2	Tuesday	62	0.1	0	57
6/3	Wednesday	75	0.0	0	NA
6/8	Monday	50	0.5	0	NA

Figure 2.5: Air Quality Data.

```
# Insert your solution here:
```

2.6 Lists

A data frame is actually a special type of another data structure called a **list**, which is a collection of objects under the same name. These objects can be vectors, matrices, data frames, or even other lists! There does not have to be any relation in size, type, or other attribute between different members of the list. We create an example list using the list() function, which takes in a series of objects. What are the types of each element of the following list?

```
ex_list <- list("John", c("ibuprofen", "metformin"),
                c(136, 142, 159))
print(ex_list)
#> [[1]]
#> [1] "John"
#>
#> [[2]]
#> [1] "ibuprofen" "metformin"
#>
#> [[3]]
#> [1] 136 142 159
```

We can access each element using the index. Note unlike indexing vectors, using single brackets will return another list which is a sub-list containing the object at that index.

```
print(class(ex_list[2]))
#> [1] "list"
ex_list[2]
#> [[1]]
#> [1] "ibuprofen" "metformin"
```

We can access the actual numeric vector at this index using double brackets.

```
ex_list[[2]]
#> [1] "ibuprofen" "metformin"
```

More often, however, it is useful to name the elements of the list for easier access. Let's create this list again but, this time, give names to each object.

```
ex_list <- list(name="John",
                medications = c("ibuprofen", "metformin"),
                past_weights = c(136, 142, 159))
print(ex_list)
#> $name
#> [1] "John"
#>
#> $medications
```

```
#> [1] "ibuprofen" "metformin"
#>
#> $past_weights
#> [1] 136 142 159
ex_list$medications
#> [1] "ibuprofen" "metformin"
```

To edit a list, we can use indexing to access different objects in the list and then assign them to new values. Additionally, we can add objects to the list using the $ accessor.

```
ex_list$supplements <- c("vitamin D", "biotin")
ex_list$supplements[2] <- "collagen"
ex_list
#> $name
#> [1] "John"
#>
#> $medications
#> [1] "ibuprofen" "metformin"
#>
#> $past_weights
#> [1] 136 142 159
#>
#> $supplements
#> [1] "vitamin D" "collagen"
```

2.7 Exercises

1. Recreate the data frame in Figure 2.6 in R, where temperature and co2 represent the average temperature in Fahrenheit and the average CO_2 concentrations in mg/m^3 for the month of January 2008, and name it city_air_quality.

2. Create a character vector named precipitation with entries Yes or No indicating whether or not there was more precipitation than average in January 2008 in these cities (you can make this information up yourself). Then, append this vector to the city_air_quality data frame as a new column.

A data.frame: 7 × 4

city	country	temperature	co2
<chr>	<chr>	<dbl>	<dbl>
Beijing	China	30	417.0
Shanghai	China	40	405.0
Paris	France	37	401.2
Rome	Italy	54	398.7
London	United Kingdom	43	412.3
San Francisco	United States	52	419.0
Toronto	Canada	25	399.4

Figure 2.6: City Air Quality Data.

3. Convert the categorical column `precipitation` to a factor. Then, add a row to the data frame `city_air_quality` using the `rbind()` function to match Figure 2.7.

Reykjavik	Iceland	29	402.1	No

Figure 2.7: Updated City Air Quality Data.

4. Use single square brackets to access the precipitation and CO_2 concentration entries for San Francisco and Paris in your data frame. Then, create a list `city_list` which contains two lists, one for San Francisco and one for Paris, where each inner list contains the city name, precipitation, and CO_2 concentration information for that city.

3

Working with Data Files in R

In this chapter, we work with data in R. To start, we need to load our data into R; this requires identifying the type of data file we have (e.g., .csv, .xlsx, .dta, .txt) and finding the appropriate function to load in the data. This creates a data frame object containing the information from the file. After demonstrating how to load in such data, this chapter shows you how to find information about data columns, including finding missing values, summarizing columns, and subsetting the data. Additionally, we look at how to create new columns through some simple transformations.

In this chapter and all future chapters, we load in the required libraries at the start of the chapter; for example, in this particular chapter, we need a single package **HDSinRdata** that contains the sample datasets used in this book.

```
library(HDSinRdata)
```

3.1 Importing and Exporting Data

The data we use in this chapter contains information about patients who visited one of the University of Pittsburgh's seven pain management clinics. This includes patient-reported pain assessments using the Collaborative Health Outcomes Information Registry (CHOIR) at baseline and at a 3-month follow-up (Alter et al. 2021). You can use the help operator ?pain to learn more about the source of this data and to read its column descriptions. Since this data is available in our R package, we can use the data() function to load this data into our environment. Note that this data has 21,659 rows and 92 columns.

```
data(pain)
dim(pain)
#> [1] 21659     92
```

In general, the data you will be using is not available in R packages and will instead exist in one or more data files on your personal computer. In order to load in this data to R, you need to use the function that corresponds to the file type you have. For example, you can load a .csv file using the read.csv() function in base R or using the read_csv() function from the **readr** package, both of which were shown in Chapter 1. As an example, we load the fake_names.csv dataset using both of these functions. Looking at the print output, we can see that there is a slight difference in the data structure and data types storing the data between these two functions. The function read.csv() loads the data as a data frame, whereas the function read_csv() loads the data as a spec_tbl_df, a special type of data frame called a **tibble** that is used by the **tidyverse** packages. We cover this data structure in more detail in Chapter 5. For now, note that you can use either function to read in a .csv file.

```
read.csv("data/fake_names.csv")
#>                   Name Age     DOB           City State
#> 1          Ken Irwin  37 6/28/85      Providence    RI
#> 2 Delores Whittington  56 4/28/67      Smithfield    RI
#> 3      Daniel Hughes  41 5/22/82      Providence    RI
#> 4        Carlos Fain  83  2/2/40          Warren    RI
#> 5       James Alford  67 2/23/56 East Providence    RI
#> 6       Ruth Alvarez  34 9/22/88      Providence    RI
```

```
readr::read_csv("data/fake_names.csv", show_col_types=FALSE)
#> # A tibble: 6 x 5
#>   Name                  Age DOB     City            State
#>   <chr>               <dbl> <chr>   <chr>           <chr>
#> 1 Ken Irwin              37 6/28/85 Providence      RI
#> 2 Delores Whittington    56 4/28/67 Smithfield      RI
#> 3 Daniel Hughes          41 5/22/82 Providence      RI
#> 4 Carlos Fain            83 2/2/40  Warren          RI
#> 5 James Alford           67 2/23/56 East Providence RI
#> 6 Ruth Alvarez           34 9/22/88 Providence      RI
```

In addition to loading data into R, you may also want to save data from R into a data file you can access later or share with others. To write a data frame from R to a .csv file, you can use the write.csv() function. This function has three key arguments: the first argument is the data frame in R that you want to write to a file, the second argument is the file name or the full file path where you want to write the data, and the third argument is whether or not you want to include the row names as an extra column. In this case, we do not include row names. If you do not specify a file path, R saves the file in our current working directory.

```
df <- data.frame(x = c( 1, 0, 1), y = c("A", "B", "C"))
write.csv(df, "data/test.csv", row.names=FALSE)
```

If your data is not in a .csv file, you may need to use another package to read in the file. The two most common packages are the **readxl** package (Wickham and Bryan 2023), which makes it easy to read in Excel files, and the **haven** package (Wickham, Miller, and Smith 2023), which can import SAS, SPSS, and Stata files. For each function, you need to specify the file path to the data file.

- **Tab-Delimited Files**: You can read in a tab-separated .txt file using the `read.delim()` function in base R.

- **Excel Files**: You can read in a .xls or .xlsx file using `readxl::read_excel()`, which allows you to specify a sheet and/or cell range within a file (e.g., `read_excel('test.xlsx', sheet="Sheet1"))`.

- **SAS**: `haven::read_sas()` reads in .sas7bdat or .sas7bcat files, `haven::read_xpt()` reads in SAS transport files.

- **Stata**: `haven::read_dta()` reads in .dta files.

- **SPSS**: `haven::read_spss()` reads in .spss files.

3.2 Summarizing and Creating Data Columns

We now look at the data we have loaded into the data frame called `pain`. We use the `head()` function to print the first six rows. However, note that we have so many columns that not all of the columns are displayed! For those that are displayed, we can see the data type for each column under the column name. For example, we can see that the column `PATIENT_NUM` is a numeric column of type `dbl`. Because patients identification numbers are technically nominal in nature, we might consider whether we should make convert this column to a factor or a character representation later on. We can use the `names()` function to print all the column names. Note that columns `X101` to `X238` correspond to numbers on a body pain map (see the data documentation for the image of this map). Each of these columns has a 1 if the patient indicated that they have pain in that corresponding body part and a 0 otherwise.

```
head(pain)
#> # A tibble: 6 x 92
#>   PATIENT_NUM  X101  X102  X103  X104  X105  X106  X107  X108  X109
#>         <dbl> <dbl> <dbl> <dbl> <dbl> <dbl> <dbl> <dbl> <dbl> <dbl>
#> 1       13118     0     0     0     0     0     0     0     0     0
#> 2       21384     0     0     0     0     0     0     0     0     0
#> 3        6240     0     0     0     0     0     0     0     0     0
#> 4        1827     0     0     0     0     0     0     0     0     0
#> 5       11309     0     0     0     0     0     0     0     0     0
#> 6       11093     0     0     0     0     0     0     0     0     0
#> # i 82 more variables: X110 <dbl>, X111 <dbl>, X112 <dbl>, X113
#> ↳  <dbl>,
#> #   X114 <dbl>, X115 <dbl>, X116 <dbl>, X117 <dbl>, X118 <dbl>,
#> #   X119 <dbl>, X120 <dbl>, X121 <dbl>, X122 <dbl>, X123 <dbl>,
#> #   X124 <dbl>, X125 <dbl>, X126 <dbl>, X127 <dbl>, X128 <dbl>,
#> #   X129 <dbl>, X130 <dbl>, X131 <dbl>, X132 <dbl>, X133 <dbl>,
#> #   X134 <dbl>, X135 <dbl>, X136 <dbl>, X201 <dbl>, X202 <dbl>,
#> #   X203 <dbl>, X204 <dbl>, X205 <dbl>, X206 <dbl>, X207 <dbl>, ...
names(pain)
#>  [1] "PATIENT_NUM"
#>  [2] "X101"
#>  [3] "X102"
#>  [4] "X103"
#>  [5] "X104"
#>  [6] "X105"
#>  [7] "X106"
#>  [8] "X107"
#>  [9] "X108"
#> [10] "X109"
#> [11] "X110"
#> [12] "X111"
#> [13] "X112"
#> [14] "X113"
#> [15] "X114"
#> [16] "X115"
#> [17] "X116"
#> [18] "X117"
#> [19] "X118"
#> [20] "X119"
#> [21] "X120"
#> [22] "X121"
#> [23] "X122"
#> [24] "X123"
```

```
#> [25] "X124"
#> [26] "X125"
#> [27] "X126"
#> [28] "X127"
#> [29] "X128"
#> [30] "X129"
#> [31] "X130"
#> [32] "X131"
#> [33] "X132"
#> [34] "X133"
#> [35] "X134"
#> [36] "X135"
#> [37] "X136"
#> [38] "X201"
#> [39] "X202"
#> [40] "X203"
#> [41] "X204"
#> [42] "X205"
#> [43] "X206"
#> [44] "X207"
#> [45] "X208"
#> [46] "X209"
#> [47] "X210"
#> [48] "X211"
#> [49] "X212"
#> [50] "X213"
#> [51] "X214"
#> [52] "X215"
#> [53] "X216"
#> [54] "X217"
#> [55] "X218"
#> [56] "X219"
#> [57] "X220"
#> [58] "X221"
#> [59] "X222"
#> [60] "X223"
#> [61] "X224"
#> [62] "X225"
#> [63] "X226"
#> [64] "X227"
#> [65] "X228"
#> [66] "X229"
#> [67] "X230"
```

```
#>  [68]  "X231"
#>  [69]  "X232"
#>  [70]  "X233"
#>  [71]  "X234"
#>  [72]  "X235"
#>  [73]  "X236"
#>  [74]  "X237"
#>  [75]  "X238"
#>  [76]  "PAIN_INTENSITY_AVERAGE"
#>  [77]  "PROMIS_PHYSICAL_FUNCTION"
#>  [78]  "PROMIS_PAIN_BEHAVIOR"
#>  [79]  "PROMIS_DEPRESSION"
#>  [80]  "PROMIS_ANXIETY"
#>  [81]  "PROMIS_SLEEP_DISTURB_V1_0"
#>  [82]  "PROMIS_PAIN_INTERFERENCE"
#>  [83]  "GH_MENTAL_SCORE"
#>  [84]  "GH_PHYSICAL_SCORE"
#>  [85]  "AGE_AT_CONTACT"
#>  [86]  "BMI"
#>  [87]  "CCI_TOTAL_SCORE"
#>  [88]  "PAIN_INTENSITY_AVERAGE.FOLLOW_UP"
#>  [89]  "PAT_SEX"
#>  [90]  "PAT_RACE"
#>  [91]  "CCI_BIN"
#>  [92]  "MEDICAID_BIN"
```

Recall that the $ operator can be used to access a single column. Alternatively, we can use double brackets [[]] to select a column. We demonstrate both ways to print the first five values in the column with the patient's average pain intensity.

```
pain$PAIN_INTENSITY_AVERAGE[1:5]
#> [1] 7 5 4 7 8
pain[["PAIN_INTENSITY_AVERAGE"]][1:5]
#> [1] 7 5 4 7 8
```

3.2.1 Column Summaries

To explore the range and distribution of a column's values, we can use some of the base R functions. For example, the summary() function is a useful way to summarize a numeric column's values. We can see that the pain intensity values range from 0 to 10 with a median value of 7 and that there is a NA value.

```
summary(pain$PAIN_INTENSITY_AVERAGE)
#>    Min. 1st Qu.  Median    Mean 3rd Qu.    Max.    NA's
#>    0.00    5.00    7.00    6.49    8.00   10.00       1
```

We have already seen the max(), min(), mean(), and median() functions that could have computed some of these values for us separately. Since we do have an NA value, we add the na.rm=TRUE argument to these functions. Without this argument, the returned value for all of the functions is NA.

```
min(pain$PAIN_INTENSITY_AVERAGE, na.rm=TRUE)
#> [1] 0
max(pain$PAIN_INTENSITY_AVERAGE, na.rm=TRUE)
#> [1] 10
mean(pain$PAIN_INTENSITY_AVERAGE, na.rm=TRUE)
#> [1] 6.49
median(pain$PAIN_INTENSITY_AVERAGE, na.rm=TRUE)
#> [1] 7
```

Additionally, the following functions are helpful for summarizing quantitative columns.

- range() - returns the minimum and maximum values for a numeric vector x.
- quantile() - returns the sample quantiles for a numeric vector.
- IQR() - returns the interquartile range for a numeric vector.

By default, the quantile() function returns the sample quantiles.

```
quantile(pain$PAIN_INTENSITY_AVERAGE, na.rm = TRUE)
#>    0%   25%   50%   75%  100%
#>     0     5     7     8    10
```

However, we can pass in a list of probabilities to use instead. For example, in the following code we find the 0.1 and 0.9 quantiles. Again, we add the na.rm=TRUE argument.

```
quantile(pain$PAIN_INTENSITY_AVERAGE, probs = c(0.1, 0.9), na.rm=TRUE)
#> 10% 90%
#>   4   9
```

We can also plot a histogram of the sample distribution using the `hist()` function. We look more in depth at how to change aspects of this histogram in Chapter 4.

```
hist(pain$PAIN_INTENSITY_AVERAGE)
```

Histogram of pain$PAIN_INTENSITY_AVERAGE

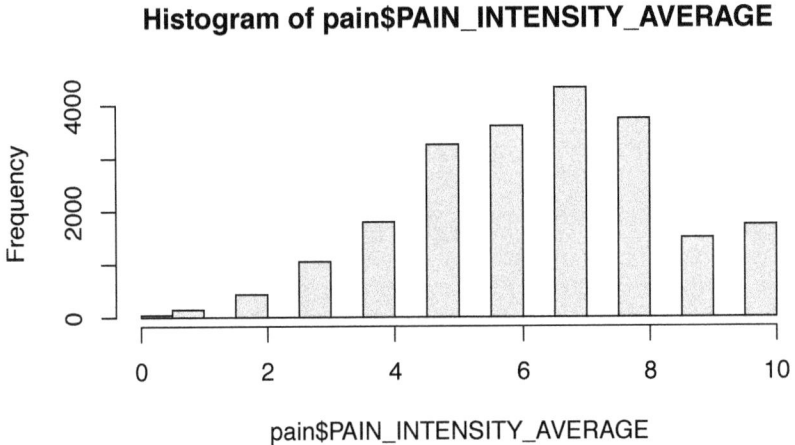

pain$PAIN_INTENSITY_AVERAGE

3.2.2 Practice Question

Summarize the `PROMIS_SLEEP_DISTURB_V1_0` column both numerically and visually. Your results should look like the results in Figure 3.1.

```
# Insert your solution here:
```

We can also use the `summary()` function for categorical variables. In this case, R finds the counts for each level.

```
summary(pain$PAT_SEX)
#>    Length     Class      Mode
#>     21659 character character
```

For categorical columns, it is also useful to use the `table()` function, which returns the counts for each possible value, instead of the `summary()` function. By default, `table()` ignores NA values. However, we can set `useNA="always"` if we also want to display the number of NA values in the table output. Ad-

```
  Min. 1st Qu.   Median    Mean 3rd Qu.     Max.    NA's
 26.35   54.33    59.57   59.67   65.25    83.79      87
```

Histogram of pain$PROMIS_SLEEP_DISTURB_V1_0

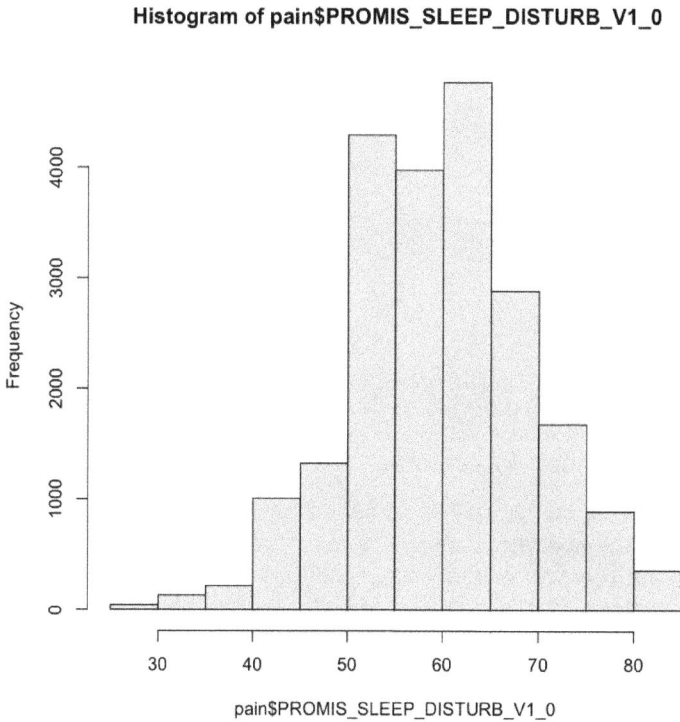

Figure 3.1: Summarizing a Column.

ditionally, we can use the `prop.table()` function to convert the counts to proportions. Using these functions, we can see that the column PAT_SEX column, which corresponds to the reported patient sex, has a single missing value, and we can also see that around 60% of patients are female.

```
table(pain$PAT_SEX, useNA="always")
#>
#> female    male    <NA>
#>  13102    8556       1


prop.table(table(pain$PAT_SEX))
#>
```

```
#> female    male
#>  0.605   0.395
```

Note that this column is not actually a factor column yet, which we can check using the is.factor() function. We can convert it to one using as.factor().

```
is.factor(pain$PAT_SEX)
#> [1] FALSE
```

```
pain$PAT_SEX <- as.factor(pain$PAT_SEX)
is.factor(pain$PAT_SEX)
#> [1] TRUE
```

3.2.3 Other Summary Functions

Sometimes we want to summarize information across multiple columns or rows. We can use the rowSums() and colSums() functions to sum over the rows or columns of a matrix or data frame. We first subset the data to the body pain map regions. In the first line of code, I select the column names pertaining to these columns. This allows me to select those columns in the second line of code and store this subset of the data as a new data frame called pain_body_map.

```
body_map_cols <- names(pain)[2:75]
pain_body_map <- pain[, body_map_cols]
head(pain_body_map)
#> # A tibble: 6 x 74
#>     X101  X102  X103  X104  X105  X106  X107  X108  X109  X110  X111
#>    <dbl> <dbl> <dbl> <dbl> <dbl> <dbl> <dbl> <dbl> <dbl> <dbl> <dbl>
#> 1      0     0     0     0     0     0     0     0     0     0     0
#> 2      0     0     0     0     0     0     0     0     0     0     0
#> 3      0     0     0     0     0     0     0     0     0     0     0
#> 4      0     0     0     0     0     0     0     0     0     0     0
#> 5      0     0     0     0     0     0     0     0     0     0     0
#> 6      0     0     0     0     0     0     0     0     0     1     0
#> # i 63 more variables: X112 <dbl>, X113 <dbl>, X114 <dbl>, X115
#>  ↵ <dbl>,
#> #    X116 <dbl>, X117 <dbl>, X118 <dbl>, X119 <dbl>, X120 <dbl>,
#> #    X121 <dbl>, X122 <dbl>, X123 <dbl>, X124 <dbl>, X125 <dbl>,
#> #    X126 <dbl>, X127 <dbl>, X128 <dbl>, X129 <dbl>, X130 <dbl>,
```

```
#> #    X131 <dbl>, X132 <dbl>, X133 <dbl>, X134 <dbl>, X135 <dbl>,
#> #    X136 <dbl>, X201 <dbl>, X202 <dbl>, X203 <dbl>, X204 <dbl>,
#> #    X205 <dbl>, X206 <dbl>, X207 <dbl>, X208 <dbl>, X209 <dbl>, ...
```

I now compute the row sums and column sums on this subset of data. The
row sum for each patient is the total number of body parts in which they
experience pain, whereas the column sum for each pain region is the total
number of patients who experience pain in that area. The following histogram
shows that most people select a low number of total regions.

```
hist(rowSums(pain_body_map))
```

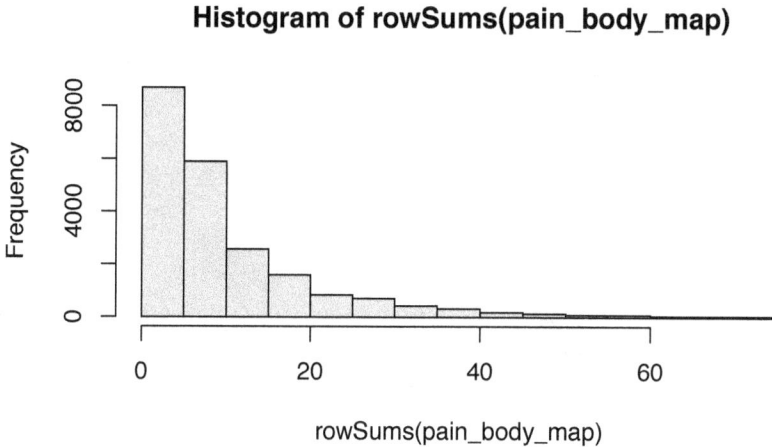

Histogram of rowSums(pain_body_map)

We can also see that some body parts are more often selected than others. We
create a vector called `perc_patients` by finding the number of patients who
selected each region divided by the total number of patients. The histogram
shows that some body regions are selected by over 50% of patients!

```
perc_patients <- colSums(pain_body_map, na.rm=TRUE) /
  nrow(pain_body_map)
hist(perc_patients)
```

Histogram of perc_patients

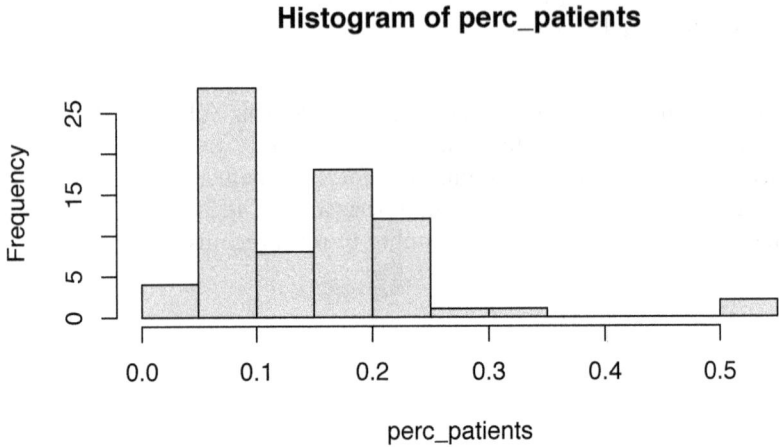

We use the `which.max()` function to see that the 55th region X219 is selected the most number of times. This corresponds to lower back pain.

```
which.max(perc_patients)
#> X219
#>    55
```

Another pair of useful functions are `pmin()` and `pmax()`. These functions take at least two vectors and find the pairwise minimum or maximum across those vectors, as shown in the subsequent code.

```
v1 = c(5, 9, 12)
v2 = c(2, 18, 4)
pmax(v1, v2)
#> [1]  5 18 12
```

Looking back at the `pain` data, if we want to create a new column `lower_back_pain` that corresponds to whether someone selects *either* X218 or X219 we can use the `pmax()` function to find the maximum value between columns X218 and X219. We can see that almost 60% of patients select at least one of these regions.

```
lower_back <- pmax(pain_body_map$X218, pain_body_map$X219)
prop.table(table(lower_back))
#> lower_back
```

```
#>      0     1
#> 0.405 0.595
```

We might want to store the total number of pain regions and our indicator of whether or not a patient has lower back pain as new columns. We create new columns in the pain data using the $ operator in the previous code chunk. To be consistent with the column naming in the data, we use all uppercase for our column names. The dim() function shows that our data has grown by two columns, as expected.

```
pain$NUM_REGIONS <- rowSums(pain_body_map)
pain$LOWER_BACK <- lower_back
dim(pain)
#> [1] 21659    94
```

Another useful function that allows us to perform computations over the rows or columns of a matrix or data frame is the apply(X, MARGIN, FUN) function, which takes in three arguments. The first argument is a data frame or matrix X, the second argument MARGIN indicates whether to compute over the rows (1) or columns (2), and the last argument is the function FUN to apply across that margin. The subsequent code finds the maximum value for each row in the data frame pain_body_map. Taking the minimum value of the row maximum values shows that every patient selected at least one body map region.

```
any_selected <- apply(pain_body_map, 1, max)
min(any_selected, na.rm=TRUE)
#> [1] 1
```

In a second example, we find the sum of the body pain regions over the columns, which is equivalent to the previous example using colSums(). In this case, we added the na.rm=TRUE argument. The apply() function passes any additional arguments to the function FUN.

```
perc_patients <- apply(pain_body_map, 2, sum, na.rm=TRUE) /
  nrow(pain_body_map)
summary(perc_patients)
#>    Min. 1st Qu.  Median    Mean 3rd Qu.    Max.
#>   0.032   0.070   0.136   0.144   0.181   0.542
```

3.2.4   Practice Question

Find the sum of each of the PROMIS measures across all patients using ap-ply() and then using colSums(). Verify that these two methods return the same result, which is given in Figure 3.2.

PROMIS_PHYSICAL_FUNCTION: 763930.939999992 PROMIS_PAIN_BEHAVIOR: 933907.940000042 PROMIS_DEPRESSION: 1191575.03999999
PROMIS_ANXIETY: 1213957.77000006 PROMIS_SLEEP_DISTURB_V1_0: 1287215.15999999 PROMIS_PAIN_INTERFERENCE: 1427380.18000004

Figure 3.2: Summing Across Columns.

```
# Insert your solution here:
```

3.2.5   Missing, Infinite, and NaN Values

As we have seen, this data contains some missing values, which are represented as NA in R. R treats these values as if they were unknown, which is why we have to add the na.rm=TRUE argument to functions like sum() and max(). In the following example, we can see that R figures out that 1 plus an unknown number is also unknown!

```
NA+1
#> [1] NA
```

We can determine whether a value is missing using the function is.na(). This function returns TRUE if the value is NA, and FALSE otherwise. We can then sum up these values for a single column since each TRUE value corresponds to a value of 1, and each FALSE corresponds to a value of 0. We observe that there is a single NA value for the column PATIENT_NUM, which is the patient ID number.

```
sum(is.na(pain$PATIENT_NUM))
#> [1] 1
```

If we want to calculate the sum of NA values for each column instead of just a single column, we can use the apply() function. Since we want to apply this computation over the columns, the second argument has value 2. Recall that the last argument is the function we want to call for each column. In this case, we want to apply the combination of the sum() and is.na() function. To do so, we have to specify this function ourselves. This is called an **anonymous function** , since it doesn't have a name.

```
num_missing_col <- apply(pain, 2, function(x) sum(is.na(x)))
min(num_missing_col)
#> [1] 1
```

Interestingly, we can see that there is at least one missing value in each column. It might be the case that there is a row with all NA values. Let's apply the same function by row. Taking the maximum, we can see that row 11749 has all NA values.

```
num_missing_row <- apply(pain, 1, function(x) sum(is.na(x)))
max(num_missing_row)
#> [1] 94
which.max(num_missing_row)
#> [1] 11749
```

We remove that row and then find the percentage of missing values by column. We can see that the column with the highest percentage of missing values is the pain intensity at follow-up. In fact, only 33% of patients have a recorded follow-up visit.

```
pain <- pain[-11749, ]
num_missing_col <- apply(pain, 2,
                    function(x) sum(is.na(x))/nrow(pain))
num_missing_col
#>                    PATIENT_NUM                      X101
#>                        0.00000                   0.00000
#>                           X102                      X103
#>                        0.00000                   0.00000
#>                           X104                      X105
#>                        0.00000                   0.00000
#>                           X106                      X107
#>                        0.00000                   0.00000
#>                           X108                      X109
#>                        0.00000                   0.00000
#>                           X110                      X111
#>                        0.00000                   0.00000
#>                           X112                      X113
#>                        0.00000                   0.00000
#>                           X114                      X115
#>                        0.00000                   0.00000
#>                           X116                      X117
#>                        0.00000                   0.00000
```

```
#>                        X118                        X119
#>                     0.00000                     0.00000
#>                        X120                        X121
#>                     0.00000                     0.00000
#>                        X122                        X123
#>                     0.00000                     0.00000
#>                        X124                        X125
#>                     0.00000                     0.00000
#>                        X126                        X127
#>                     0.00000                     0.00000
#>                        X128                        X129
#>                     0.00000                     0.00000
#>                        X130                        X131
#>                     0.00000                     0.00000
#>                        X132                        X133
#>                     0.00000                     0.00000
#>                        X134                        X135
#>                     0.00000                     0.00000
#>                        X136                        X201
#>                     0.00000                     0.00000
#>                        X202                        X203
#>                     0.00000                     0.00000
#>                        X204                        X205
#>                     0.00000                     0.00000
#>                        X206                        X207
#>                     0.00000                     0.00000
#>                        X208                        X209
#>                     0.00000                     0.00000
#>                        X210                        X211
#>                     0.00000                     0.00000
#>                        X212                        X213
#>                     0.00000                     0.00000
#>                        X214                        X215
#>                     0.00000                     0.00000
#>                        X216                        X217
#>                     0.00000                     0.00000
#>                        X218                        X219
#>                     0.00000                     0.00000
#>                        X220                        X221
#>                     0.00000                     0.00000
#>                        X222                        X223
#>                     0.00000                     0.00000
#>                        X224                        X225
```

```
#>                       0.00000                       0.00000
#>                          X226                          X227
#>                       0.00000                       0.00000
#>                          X228                          X229
#>                       0.00000                       0.00000
#>                          X230                          X231
#>                       0.00000                       0.00000
#>                          X232                          X233
#>                       0.00000                       0.00000
#>                          X234                          X235
#>                       0.00000                       0.00000
#>                          X236                          X237
#>                       0.00000                       0.00000
#>                          X238          PAIN_INTENSITY_AVERAGE
#>                       0.00000                       0.00000
#>      PROMIS_PHYSICAL_FUNCTION            PROMIS_PAIN_BEHAVIOR
#>                       0.00000                       0.29412
#>             PROMIS_DEPRESSION                  PROMIS_ANXIETY
#>                       0.00402                       0.00402
#>      PROMIS_SLEEP_DISTURB_V1_0       PROMIS_PAIN_INTERFERENCE
#>                       0.00402                       0.00697
#>               GH_MENTAL_SCORE               GH_PHYSICAL_SCORE
#>                       0.13602                       0.13602
#>               AGE_AT_CONTACT                             BMI
#>                       0.00000                       0.26004
#>               CCI_TOTAL_SCORE PAIN_INTENSITY_AVERAGE.FOLLOW_UP
#>                       0.00000                       0.67042
#>                       PAT_SEX                        PAT_RACE
#>                       0.00000                       0.00651
#>                       CCI_BIN                    MEDICAID_BIN
#>                       0.00000                       0.01385
#>                   NUM_REGIONS                      LOWER_BACK
#>                       0.00000                       0.00000
```

We create two new columns: first, we create a column for the change in pain at follow-up, and second, we create a column for the percent change in pain at follow-up.

```
pain$PAIN_CHANGE <- pain$PAIN_INTENSITY_AVERAGE.FOLLOW_UP -
  pain$PAIN_INTENSITY_AVERAGE
hist(pain$PAIN_CHANGE)
```

Histogram of pain$PAIN_CHANGE

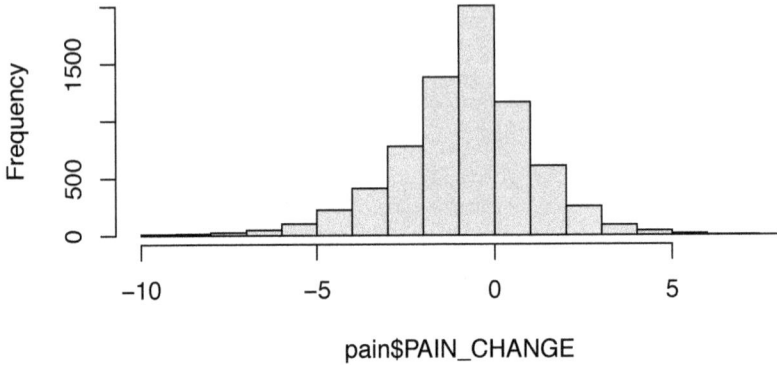

pain$PAIN_CHANGE

```
pain$PERC_PAIN_CHANGE <- pain$PAIN_CHANGE /
  pain$PAIN_INTENSITY_AVERAGE
summary(pain$PERC_PAIN_CHANGE)
#>    Min. 1st Qu.  Median    Mean 3rd Qu.    Max.    NA's
#>      -1       0       0     Inf       0     Inf   14520
```

In the summary of the percent change, we can see that the maximum value is Inf. This is R's representation of infinity. This occurred because some patients have an initial pain score of 0, which creates infinite values when we divide through by this value to find the percent change. We can test whether something is infinite using the is.infinite() or is.finite() functions. This shows that there were three patients with infinite values. The value -Inf is used to represent negative infinity.

```
sum(is.infinite(pain$PERC_PAIN_CHANGE))
#> [1] 3
```

Another special value in R is NaN, which stands for "Not a Number". For example, 0/0 results in a NaN value. We can test for NaN values using the is.nan() function.

```
0/0
#> [1] NaN
```

Looking back at the missing values, there are two useful functions for selecting the complete cases in a data frame. The na.omit() function returns the
data frame with incomplete cases removed, whereas complete.cases() returns
TRUE/FALSE values for each row indicating whether each row is complete,
which we can then use to select the rows with TRUE values. In the following
code, we see that both approaches select the same number of rows.

```
pain_sub1 <- na.omit(pain)
pain_sub2 <- pain[complete.cases(pain), ]
dim(pain_sub1)
#> [1] 2413    96
dim(pain_sub2)
#> [1] 2413    96
```

3.2.6 Dates in R

The columns in the pain data contain character and numeric values. One special type of character column that is not present is a column that corresponds
to a date or date-time. By default, read.csv() reads these columns in as character columns, whereas the read_csv() function from the **readr** package in
the **tidyverse** family recognizes common date formats. If we have a character column, we can convert to a date object using as.Date() for date columns
and as.POSIXct() for date-time columns. For columns with only a time but no
date, you can add a date or use the **hms** package (Müller 2023), which is not
demonstrated here. These functions automatically try to detect the format of
the inputted string, but it is often helpful to provide the format and time zone
tz. To input our format we use the following key.

Symbol	Description
%Y	Four-digit year.
%y	Two-digit year.
%m	Numeric month.
%b%	Abbreviated name of month.
%B	Full name of month.
%d	Numeric day of the month.
%H	Military time hour (24 hours).
%I	Imperial time hour (12 hours).
%M	Minute.
%S	Seconds.
%p	AM/PM

```
date_example <- data.frame(x = c("2020-01-15", "2021-11-16",
                                 "2019-08-01"),
                           y = c("2020-01-15 3:14 PM",
                                 "2021-11-16 5:00 AM",
                                 "2019-08-01 3:00 PM"),
                           z = c("04:10:00", "11:35:11", "18:00:45"))

# Convert date and date times using formats
date_example$x <- as.Date(date_example$x, format = "%Y-%m-%d",
                          tz = "EST")
date_example$y <- as.POSIXct(date_example$y,
                             format = "%Y-%m-%d %I:%M %p")

# Add date to z and convert
date_example$z <- paste("2024-06-24", date_example$z)
date_example$z <- as.POSIXct(date_example$z,
                             format = "%Y-%m-%d %H:%M:%S")
date_example
#>           x                   y                   z
#> 1 2020-01-15 2020-01-15 15:14:00 2024-06-24 04:10:00
#> 2 2021-11-16 2021-11-16 05:00:00 2024-06-24 11:35:11
#> 3 2019-08-01 2019-08-01 15:00:00 2024-06-24 18:00:45
```

By recognizing these columns as dates, we can find the time between two dates using the `difftime()` function. This function takes in two times `time1` and `time2` and finds the difference `time1 - time2` in the given `units`.

```
difftime(date_example$x[2], date_example$x[1], units = "days")
#> Time difference of 671 days
```

Additionally, we can use the `seq()` function to add or subtract time by specifying a unit for `by`.

```
seq(date_example$x[1], by = "month", length = 3)
#> [1] "2020-01-15" "2020-02-15" "2020-03-15"
```

For those interested in doing more manipulations with dates, the **lubridate** package (Spinu, Grolemund, and Wickham 2023) in the **tidyverse** expands upon the base functionality of R for working with dates. This package uses its own date-time class and includes functions to easily extract information from and manipulate dates.

3.3 Using Logic to Subset, Summarize, and Transform

We have already seen how to use TRUE/FALSE values to select rows in a data frame. The following logic operators in R allow us to expand on this capability to write more complex logic.

- < less than
- <= less than or equal to
- > greater than
- >= greater than or equal to
- == equal to
- != not equal to
- a %in% b a's value is in a vector of values b

The first six operators are a direct comparison between two values.

```
2 < 2
#> [1] FALSE
2 <= 2
#> [1] TRUE
3 > 2
#> [1] TRUE
3 >= 2
#> [1] TRUE
"A" == "B"
#> [1] FALSE
"A" != "B"
#> [1] TRUE
```

The operators assume there is a natural ordering or comparison between values. For example, for strings the ordering is alphabetical and for logical operators we use their numeric interpretation (TRUE = 1, FALSE = 0).

```
"A" < "B"
#> [1] TRUE
TRUE < FALSE
#> [1] FALSE
```

The %in% operator is slightly different. This operator checks whether a value is in a set of possible values. For example, we can check whether values are in the set c(4,1,2).

```
1 %in% c(4, 1, 2)
#> [1] TRUE
c(0, 1, 5) %in% c(4, 1, 2)
#> [1] FALSE  TRUE FALSE
```

Additionally, we can use the following operators, which allow us to negate or combine logical operators.

- !x - the **NOT** operator ! reverses TRUE/FALSE values
- x | y - the **OR** operator | checks whether *either* x or y is equal to TRUE
- x & y - the **AND** operator & checks whether *both* x and y are equal to TRUE
- xor(x,y) - the **xor** function checks whether exactly one of x or y is equal to TRUE (called exclusive or)
- any(x) - the **any** function checks whether any value in x is TRUE (equivalent to using an OR operator | between all values)
- all(x) - the **all** function checks whether all values in x are TRUE (equivalent to using an AND operator & between all values)

Some simple examples for each are given in the following code chunk.

```
!(2 < 3)
#> [1] FALSE
("Alice" < "Bob") | ("Alice" < "Aaron")
#> [1] TRUE
("Alice" < "Bob") & ("Alice" < "Aaron")
#> [1] FALSE
xor(TRUE, FALSE)
#> [1] TRUE
any(c(FALSE, TRUE, TRUE))
#> [1] TRUE
all(c(FALSE, TRUE, TRUE))
#> [1] FALSE
```

Let's demonstrate these operators on the pain data. We first update the Medicaid column by making the character values more informative. The logic on the left-hand side selects those who do or do not have Medicaid and then assigns those values to the new ones.

```
pain$MEDICAID_BIN[pain$MEDICAID_BIN == "no"] <- "No Medicaid"
pain$MEDICAID_BIN[pain$MEDICAID_BIN == "yes"] <- "Medicaid"
table(pain$MEDICAID_BIN)
#>
```

```
#>    Medicaid No Medicaid
#>       4601       16757
```

Additionally, we could subset the data to only those who have a follow-up. The not operator ! reverses the TRUE/FALSE values returned from the is.na() function. Therefore, the new value is TRUE if the follow-up value is *not* NA.

```
pain_follow_up <- pain[!is.na(pain$PAIN_INTENSITY_AVERAGE.FOLLOW_UP),
  ↳ ]
```

Earlier, we created a column indicating whether or not a patient has lower back pain. We now use the any() function to check whether a patient has general back pain. If at least one of these values is equal to 1, then the function returns TRUE. If we had used the all() function instead, this would check whether all values are equal to 1, indicating that a patient has pain in their whole back.

```
pain$BACK <- any(pain$X208==1, pain$X209==1, pain$X212==1,
                 pain$X213==1, pain$X218==1, pain$X219==1)
```

3.3.1 Practice Question

Subset the pain data to those who have a follow-up and have an initial average pain intensity of 5 or above. Name this subset of the data pain_subset. Print the head of this data. The first six patient IDs in this new dataset should be 13118, 21384, 1827, 11309, 11093, and 14667.

```
# Insert your solution here:
```

Lastly, we look at the column for patient race PAT_RACE. The table() function shows that most patients are WHITE or BLACK. Given how few observations are in the other categories, we may want to combine some of these levels into one.

```
table(pain$PAT_RACE)
#>
#>       ALASKA NATIVE    AMERICAN INDIAN              BLACK
#>                   2                 58               3229
#>             CHINESE           DECLINED           FILIPINO
#>                  21                121                  6
#>       GUAM/CHAMORRO           HAWAIIAN     INDIAN (ASIAN)
```

```
#>                    1                        1                    49
#>             JAPANESE                   KOREAN        NOT SPECIFIED
#>                    9                       10                     4
#>                OTHER        OTHER ASIAN OTHER PACIFIC ISLANDER
#>                    1                       47                    12
#>           VIETNAMESE                    WHITE
#>                    6                    17940
```

Another way we could have found all possible values for this column is to use the `unique()` function. This function takes in a data frame or vector x and returns x with all duplicate rows or values removed.

```
unique(pain$PAT_RACE)
#>  [1] "WHITE"                "BLACK"
#>  [3] "DECLINED"             "AMERICAN INDIAN"
#>  [5] "INDIAN (ASIAN)"       "ALASKA NATIVE"
#>  [7] NA                     "FILIPINO"
#>  [9] "JAPANESE"             "VIETNAMESE"
#> [11] "KOREAN"               "CHINESE"
#> [13] "OTHER ASIAN"          "NOT SPECIFIED"
#> [15] "HAWAIIAN"             "OTHER PACIFIC ISLANDER"
#> [17] "OTHER"                "GUAM/CHAMORRO"
```

To combine some of these levels, we can use the `%in%` operator. We first create an Asian, Asian American, or Pacific Islander race category and then create an American Indian or Alaska Native category.

```
aapi_values <- c("CHINESE", "HAWAIIAN", "INDIAN (ASIAN)", "FILIPINO",
                 "VIETNAMESE", "JAPANESE", "KOREAN", "GUAM/CHAMORRO",
                 "OTHER ASIAN", "OTHER PACIFIC ISLANDER")
pain$PAT_RACE[pain$PAT_RACE %in% aapi_values] <- "AAPI"
pain$PAT_RACE[pain$PAT_RACE %in%
              c("ALASKA NATIVE", "AMERICAN INDIAN")] <- "AI/AN"
table(pain$PAT_RACE)
#>
#>      AAPI      AI/AN      BLACK   DECLINED NOT SPECIFIED
#>       162         60       3229        121             4
#>     OTHER      WHITE
#>         1      17940
```

3.3.2   Other Selection Functions

In the previous code, we selected rows using TRUE/FALSE Boolean values. Instead, we could have also used the `which()` function. This function takes TRUE/FALSE values and returns the index values for all the TRUE values. We use this to treat those with race given as DECLINED as not specified.

```
pain$PAT_RACE[which(pain$PAT_RACE == "DECLINED")] <- "NOT SPECIFIED"
```

Another selection function is the `subset()` function. This function takes in two arguments. The first is the vector, matrix, or data frame to select from, and the second is a vector of TRUE/FALSE values to use for row selection. We use this to find the observation with race marked as OTHER. We then update this race to also be marked as not specified.

```
subset(pain, pain$PAT_RACE == "OTHER")
#> # A tibble: 1 x 97
#>   PATIENT_NUM  X101  X102  X103  X104  X105  X106  X107  X108  X109
#>         <dbl> <dbl> <dbl> <dbl> <dbl> <dbl> <dbl> <dbl> <dbl> <dbl>
#> 1        3588     1     1     1     0     1     1     1     0     0
#> # i 87 more variables: X110 <dbl>, X111 <dbl>, X112 <dbl>, X113
#> ↳  <dbl>,
#> #   X114 <dbl>, X115 <dbl>, X116 <dbl>, X117 <dbl>, X118 <dbl>,
#> #   X119 <dbl>, X120 <dbl>, X121 <dbl>, X122 <dbl>, X123 <dbl>,
#> #   X124 <dbl>, X125 <dbl>, X126 <dbl>, X127 <dbl>, X128 <dbl>,
#> #   X129 <dbl>, X130 <dbl>, X131 <dbl>, X132 <dbl>, X133 <dbl>,
#> #   X134 <dbl>, X135 <dbl>, X136 <dbl>, X201 <dbl>, X202 <dbl>,
#> #   X203 <dbl>, X204 <dbl>, X205 <dbl>, X206 <dbl>, X207 <dbl>, ...
```

```
pain$PAT_RACE[pain$PATIENT_NUM==3588] <- "NOT SPECIFIED"
table(pain$PAT_RACE)
#>
#>          AAPI         AI/AN    BLACK  NOT SPECIFIED        WHITE
#>           162            60     3229            126        17940
```

3.4   Exercises

For these exercises, we use the `pain` data from the **HDSinRdata** package.

1. Print summary statistics for the PROMIS_PHYSICAL_FUNCTION and PROMIS_ANXIETY columns in this dataset. Read the data documentation for these two columns, which both have range 0 to 100, and then comment on the distributions of these columns.

2. Create frequency tables for the values of PAT_SEX and PAT_RACE and summarize what these tables tell you about the distributions of these demographic characteristics.

3. Create a new data frame called pain.new that doesn't contain patients with NA values for both GH_MENTAL_SCORE and GH_PHYSICAL_SCORE, which are the PROMIS global mental and physical scores, respectively.

4. Create a vector of the proportion of patients who reported pain in each of the pain regions. Then, find the minimum, median, mean, maximum, standard deviation, and variance of this vector.

5. Calculate the median and interquartile range of the distribution of the total number of painful **leg** regions selected for each patient. Then, write a few sentences explaining anything interesting you observe about this distribution in the context of this dataset.

6. Look at the distribution of average pain intensity between patients with only one pain region selected vs. those with more than one region selected. What do you notice?

7. Create a histogram to plot the distribution of the PAIN_INTENSITY_AVERAGE.FOLLOW_UP column. Then, create a table summarizing how many patients had missing values in this column. Finally, choose two columns to compare the distribution between those with and without missing follow-up. What do you notice?

Part II

Exploratory Analysis

4

Intro to Exploratory Data Analysis

In the last chapter, we learned about loading data into R and practiced selecting and summarizing columns and rows of the data. In this chapter, we learn how to conduct more exploratory analysis, focusing on the univariate and bivariate sample distributions of the data. The first half focuses on using base R to create basic plots and summaries. In the second half, we show how to create summary plots using the **GGally** package (Schloerke et al. 2021) and tables using the **gt** (Iannone et al. 2023) and **gtsummary** (Sjoberg et al. 2023) packages.

```
library(HDSinRdata)
library(GGally)
library(gt)
library(gtsummary)
```

4.1 Univariate Distributions

In this chapter, we use a sample of the National Health and Nutrition Examination Survey (Centers for Disease Control and Prevention (CDC) 1999-2018) containing lead, blood pressure, BMI, smoking status, alcohol use, and demographic variables from NHANES 1999-2018. Variable selection and feature engineering followed the analysis in Huang (2022). There are 31,625 observations in this sample. Use the help operator `?NHANESsample` to read the column descriptions.

```
data(NHANESsample)
dim(NHANESsample)
#> [1] 31265      21
names(NHANESsample)
#>  [1] "ID"          "AGE"         "SEX"         "RACE"
#>  [5] "EDUCATION"   "INCOME"      "SMOKE"       "YEAR"
```

```
#>   [9] "LEAD"          "BMI_CAT"       "LEAD_QUANTILE" "HYP"
#>  [13] "ALC"           "DBP1"          "DBP2"          "DBP3"
#>  [17] "DBP4"          "SBP1"          "SBP2"          "SBP3"
#>  [21] "SBP4"
```

To start our exploration, we look at whether there are any missing values. We use the `complete.cases()` function to observe that there are no complete cases. We also see that the subsequent blood pressure measurements and alcohol use have the highest percentage of missing values. For demonstration, we choose to only keep the first systolic and diastolic blood pressure measurements and do a complete case analysis using the `na.omit()` function to define our complete data frame `nhanes_df`.

```
sum(complete.cases(NHANESsample))
#> [1] 0
apply(NHANESsample, 2, function(x) sum(is.na(x)))/nrow(NHANESsample)
#>            ID           AGE           SEX          RACE     EDUCATION
#>      0.000000      0.000000      0.000000      0.000000      0.000672
#>        INCOME         SMOKE          YEAR          LEAD       BMI_CAT
#>      0.000000      0.000000      0.000000      0.000000      0.000000
#> LEAD_QUANTILE           HYP           ALC          DBP1          DBP2
#>      0.000000      0.000000      0.026867      0.060035      0.063905
#>          DBP3          DBP4          SBP1          SBP2          SBP3
#>      0.070974      0.891124      0.060035      0.063905      0.070942
#>          SBP4
#>      0.891124
```

```
nhanes_df <- na.omit(subset(NHANESsample,
                     select = -c(SBP2, SBP3, SBP4, DBP2, DBP3,
                                 DBP4)))
```

In the last chapter, we introduced the `table()` and `summary()` functions to quickly summarize categorical and quantitative vectors. We can observe that over half of the observations never smoked and that the most recent NHANES cycle in the data is 2017-2018.

```
table(nhanes_df$SMOKE)
#>
#> NeverSmoke  QuitSmoke StillSmoke
#>      13774       8019       6799
summary(nhanes_df$YEAR)
```

```
#>     Min. 1st Qu.  Median   Mean 3rd Qu.   Max.
#>     1999    2003    2007    2008    2011   2017
```

We decide to select the most recent observations from NHANES 2017-2018 for our analysis in this chapter. We use the `subset()` function to select these rows.

```
nhanes_df <- subset(nhanes_df, nhanes_df$YEAR == 2017)
```

As shown, smoking status has been coded into three categories: "NeverSmoke", "QuitSmoke", and "StillSmoke". We want to create a new column to represent whether someone has ever smoked. To do so, we use the `ifelse()` function, which allows us to create a new vector using logic. The logic captured by this function is that we want to use one value if we meet some condition, and we want to use a second value if the condition is not met. The first argument is a vector of TRUE/FALSE values representing the conditions, the next argument is the value or vector to use if we meet the condition(s), and the last argument is the value or vector to use otherwise. We use this function to create a new vector `EVER_SMOKE` that is equal to "Yes" for those who are either still smoking or quit smoking and equal to "No" otherwise.

```
nhanes_df$EVER_SMOKE <- ifelse(nhanes_df$SMOKE %in% c("QuitSmoke",
                                                      "StillSmoke"),
                        "Yes", "No")
table(nhanes_df$EVER_SMOKE)
#>
#>   No  Yes
#> 1411 1173
```

If we did not want to store this new column, we could use the pipe operator `|>` to send the output directly to the `table()` function. The pipe operator takes the result on the left-hand side and passes it as the first argument to the function on the right-hand side.

```
ifelse(nhanes_df$SMOKE %in% c("QuitSmoke", "StillSmoke"),
       "Yes", "No") |>
  table()
#>
#>   No  Yes
#> 1411 1173
```

The `summary()` and `table()` functions allow us to summarize the univariate sample distributions of columns. We may also want to plot these distributions. We saw in Chapter 3 that the `hist()` function creates a histogram plot. We use this function to plot a histogram of the log transformation of the lead column.

```
hist(log(nhanes_df$LEAD))
```

Histogram of log(nhanes_df$LEAD)

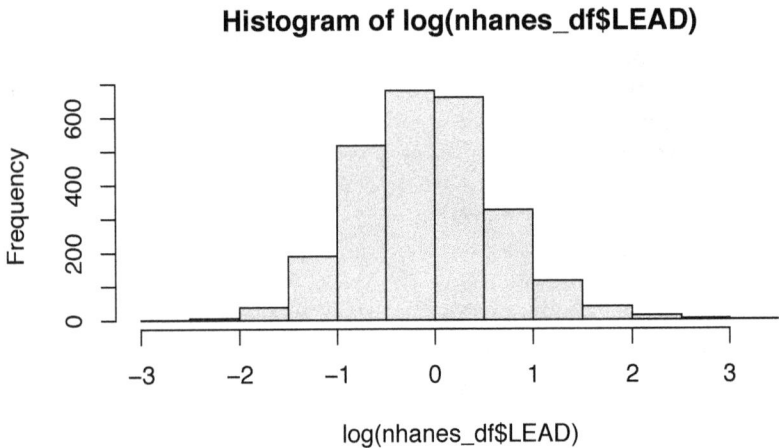

If we want to polish this figure, we can use some of the other optional arguments to the `hist()` function. For example, we may want to update the text `log(nhanes_df$lead)` in the title and x-axis. In the following code, we update the color, labels, and number of bins for the plot. The function `colors()` returns all recognized colors in R. The argument `breaks` specifies the number of bins to use to create the histogram, `col` specifies the color, `main` specifies the title of the plot, and `xlab` specifies the x-axis label (using `ylab` would specify the y-axis label). Read the documentation `?hist` for the full list of arguments available.

```
hist(log(nhanes_df$LEAD), breaks = 30, col = "blue",
     main = "Histogram of Log Blood Lead Level",
     xlab = "Log Blood Lead Level")
```

Histogram of Log Blood Lead Level

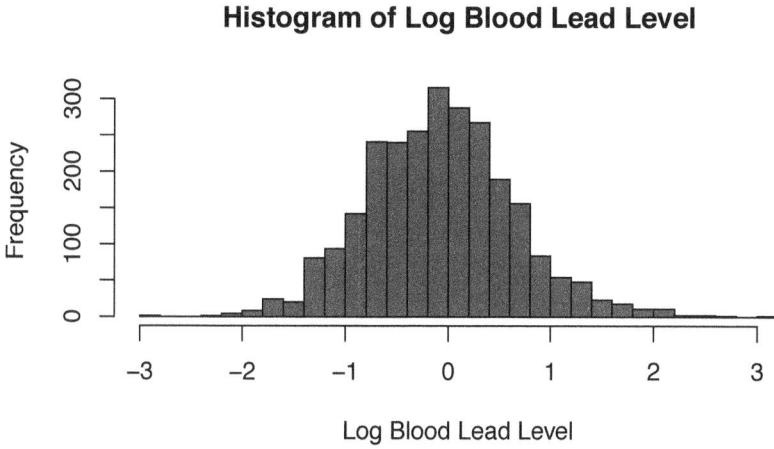

For categorical columns, we may want to plot the counts in each category using a barplot. The function `barplot()` asks us to specify the `names` and `heights` of the bars. To do so, we need to store the counts for each category. Again, we update the color and labels.

```
smoke_counts <- table(nhanes_df$SMOKE)
barplot(height = smoke_counts, names = names(smoke_counts),
        col = "violetred", xlab="Smoking Status", ylab="Frequency")
```

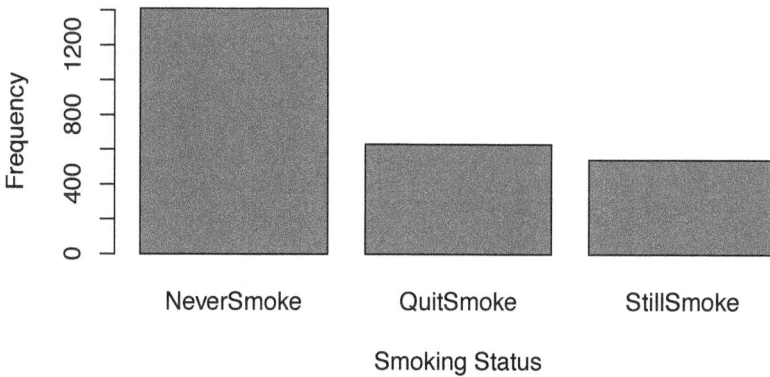

With a barplot, we can even specify a different color for each bar. To do so, col must be a vector of specified colors with the same length as the number of categories.

```
barplot(height = smoke_counts, names = names(smoke_counts),
        col = c("orange", "violetred", "blue"),
        xlab = "Smoking Status", ylab = "Frequency")
```

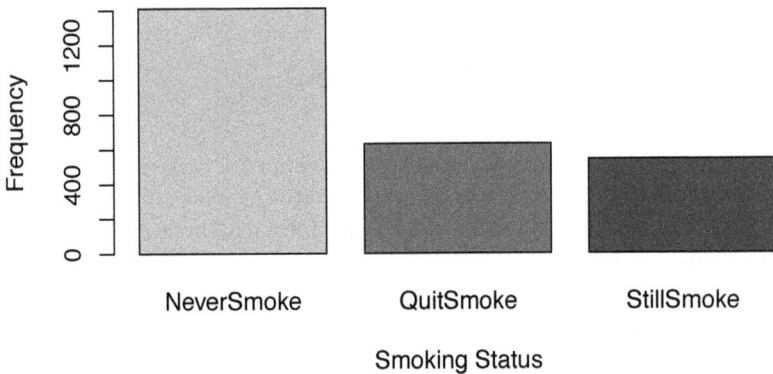

4.1.1 Practice Question

Recreate the barplot in Figure 4.1 below showing the proportion of values in each LEAD_QUANTILE category.

```
# Insert your solution here:
```

4.2 Bivariate Distributions

We now turn our attention to relationships among multiple columns. When we have two categorical columns, we can use the table() function to find the counts across all combinations. For example, we look at the distribution of smoking status levels by sex. We observe that a higher percentage of female participants have never smoked.

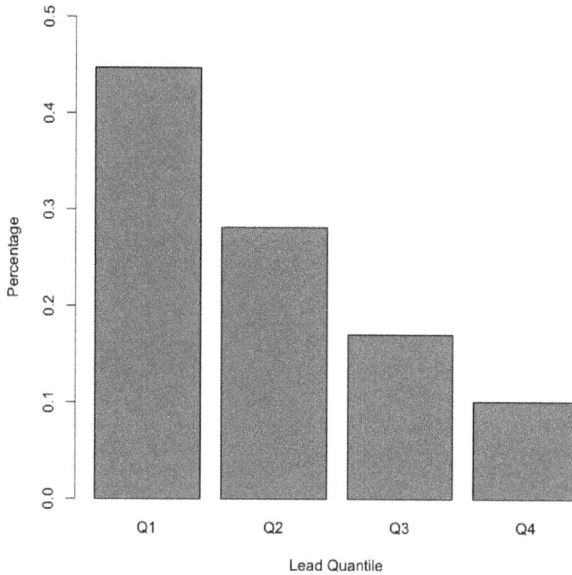

Figure 4.1: Lead Quantile Barplot.

```
table(nhanes_df$SMOKE, nhanes_df$SEX)
#>
#>                  Male Female
#>    NeverSmoke    596    815
#>    QuitSmoke     390    241
#>    StillSmoke    324    218
```

To look at the sample distribution of a continuous column stratified by a categorical column, we can call the summary() function for each subset of the data. In the subsequent code, we look at the distribution of blood lead level by sex and observe higher blood lead levels in male observations.

```
summary(nhanes_df$LEAD[nhanes_df$SEX == "Female"])
#>    Min. 1st Qu.  Median    Mean 3rd Qu.    Max.
#>    0.10    0.47    0.77    0.98    1.21    8.67
summary(nhanes_df$LEAD[nhanes_df$SEX == "Male"])
#>    Min. 1st Qu.  Median    Mean 3rd Qu.    Max.
#>    0.05    0.70    1.09    1.46    1.66   22.01
```

We can also observe this visually through a boxplot. When given one categorical column and one continuous column, the plot() function creates a boxplot.

By default, the first argument is the x-axis and the second argument is the y-axis.

```
plot(nhanes_df$SEX, log(nhanes_df$LEAD), ylab = "Log Blood Lead
 ↪ Level",
     xlab = "Sex")
```

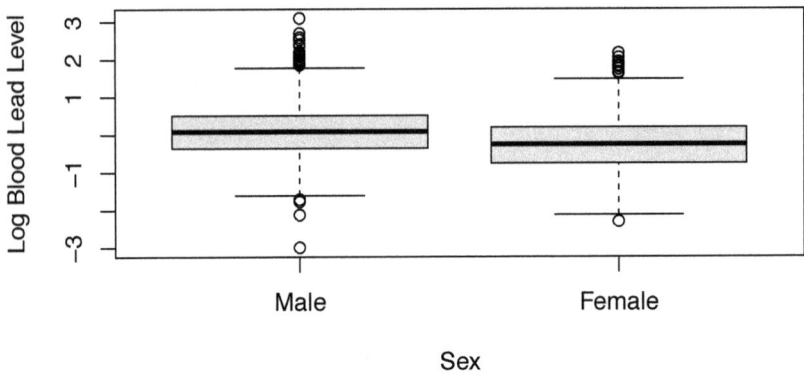

Alternatively, we can use the boxplot() function, which can be passed a formula. A formula is a string representation of how to group the data, where the left-hand side is the continuous column, and the right-hand side is one or more categorical columns to group by. In the following case, we group by multiple columns, SEX and EVER_SMOKE, so our formula is log(LEAD) ~ SEX + EVER_SMOKE. The second argument to the function specifies the data. We specify the column colors to show the link between the boxplots shown.

```
boxplot(log(LEAD) ~ SEX + EVER_SMOKE, data = nhanes_df,
        col=c("orange", "blue", "orange", "blue"),
        xlab = "Sex : Ever Smoked", ylab = "Log Blood Lead Level")
```

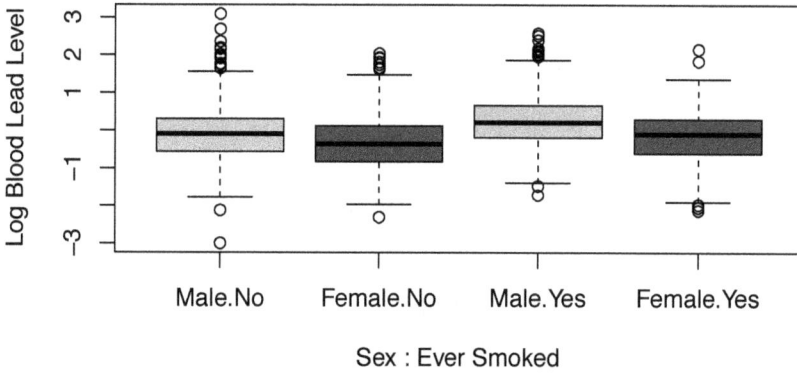

To visualize the bivariate distributions between two continuous columns, we can use scatter plots. To create a scatter plot, we use the `plot()` function again. We use this function to show the relationship between systolic and diastolic blood pressure.

```
plot(nhanes_df$SBP1, nhanes_df$DBP1, col = "blue",
    xlab = "Systolic Blood Pressure",
    ylab = "Diastolic Blood Pressure")
```

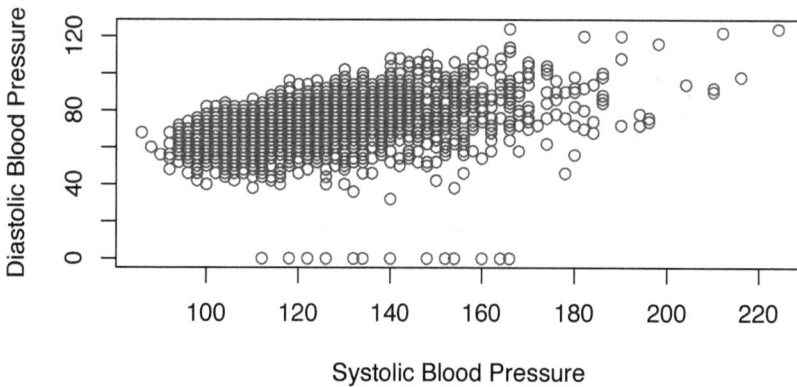

The two measures of blood pressure look highly correlated. We can calculate
their Pearson and Spearman correlation using the cor() function. The default
method is the Pearson correlation, but we can also calculate the Kendall or
Spearman correlation by specifying the method.

```
cor(nhanes_df$SBP1, nhanes_df$DBP1)
#> [1] 0.417
cor(nhanes_df$SBP1, nhanes_df$DBP1, method = "spearman")
#> [1] 0.471
```

We may also want to add some extra information to our plot. This time,
instead of specifying the color manually, we use the column hyp, an indicator
for hypertension, to specify the color. We have to make sure this vector is
a factor for R to color by group. Additionally, we add a blue vertical and
horizontal line using the abline() function to mark cutoffs for hypertension.
Even though this function is called after plot(), the lines are automatically
added to the current plot. We can see that most of those with hypertension
have systolic or diastolic blood pressure measurements above this threshold.

```
plot(nhanes_df$SBP1, nhanes_df$DBP1, col = as.factor(nhanes_df$HYP),
     xlab = "Systolic Blood Pressure",
     ylab = "Diastolic Blood Pressure")
abline(v = 130, col = "blue")
abline(h = 80, col = "blue")
```

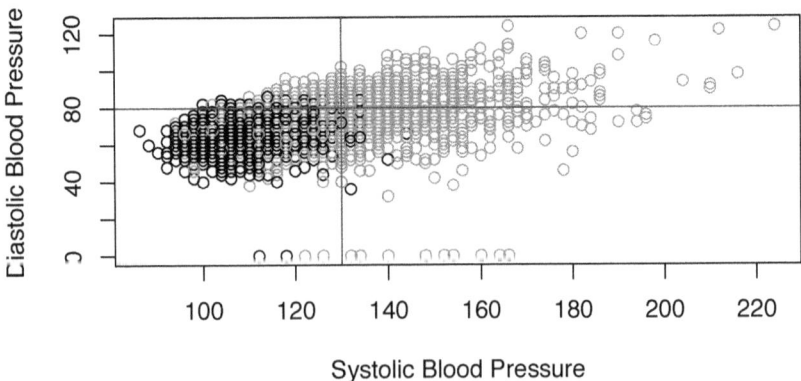

The previous plots are all displayed as a single figure. If we want to display multiple plots next to each other, we can specify the graphical parameters using the `par()` function by updating the argument `mfrow = c(nrow, ncol)` with the number of columns and rows we would like to use for our figures. We use this to display the distribution of log blood lead level between those with and without hypertension next to the previous plot.

```
par(mfrow = c(1, 2))

# boxplot
boxplot(log(LEAD) ~ HYP, data = nhanes_df, xlab = "Hypertension",
        ylab = "Log Blood Lead Level")

# scatter plot
plot(nhanes_df$SBP1, nhanes_df$DBP1, col = as.factor(nhanes_df$HYP),
     xlab = "Systolic Blood Pressure",
     ylab = "Diastolic Blood Pressure")
abline(v = 130, col = "blue")
abline(h = 80, col = "blue")
```

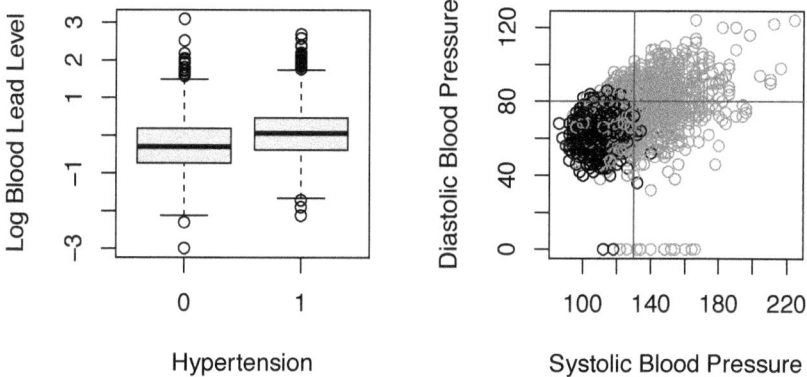

We then reset to only display a single plot for future images using the `par()` function again.

```
par(mfrow = c(1, 1))
```

4.2.1 Practice Question

Recreate the three boxplots in Figure 4.2 (one for each education level) of income by BMI category and arrange them next to each other using the par() function.

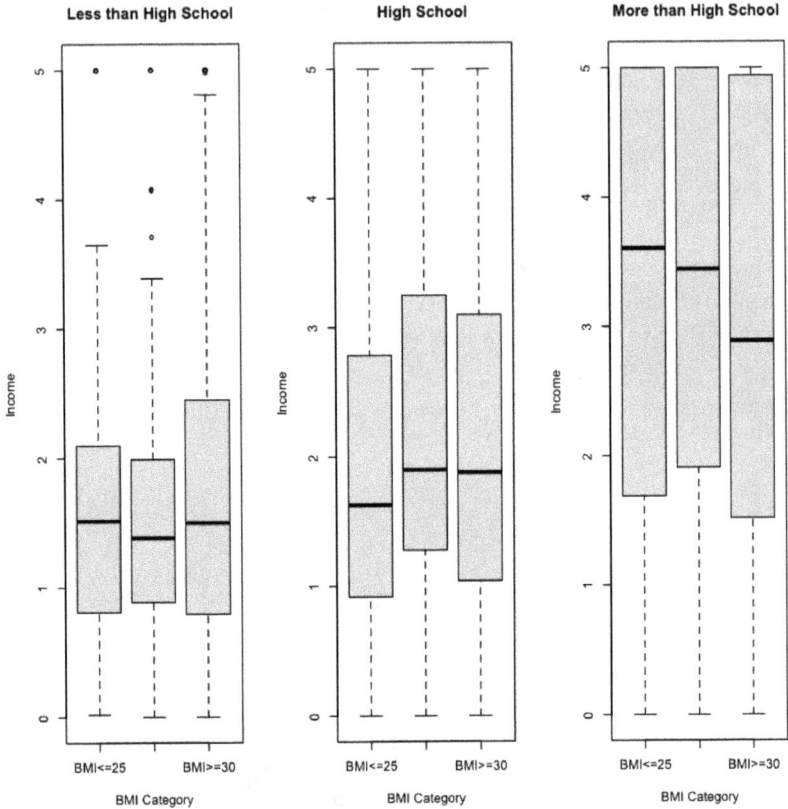

Figure 4.2: Boxplot Example.

```
# Insert your solution here:
```

4.3 Autogenerated Plots

In the previous sections, we learned some new functions for visualizing the relationship between columns. The **GGally** package contains some useful functions for looking at multiple univariate and bivariate relationships at the same time, such as the `ggpairs()` function. The function `ggpairs()` takes the data as its first argument. By default, it plots the pairwise distributions for all columns, but we can also specify to only select a subset of columns using the `columns` argument. You can see in the following example that it plots barplots and density plots for each univariate sample distribution. It then plots the bivariate distributions and calculates the Pearson correlation for all pairs of continuous columns. That's a lot of information!

```
ggpairs(nhanes_df, columns = c("SEX", "AGE", "LEAD", "SBP1", "DBP1"))
```

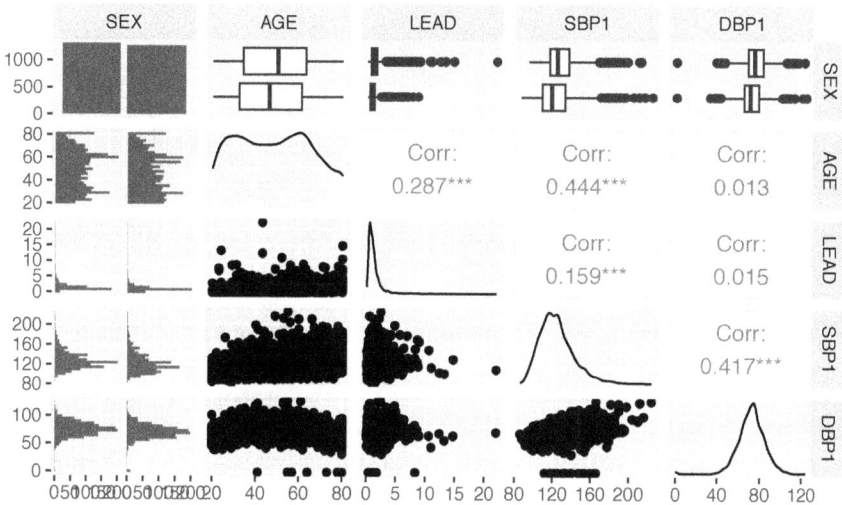

Another useful function in this package is the `ggcorr()` function. This function takes in a data frame with only numeric columns and displays the correlation between all pairs of columns, where the color of each grid cell indicates the strength of the correlation. The additional argument `label=TRUE` prints the actual correlation value on each grid cell. This is a useful way to identify pairs of strongly correlated columns. Note that we used the pipe operator again to find the correlation on the continuous columns without saving this subset of data.

```
nhanes_df[, c("AGE", "LEAD", "SBP1", "DBP1")] |>
  ggcorr(label = TRUE)
```

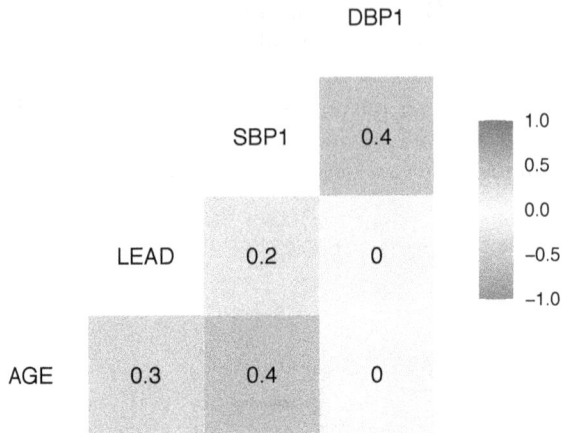

4.4 Tables

Another useful way to display information about your data is through tables. For example, it is standard practice in articles to have the first table in the paper give information about the study sample, such as the mean and standard deviation for all continuous columns and the proportions for categorical columns. The **gt** package is designed to create polished tables that can include footnotes, titles, column labels, etc. The **gtsummary** package is an extension of this package that can create summary tables. We focus on the latter but come back to creating nice tables in Chapter 22.

To start, we create a gt object (a special type of table) of the first six rows of our data using the `gt()` function. You can see the difference in the formatting as opposed to printing the data.

```
gt(head(nhanes_df[, c("ID", "AGE", "SEX", "RACE")]))
```

ID	AGE	SEX	RACE
93711	56	Male	Other Race
93713	67	Male	Non-Hispanic White
93716	61	Male	Other Race
93717	22	Male	Non-Hispanic White
93721	60	Female	Mexican American
93722	60	Female	Non-Hispanic White

We now show you how to use the `tbl_summary()` function in the **gtsummary** package. The first argument to this function is again the data frame. By default, this function summarizes all the columns in the data. Instead, we use the `include` argument to specify a list of columns to include. We then pipe this output to the function `as_gt()`, which creates a gt table from the summary output. Note that the table computes the total number of observations and the proportions for categorical columns and the median and interquartile range for continuous columns.

```
tbl_summary(nhanes_df,
            include = c("SEX", "RACE", "AGE", "EDUCATION", "SMOKE",
                        "BMI_CAT", "LEAD", "SBP1", "DBP1", "HYP")) |>
  as_gt()
```

Characteristic	N = 2,584[1]
SEX	
Male	1,310 (51%)
Female	1,274 (49%)
RACE	
Mexican American	358 (14%)
Other Hispanic	225 (8.7%)
Non-Hispanic White	992 (38%)
Non-Hispanic Black	568 (22%)
Other Race	441 (17%)
AGE	48 (33, 62)
EDUCATION	
LessThanHS	373 (14%)
HS	593 (23%)
MoreThanHS	1,618 (63%)
SMOKE	
NeverSmoke	1,411 (55%)
QuitSmoke	631 (24%)
StillSmoke	542 (21%)
BMI_CAT	
BMI<=25	663 (26%)
25<BMI<30	808 (31%)
BMI>=30	1,113 (43%)
LEAD	0.93 (0.56, 1.44)
SBP1	122 (112, 134)
DBP1	72 (66, 80)
HYP	1,451 (56%)

[1]n (%); Median (IQR)

We can update our table by changing some of its arguments. This time, we specify that we want to stratify our table by hypertension status so that the table summarizes the data by this grouping. Additionally, we change how continuous columns are summarized by specifying that we want to report the mean and standard deviation instead of the median and interquartile range. We do this using the `statistic` argument. The documentation for the `tbl_summary()` function can help you format this argument depending on which statistics you would like to display.

```
tbl_summary(nhanes_df,
            include = c("SEX", "RACE", "AGE", "EDUCATION", "SMOKE",
                        "BMI_CAT", "LEAD", "SBP1", "DBP1", "HYP"),
            by = "HYP",
            statistic = list(all_continuous() ~ "{mean} ({sd})")) |>
as_gt()
```

Characteristic	0, N = 1,133[1]	1, N = 1,451[1]
SEX		
Male	472 (42%)	838 (58%)
Female	661 (58%)	613 (42%)
RACE		
Mexican American	186 (16%)	172 (12%)
Other Hispanic	104 (9.2%)	121 (8.3%)
Non-Hispanic White	429 (38%)	563 (39%)
Non-Hispanic Black	203 (18%)	365 (25%)
Other Race	211 (19%)	230 (16%)
AGE	40 (15)	55 (16)
EDUCATION		
LessThanHS	151 (13%)	222 (15%)
HS	250 (22%)	343 (24%)
MoreThanHS	732 (65%)	886 (61%)
SMOKE		
NeverSmoke	678 (60%)	733 (51%)
QuitSmoke	220 (19%)	411 (28%)
StillSmoke	235 (21%)	307 (21%)
BMI_CAT		
BMI<=25	392 (35%)	271 (19%)
25<BMI<30	351 (31%)	457 (31%)
BMI>=30	390 (34%)	723 (50%)
LEAD	1.03 (1.15)	1.37 (1.25)
SBP1	112 (10)	134 (18)
DBP1	67 (9)	77 (14)

[1]n (%); Mean (SD)

Outside of the **gt** and **gtsummary** packages, another common package used to create summary tables is the **tableone** package (Yoshida and Bartel 2022), which is not covered in this book.

4.5 Exercises

For these exercises, we continue using the nhanes_df data.

1. Using both numerical and graphical summaries, describe the distribution of the first diastolic blood pressure reading DBP1 among study participants. Then, create a column called INCOME_CAT with two categories: "low" for those whose income is at most 2 and "not low" otherwise, and examine the bivariate distribution of DBP1 and INCOME_CAT. Arrange the two plots next to each other. What do you notice?

2. Create a subset of the data containing only adults between the ages of 20 and 55, inclusive. Then, explore how blood pressure varies by age and gender among this age group. Is there a visible trend in blood pressure with increasing age among either sex?

3. For males between the ages of 50 and 59, compare blood pressure across race as reported in the race column. Then, create a summary table stratified by the race column and report the mean, standard deviation, minimum, and maximum values for all continuous columns.

4. Recreate the plots in Figure 4.3 and Figure 4.4. Based on these plots, what trend do you expect to see in blood lead levels over time? Check your answer to the previous question by plotting these two columns against each other.

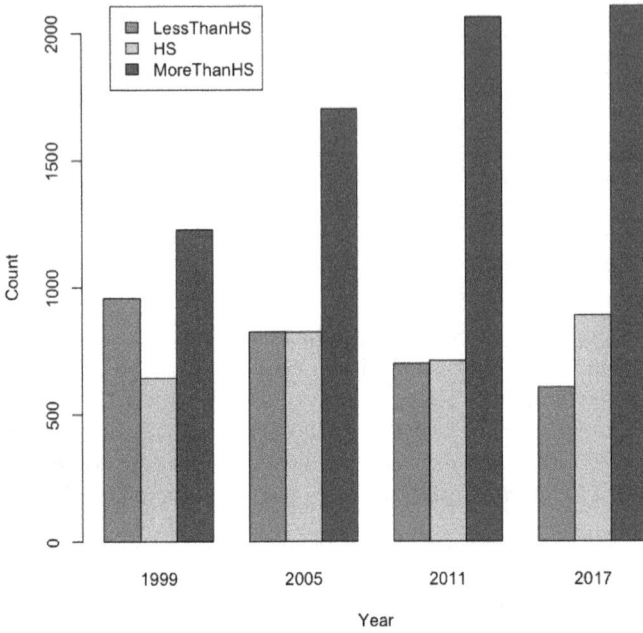

Figure 4.3: Education Levels Over Time.

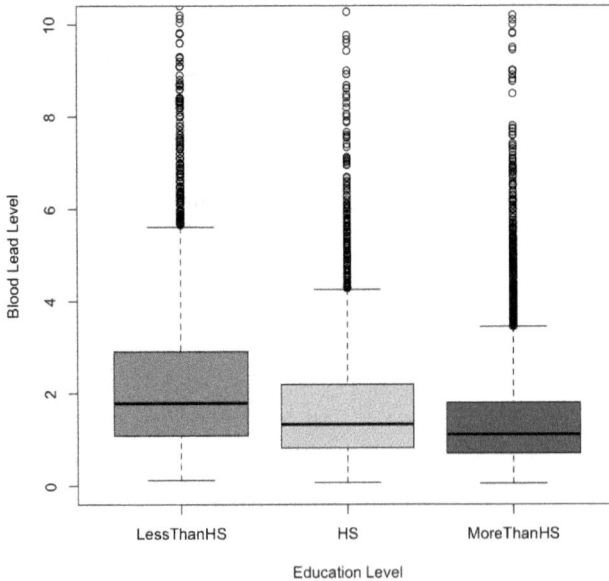

Figure 4.4: Blood Lead Level by Education Level.

5

Data Transformations and Summaries

In this chapter, we introduce the **dplyr** package (Wickham et al. 2023), which is part of the **tidyverse** group of packages, to expand our tools in exploring and transforming our data. We learn how to do some basic manipulations of data (e.g., adding or removing columns, filtering data, arranging by one or multiple columns) as well as how to summarize data (e.g., grouping by values, calculating summary statistics). We also practice combining these operations using the pipe operator %>% from the **tidyverse**. We use the same sample of the National Health and Nutrition Examination Survey (Centers for Disease Control and Prevention (CDC) 1999-2018) as in Chapter 4.

```
library(HDSinRdata)
library(tidyverse)

data(NHANESsample)
```

5.1 Tibbles and Data Frames

Take a look at the class of NHANESsample. As we might expect, the data is stored as a data frame.

```
class(NHANESsample)
#> [1] "data.frame"
```

However, **tidyverse** packages also work with another data structure called a **tibble**. A **tibble** has all the properties of data frames that we have learned so far, but they are a more modern version of a data frame. To convert our data to this data structure, we use the as_tibble() function. In practice, there are only very slight differences between the two data structures, and you generally do not need to convert data frames to tibbles. In the following code chunks, we convert our data from a data frame to a tibble and print the head of the data before converting it back to a data frame and repeating. You can see the

two structures have a slightly different print statement but are otherwise very
similar.

```
nhanes_df <- as_tibble(NHANESsample)
print(head(nhanes_df))
#> # A tibble: 6 x 21
#>       ID   AGE SEX    RACE      EDUCATION INCOME SMOKE  YEAR  LEAD
#>    ↳ BMI_CAT
#>    <dbl> <dbl> <fct>  <fct>     <fct>      <dbl> <fct> <dbl> <dbl>
#>    ↳ <fct>
#> 1     2    77 Male   Non-His~ MoreThan~      5  Neve~  1999  5
#>    ↳ BMI<=25
#> 2     5    49 Male   Non-His~ MoreThan~      5  Quit~  1999  1.6
#>    ↳ 25<BMI~
#> 3    12    37 Male   Non-His~ MoreThan~   4.93 Neve~  1999  2.4
#>    ↳ BMI>=30
#> 4    13    70 Male   Mexican~ LessThan~   1.07 Quit~  1999  1.6
#>    ↳ 25<BMI~
#> 5    14    81 Male   Non-His~ LessThan~   2.67 Stil~  1999  5.5
#>    ↳ 25<BMI~
#> 6    15    38 Female Non-His~ MoreThan~   4.52 Stil~  1999  1.5
#>    ↳ 25<BMI~
#> # i 11 more variables: LEAD_QUANTILE <fct>, HYP <dbl>, ALC <chr>,
#> #   DBP1 <dbl>, DBP2 <dbl>, DBP3 <dbl>, DBP4 <dbl>, SBP1 <dbl>,
#> #   SBP2 <dbl>, SBP3 <dbl>, SBP4 <dbl>
```

```
nhanes_df <- as.data.frame(nhanes_df)
print(head(nhanes_df))
#>    ID AGE    SEX              RACE EDUCATION INCOME      SMOKE YEAR
#> 1   2  77   Male Non-Hispanic White MoreThanHS   5.00 NeverSmoke 1999
#> 2   5  49   Male Non-Hispanic White MoreThanHS   5.00  QuitSmoke 1999
#> 3  12  37   Male Non-Hispanic White MoreThanHS   4.93 NeverSmoke 1999
#> 4  13  70   Male   Mexican American LessThanHS   1.07  QuitSmoke 1999
#> 5  14  81   Male Non-Hispanic White LessThanHS   2.67 StillSmoke 1999
#> 6  15  38 Female Non-Hispanic White MoreThanHS   4.52 StillSmoke 1999
#>    LEAD   BMI_CAT LEAD_QUANTILE HYP ALC DBP1 DBP2 DBP3 DBP4 SBP1 SBP2
#> 1   5.0   BMI<=25            Q4   0 Yes   58   56   56   NA  106   98
#> 2   1.6 25<BMI<30            Q3   1 Yes   62   64   62   NA  122  122
#> 3   2.4   BMI>=30            Q4   1 Yes  108   98  100   NA  182  172
#> 4   1.6 25<BMI<30            Q3   1 Yes   78   62   70   NA  140  130
#> 5   5.5 25<BMI<30            Q4   1 Yes   56   NA   58   64  142   NA
#> 6   1.5 25<BMI<30            Q3   0 Yes   68   68   70   NA  106  112
#>    SBP3 SBP4
```

```
#> 1    98    NA
#> 2   122    NA
#> 3   176    NA
#> 4   130    NA
#> 5   134   138
#> 6   106    NA
```

We mention tibbles here since some functions in the **tidyverse** convert data frames to tibbles in their output. In particular, when we later summarize over groups we can expect a tibble to be returned. It is useful to be aware that our data may change data structure with such functions and to know that we can always convert back if needed.

5.2 Subsetting Data

In earlier chapters, we have seen how to select and filter data using row and column indices as well as using the `subset()` function. The **dplyr** package has its own functions that are useful for subsetting data. The `select()` function allows us to select a subset of columns: this function takes in the data frame (or tibble) and the names or indices of the columns we want to select. For example, if we only wanted to select the variables for race and blood lead level, we could specify these two columns. To display the result of this selection, we use the pipe operator `%>%` from the **magittr** package of the **tidyverse**. Similar to the pipe operator `|>` in base R, the pipe operator `%>%` takes the result on the left-hand side and passes it as the first argument to the function on the right-hand side. The following output shows that there are only two columns in the filtered data.

```
select(nhanes_df, c(RACE, LEAD)) %>% head()
#>                   RACE LEAD
#> 1 Non-Hispanic White  5.0
#> 2 Non-Hispanic White  1.6
#> 3 Non-Hispanic White  2.4
#> 4    Mexican American  1.6
#> 5 Non-Hispanic White  5.5
#> 6 Non-Hispanic White  1.5
```

The `select()` function can also be used to *remove* columns by adding a negative sign in front of the vector of column names in its arguments. For example, we keep all columns except `ID` and `LEAD_QUANTILE`. Note that in this case we have saved the selected data back to our data frame `nhanes_df`. Additionally, this time we used a pipe operator to pipe the data to the select function itself.

```
nhanes_df <- nhanes_df %>% select(-c(ID, LEAD_QUANTILE))
names(nhanes_df)
#>  [1] "AGE"        "SEX"        "RACE"       "EDUCATION"  "INCOME"
#>  [6] "SMOKE"      "YEAR"       "LEAD"       "BMI_CAT"    "HYP"
#> [11] "ALC"        "DBP1"       "DBP2"       "DBP3"       "DBP4"
#> [16] "SBP1"       "SBP2"       "SBP3"       "SBP4"
```

While `select()` allows us to choose a subset of columns, the `filter()` function allows us to choose a subset of rows. The `filter()` function takes a data frame as the first argument and a vector of Booleans as the second argument. This vector of Booleans can be generated using conditional statements as we used in Chapter 4. We choose to filter the data to only observations after 2008.

```
nhanes_df_recent <- nhanes_df %>% filter(YEAR >= 2008)
```

We can combine conditions by using multiple `filter()` calls, by creating a more complicated conditional statement using the & (and), | (or), and %in% (in) operators, or by separating the conditions with commas within filter. In the following code, we demonstrate these three ways to filter the data to males between 2008 and 2012. Note that the `between()` function allows us to capture the logic `YEAR >= 2008 & YEAR <= 2012`.

```
# Example 1: multiple filter calls
nhanes_df_males1 <- nhanes_df %>%
  filter(YEAR <= 2012) %>%
  filter(YEAR >= 2008) %>%
  filter(SEX == "Male")

# Example 2: combine with & operator
nhanes_df_males2 <- nhanes_df %>%
  filter((YEAR <= 2012) & (YEAR >= 2008) & (SEX == "Male"))

# Example 3: combine into one filter call with commas
nhanes_df_males3 <- nhanes_df %>%
  filter(between(YEAR, 2008, 2012), SEX == "Male")
```

The use of parentheses in the previous code is especially important in order to capture our desired logic. In all these examples, we broke our code up into multiple lines, which makes it easier to read. A good rule of thumb is to not go past 80 characters in a line, and R Studio conveniently has a vertical gray line at this limit. To create a new line, you can hit enter either after an operator (e.g., %>%, +, |) or within a set of unfinished brackets or parentheses. Either of these breaks lets R know that your code is not finished yet.

Lastly, we can subset the data using the slice() function to select a slice of rows by their index. The function takes in the dataset and a vector of indices. In the following example, we find the first and last rows of the data.

```
slice(nhanes_df, c(1, nrow(nhanes_df)))
#>    AGE  SEX                   RACE  EDUCATION INCOME       SMOKE YEAR LEAD
#> 1   77 Male Non-Hispanic White MoreThanHS   5.00 NeverSmoke 1999  5.0
#> 2   38 Male Non-Hispanic White MoreThanHS   1.56 StillSmoke 2017  0.9
#>    BMI_CAT HYP ALC DBP1 DBP2 DBP3 DBP4 SBP1 SBP2 SBP3 SBP4
#> 1 BMI<=25   0 Yes   58   56   56   NA  106   98   98   NA
#> 2 BMI>=30   1 Yes   98   92   98   NA  150  146  148   NA
```

A few other useful slice functions are slice_sample(), slice_max(), and slice_min(). The first takes in an argument n which specifies the number of *random* rows to sample from the data. For example, we could randomly sample 100 rows from our data. The latter two allow us to specify a column through the argument order_by and return the n rows with either the highest or lowest values in that column. For example, we can find the three male observations from 2007 with the highest and lowest blood lead levels and select a subset of columns to display.

```
# three male observations with highest blood lead level in 2007
nhanes_df %>%
  filter(YEAR == 2007, SEX == "Male") %>%
  select(c(RACE, EDUCATION, SMOKE, LEAD, SBP1, DBP1)) %>%
  slice_max(order_by = LEAD, n = 3)
#>                RACE  EDUCATION      SMOKE LEAD SBP1 DBP1
#> 1 Non-Hispanic Black LessThanHS NeverSmoke 33.1  106   66
#> 2     Other Hispanic LessThanHS StillSmoke 26.8  106   72
#> 3     Other Hispanic LessThanHS StillSmoke 25.7  112   60

# three male observations with lowest blood lead level in 2007
nhanes_df %>%
  filter(YEAR == 2007, SEX == "Male") %>%
  select(c(RACE, EDUCATION, SMOKE, LEAD, SBP1, DBP1)) %>%
  slice_min(order_by = LEAD, n = 3)
#>                RACE  EDUCATION      SMOKE  LEAD SBP1 DBP1
#> 1 Non-Hispanic White LessThanHS NeverSmoke 0.177  114   80
#> 2     Other Hispanic LessThanHS  QuitSmoke 0.280  122   62
#> 3  Mexican American MoreThanHS  QuitSmoke 0.320  112   66
```

5.2.1 Practice Question

Filter the data to only those with an education level of more than HS who report alcohol use. Then, select only the diastolic blood pressure variables and display the fourth and tenth rows. Your result should match the result in Figure 5.1.

A data.frame: 2 × 4

DBP1	DBP2	DBP3	DBP4
<dbl>	<dbl>	<dbl>	<dbl>
68	68	70	NA
72	64	66	NA

Figure 5.1: Filtering and Selecting Data.

```
# Insert your solution here:
```

5.3 Updating Rows and Columns

The next few functions we look at allow us to update the rows and columns in our data. For example, the rename() function allows us to change the names of columns. In the following code, we change the name of INCOME to PIR since this variable is the poverty income ratio and also update the name of SMOKE to be SMOKE_STATUS. When specifying these names, the new name is on the left of the = and the old name is on the right.

```
nhanes_df <- nhanes_df %>% rename(PIR = INCOME, SMOKE_STATUS = SMOKE)
names(nhanes_df)
#>  [1] "AGE"          "SEX"            "RACE"       "EDUCATION"
#>  [5] "PIR"          "SMOKE_STATUS"   "YEAR"       "LEAD"
#>  [9] "BMI_CAT"      "HYP"            "ALC"        "DBP1"
#> [13] "DBP2"         "DBP3"           "DBP4"       "SBP1"
#> [17] "SBP2"         "SBP3"           "SBP4"
```

In the last chapter, we created a new variable called EVER_SMOKE based on the smoking status variable using the ifelse() function. Recall that this function allows us to specify a condition, and then two alternative values based on whether we meet or do not meet this condition. We see that there are about 15,000 subjects in our data who never smoked.

```
ifelse(nhanes_df$SMOKE_STATUS == "NeverSmoke", "No", "Yes") %>%
  table()
#> .
#>    No   Yes
#> 15087 16178
```

Another useful function from the **tidyverse** is the `case_when()` function, which is an extension of the `ifelse()` function but allows to specify more than two cases. We demonstrate this function to show how we could relabel the levels of the `SMOKE_STATUS` column. For each condition, we use the right side of the ~ to specify the value to be assigned when that condition is TRUE.

```
case_when(nhanes_df$SMOKE_STATUS == "NeverSmoke" ~ "Never Smoked",
          nhanes_df$SMOKE_STATUS == "QuitSmoke" ~ "Quit Smoking",
          nhanes_df$SMOKE_STATUS ==
            "StillSmoke" ~ "Current Smoker") %>%
  table()
#> .
#> Current Smoker   Never Smoked   Quit Smoking
#>           7317          15087           8861
```

In the previous example, we did not store the columns we created. To do so, we could use the $ operator or the `cbind()` function. The **tidyverse** also includes an alternative function to add columns called `mutate()`. This function takes in a data frame and a set of columns with associated names to add to the data or update. In the subsequent example, we create the column EVER_SMOKE and update the column SMOKE_STATUS. Within the `mutate()` function, we do not have to use the $ operator to reference the column SMOKE_STATUS. Instead, we can specify just the column name, and the function interprets it as that column.

```
nhanes_df <- nhanes_df %>%
  mutate(EVER_SMOKE = ifelse(SMOKE_STATUS == "NeverSmoke",
                             "No", "Yes"),
         SMOKE_STATUS =
           case_when(SMOKE_STATUS == "NeverSmoke" ~ "Never Smoked",
                     SMOKE_STATUS == "QuitSmoke" ~ "Quit Smoking",
                     SMOKE_STATUS == "StillSmoke" ~ "Current Smoker"))
```

The last function we demonstrate in this section is the `arrange()` function, which takes in a data frame and a vector of columns used to sort the data (data is sorted by the first column with ties sorted by the second column, etc.). By default, the `arrange()` function sorts the data in increasing order, but we can use the `desc()` function to instead sort in descending order. For example, the following code filters the data to male smokers before sorting by decreasing systolic and diastolic blood pressure in descending order. That is, the value of `DBP1` is used to sort rows that have the same systolic blood pressure values.

```
nhanes_df %>%
   select(c(YEAR, SEX, SMOKE_STATUS, SBP1, DBP1, LEAD)) %>%
   filter(SEX == "Male", SMOKE_STATUS == "Current Smoker") %>%
   arrange(desc(SBP1), desc(DBP1)) %>%
   head(8)
#>    YEAR  SEX  SMOKE_STATUS SBP1 DBP1 LEAD
#> 1 2011 Male Current Smoker  230  120 5.84
#> 2 2015 Male Current Smoker  230   98 1.56
#> 3 2009 Male Current Smoker  220   80 4.84
#> 4 2001 Male Current Smoker  218  118 3.70
#> 5 2017 Male Current Smoker  212  122 2.20
#> 6 2003 Male Current Smoker  212   54 4.00
#> 7 2011 Male Current Smoker  210   92 5.37
#> 8 2007 Male Current Smoker  210   80 2.18
```

If instead we had only sorted by `SBP1`, then the rows with the same value for systolic blood pressure would appear in their original order. You can see the difference in the following output.

```
nhanes_df %>%
   select(c(YEAR, SEX, SMOKE_STATUS, SBP1, DBP1, LEAD)) %>%
   filter(SEX == "Male", SMOKE_STATUS == "Current Smoker") %>%
   arrange(desc(SBP1)) %>%
   head(8)
#>    YEAR  SEX  SMOKE_STATUS SBP1 DBP1 LEAD
#> 1 2011 Male Current Smoker  230  120 5.84
#> 2 2015 Male Current Smoker  230   98 1.56
#> 3 2009 Male Current Smoker  220   80 4.84
#> 4 2001 Male Current Smoker  218  118 3.70
#> 5 2003 Male Current Smoker  212   54 4.00
#> 6 2017 Male Current Smoker  212  122 2.20
#> 7 2007 Male Current Smoker  210   80 2.18
#> 8 2011 Male Current Smoker  210   92 5.37
```

5.3.1   Practice Question

Create a new column called DBP_CHANGE that is equal to the difference between a patient's first and fourth diastolic blood pressure readings. Then, sort the data frame by this new column in increasing order and print the first four rows. The first four DBP_CHANGE values in the head of the resulting data frame should be −66, −64, −64, and −62.

```
# Insert your solution here:
```

5.4   Summarizing and Grouping

If we want to understand how many observations there are for each given race category, we could use the table() function as we described in earlier chapters. Another similar function is the count() function. This function takes in a data frame and one or more columns and counts the number of rows for each combination of unique values in these columns. If no columns are specified, it counts the total number of rows in the data frame. In the following code, we find the total number of rows (31,265) and the number of observations by race and year. We can see that the number in each group fluctuates quite a bit!

```
count(nhanes_df)
#>         n
#> 1 31265
count(nhanes_df, RACE, YEAR)
#>                   RACE YEAR    n
#> 1     Mexican American 1999  713
#> 2     Mexican American 2001  674
#> 3     Mexican American 2003  627
#> 4     Mexican American 2005  634
#> 5     Mexican American 2007  639
#> 6     Mexican American 2009  672
#> 7     Mexican American 2011  322
#> 8     Mexican American 2013  234
#> 9     Mexican American 2015  287
#> 10    Mexican American 2017  475
#> 11      Other Hispanic 1999  181
#> 12      Other Hispanic 2001  129
#> 13      Other Hispanic 2003   80
#> 14      Other Hispanic 2005   96
```

```
#> 15       Other Hispanic 2007    395
#> 16       Other Hispanic 2009    367
#> 17       Other Hispanic 2011    337
#> 18       Other Hispanic 2013    167
#> 19       Other Hispanic 2015    214
#> 20       Other Hispanic 2017    313
#> 21 Non-Hispanic White 1999   1401
#> 22 Non-Hispanic White 2001   1882
#> 23 Non-Hispanic White 2003   1785
#> 24 Non-Hispanic White 2005   1818
#> 25 Non-Hispanic White 2007   1940
#> 26 Non-Hispanic White 2009   2169
#> 27 Non-Hispanic White 2011   1463
#> 28 Non-Hispanic White 2013    917
#> 29 Non-Hispanic White 2015    685
#> 30 Non-Hispanic White 2017   1413
#> 31 Non-Hispanic Black 1999    463
#> 32 Non-Hispanic Black 2001    542
#> 33 Non-Hispanic Black 2003    576
#> 34 Non-Hispanic Black 2005    679
#> 35 Non-Hispanic Black 2007    728
#> 36 Non-Hispanic Black 2009    661
#> 37 Non-Hispanic Black 2011    876
#> 38 Non-Hispanic Black 2013    357
#> 39 Non-Hispanic Black 2015    351
#> 40 Non-Hispanic Black 2017    808
#> 41          Other Race 1999     76
#> 42          Other Race 2001     88
#> 43          Other Race 2003    109
#> 44          Other Race 2005    122
#> 45          Other Race 2007    123
#> 46          Other Race 2009    175
#> 47          Other Race 2011    475
#> 48          Other Race 2013    223
#> 49          Other Race 2015    209
#> 50          Other Race 2017    595
```

Finding the counts like we did previously is a form of a summary statistic for our data. The `summarize()` function in the **tidyverse** is used to compute summary statistics of the data and allows us to compute multiple statistics: this function takes in a data frame and one or more summary functions based on the given column names. In the subsequent example, we find the total number of observations as well as the mean and median systolic blood pressure for Non-Hispanic Blacks. Note that the `n()` function is the function within

summarize() that finds the number of observations. In the mean() and median()
functions we set na.rm=TRUE to remove NAs before computing these values
(otherwise, we could get NA as our output).

```
nhanes_df %>%
  filter(RACE == "Non-Hispanic Black") %>%
  summarize(TOT = n(), MEAN_SBP = mean(SBP1, na.rm=TRUE),
            MEAN_DBP = mean(DBP1, na.rm=TRUE))
#>    TOT MEAN_SBP MEAN_DBP
#> 1 6041      129     72.6
```

If we wanted to repeat this for the other race groups, we would have to change
the arguments to the filter() function each time. To avoid having to repeat
our code and/or do this multiple times, we can use the group_by() function,
which takes a data frame and one or more columns with which to group the
data. In the following code, we group using the RACE variable. When we look
at printed output, it looks almost the same as it did before except that we can
see that its class is now a grouped data frame, which is printed at the top. In
fact, a grouped data frame (or grouped tibble) acts like a set of data frames:
one for each group. If we use the slice() function with index 1, it returns the
first row for each group.

```
nhanes_df %>%
  group_by(RACE) %>%
  slice(1)
#> # A tibble: 5 x 20
#> # Groups:   RACE [5]
#>     AGE SEX    RACE     EDUCATION   PIR SMOKE_STATUS  YEAR  LEAD
#> ↳   BMI_CAT
#>   <dbl> <fct> <fct>    <fct>      <dbl> <chr>        <dbl> <dbl>
#> ↳   <fct>
#> 1    70 Male   Mexican~ LessThan~  1.07 Quit Smoking  1999   1.6
#> ↳   25<BMI~
#> 2    61 Female Other H~ MoreThan~  3.33 Current Smo~  1999   2.2
#> ↳   BMI<=25
#> 3    77 Male   Non-His~ MoreThan~  5    Never Smoked  1999   5
#> ↳   BMI<=25
#> 4    38 Female Non-His~ HS         0.92 Current Smo~  1999   1.8
#> ↳   25<BMI~
#> 5    63 Female Other R~ MoreThan~  5    Never Smoked  1999   1.2
#> ↳   BMI<=25
#> # i 11 more variables: HYP <dbl>, ALC <chr>, DBP1 <dbl>, DBP2 <dbl>,
```

```
#> #    DBP3 <dbl>, DBP4 <dbl>, SBP1 <dbl>, SBP2 <dbl>, SBP3 <dbl>,
#> #    SBP4 <dbl>, EVER_SMOKE <chr>
```

Grouping data is very helpful in combination with the `summarize()` function.
Like with the `slice()` function, `summarize()` calculates the summary values
for each group. We can now find the total number of observations as well as
the mean systolic and diastolic blood pressure values for each racial group.
Note that the returned summarized data is in a tibble.

```
nhanes_df %>%
  group_by(RACE) %>%
  summarize(TOT = n(), MEAN_SBP = mean(SBP1, na.rm=TRUE),
            MEAN_DBP = mean(DBP1, na.rm=TRUE))
#> # A tibble: 5 x 4
#>   RACE                  TOT MEAN_SBP MEAN_DBP
#>   <fct>               <int>    <dbl>    <dbl>
#> 1 Mexican American     5277     124.     70.4
#> 2 Other Hispanic       2279     123.     70.1
#> 3 Non-Hispanic White  15473     125.     70.4
#> 4 Non-Hispanic Black   6041     129.     72.6
#> 5 Other Race           2195     122.     72.6
```

After summarizing, the data is no longer grouped by race. If we ever want to
remove the group structure from our data, we can use the `ungroup()` function,
which restores the data to a single data frame. After ungrouping by race, we
can see that we get a single observation returned by the `slice()` function.

```
nhanes_df %>%
  select(SEX, RACE, SBP1, DBP1) %>%
  group_by(RACE) %>%
  ungroup() %>%
  arrange(desc(SBP1)) %>%
  slice(1)
#> # A tibble: 1 x 4
#>   SEX    RACE                 SBP1  DBP1
#>   <fct>  <fct>               <dbl> <dbl>
#> 1 Female Non-Hispanic White    270   124
```

5.4.1 Practice Question

Create a data frame summarizing the percent of patients with hypertension
by smoking status. The result should look like Figure 5.2.

A grouped_df: 3 × 2

SMOKE_STATUS	PCT_HYP
<chr>	<dbl>
Current Smoker	0.5096351
Never Smoked	0.5140850
Quit Smoking	0.6559079

Figure 5.2: Grouping and Summarizing Data.

```
# Insert your solution here:
```

5.5 Exercises

The following exercises use the covidcases dataset from the **HDSinRdata** package. Before completing the exercises, be sure to read the documentation for this data (?covidcases).

```
data(covidcases)
```

1. Suppose we are interested in the distribution of weekly cases by state. First, create a new column in covidcases called region specifying whether each state is in the Northeast, Midwest, South, or West (you can either do this by hand using this list[1] of which states are in which region, or you can use state.region from the **datasets** package in R). Then, create a data frame summarizing the average and standard deviation of the weekly cases for the Northeast.

2. Now, create a data frame with the average and standard deviation summarized for each region rather than for just one selected region as in Question 1. Sort this data frame from highest to lowest average weekly cases. What other information would you need in order to

[1]https://en.wikipedia.org/wiki/List_of_regions_of_the_United_States

more accurately compare these regions in terms of their average cases?

3. Find the ten counties in the Midwest with the lowest weekly deaths in week 15 of this data ignoring ties (use `slice_min()` to find the argument needed for this). What do you notice about the minimum values? See the data documentation for why we observe these values.

4. Filter the data to include weeks 9 and 20 (around the start of the pandemic), get the total cases per county during that time frame, and then find the county in each state that had the highest number of total cases.

6

Case Study: Cleaning Tuberculosis Screening Data

In this chapter, we put some of our R skills together in a case study. This case study focuses on data cleaning and pre-processing. We use the `tb_diagnosis_raw` data from the **HDSinRdata** package. This data contains information on 1,634 patients in rural South Africa who presented at a health clinic with tuberculosis-related symptoms and were tested for tuberculosis (TB) using Xpert MTB/RIF. Our goal is to clean this data to reflect the pre-processing described in Baik et al. (2020). This paper uses this data to derive a simple risk score model for screening patients for treatment while awaiting Xpert results. We use the **tidyverse** packages as well as the summary tables from **gtsummary**.

```
library(HDSinRdata)
library(tidyverse)
library(gt)
library(gtsummary)
```

To begin, read in the data and review the description of the original columns. Some things to note in the data documentation are the ways unknown, missing, or refused values are coded as well as how some of the columns are related to each other.

```
# Read in data
data("tb_diagnosis_raw")

# Inspect variable descriptions
# ?tb_diagnosis_raw
```

To start, we select variables needed for our analysis. In particular, we drop columns related to the participation in the survey and about seeking care. Since some of these variables contain long or vague names, we also rename most of the variables.

```
# Select variables and rename
tb_df <- tb_diagnosis_raw %>%
  select(c(xpert_status_fac, age_group, sex, hiv_status_fac,
           other_conditions_fac___1, other_conditions_fac___3,
           other_conditions_fac___88, other_conditions_fac___99,
           symp_fac___1, symp_fac___2, symp_fac___3, symp_fac___4,
           symp_fac___99, length_symp_unit_fac, length_symp_days_fac,
           length_symp_wk_fac, length_symp_mnt_fac, length_symp_yr_fac,
           smk_fac, dx_tb_past_fac, educ_fac)) %>%
    rename(tb = xpert_status_fac, hiv_pos = hiv_status_fac,
           cough = symp_fac___1, fever = symp_fac___2,
           weight_loss = symp_fac___3, night_sweats = symp_fac___4,
           symptoms_missing = symp_fac___99,
           ever_smoke = smk_fac,
           past_tb = dx_tb_past_fac, education = educ_fac)
```

We then use a summary table to understand the initial distributions of the variables observed. This also highlights where we have missing or unknown data.

```
tbl_summary(tb_df) %>%
  as_gt()
```

Characteristic	N = 1,634[1]
tb	
1	765 (47%)
2	869 (53%)
age_group	
[15,25)	240 (15%)
[25,35)	333 (20%)
[35,45)	385 (24%)
[45,55)	343 (21%)
[55,99)	333 (20%)
sex	
1	830 (51%)
2	804 (49%)
hiv_pos	
1	632 (39%)
2	815 (50%)
77	139 (8.5%)
88	48 (2.9%)
other_conditions_fac___1	895 (55%)

other_conditions_fac____3		52 (3.2%)
other_conditions_fac____88		11 (0.7%)
other_conditions_fac____99		30 (1.8%)
cough		1,279 (78%)
fever		479 (29%)
weight_loss		534 (33%)
night_sweats		579 (35%)
symptoms_missing		22 (1.3%)
length_symp_unit_fac		
1		207 (14%)
2		603 (39%)
3		538 (35%)
4		83 (5.4%)
77		98 (6.4%)
Unknown		105
length_symp_days_fac		3 (3, 4)
Unknown		1,427
length_symp_wk_fac		
1		183 (30%)
2		237 (39%)
3		147 (24%)
4		15 (2.5%)
5		5 (0.8%)
6		13 (2.2%)
7		3 (0.5%)
Unknown		1,031
length_symp_mnt_fac		2 (1, 3)
Unknown		1,096
length_symp_yr_fac		2 (1, 4)
Unknown		1,551
ever_smoke		
1		294 (18%)
2		252 (15%)
3		1,072 (66%)
99		16 (1.0%)
past_tb		
1		255 (16%)
2		1,354 (83%)
77		25 (1.5%)
education		10 (7, 12)

[1]n (%); Median (IQR)

One observation from the table is that the coding of variables is inconsistent, with some using 0/1 and others using 1/2. We want to standardize how these variables are represented. To start, we update our `tb` column. Additionally, we create a column `male` from the previous column `sex` to make the reference level clear. We can then drop the `sex` column.

```
# Re-code binary variables to 0/1 instead of 1/2
tb_df$tb <- case_when(tb_df$tb == 1 ~ "TB Positive",
                      tb_df$tb == 2 ~ "TB Negative")

tb_df$male <- case_when(tb_df$sex == 1 ~ 1,
                        tb_df$sex == 2 ~ 0)
tb_df <- tb_df %>% select(-c(sex))
```

Diabetes is another variable that should be coded this way. In the raw data, several columns correspond to this question about other medical conditions. Therefore, we need to use the columns `other_conditions_fac___88` and `other_conditions_fac___99` to check whether the participant did not answer the question when interpreting the 0/1 value for diabetes.

```
# Re-code diabetes to check if missing
tb_df$diabetes <- case_when(tb_df$other_conditions_fac___3 == 1 ~ 1,
                            tb_df$other_conditions_fac___1 == 1 ~ 0,
                            tb_df$other_conditions_fac___88 == 1 ~ NA,
                            tb_df$other_conditions_fac___99 == 1 ~ NA,
                            TRUE ~ 0)
tb_df <- tb_df %>% select(-c(other_conditions_fac___1,
                             other_conditions_fac___3,
                             other_conditions_fac___88,
                             other_conditions_fac___99))
table(tb_df$diabetes)
#>
#>     0    1
#> 1541   52
```

Next, we similarly code our variables about HIV status, smoking, and whether the patient has ever been diagnosed with tuberculosis before. For these variables, if the patient answered that they did not know their HIV status or if they had tested positive for TB, we code these as 0 to be consistent with the paper.

```
# Re-code variables with missing or refused values
tb_df$hiv_pos <- case_when((tb_df$hiv_pos == 1) ~ 1,
                           tb_df$hiv_pos %in% c(2,77) ~ 0,
                           tb_df$hiv_pos == 88 ~ NA)
```

```r
tb_df$ever_smoke <- case_when(tb_df$ever_smoke %in% c(1,2) ~ 1,
                              tb_df$ever_smoke == 3 ~ 0,
                              tb_df$ever_smoke == 99 ~ NA)

tb_df$past_tb <- case_when(tb_df$past_tb == 1 ~ 1,
                           tb_df$past_tb %in% c(2,77) ~ 0)
```

The next variable we clean is `education`. First, we need to code NA values correctly. We can then observe the distribution of years of education.

```r
# Code NA values and look at education distribution
tb_df$education[tb_df$education == 99] <- NA
hist(tb_df$education, xlab = "Years of Education",
     main = "Histogram of Education Years")
```

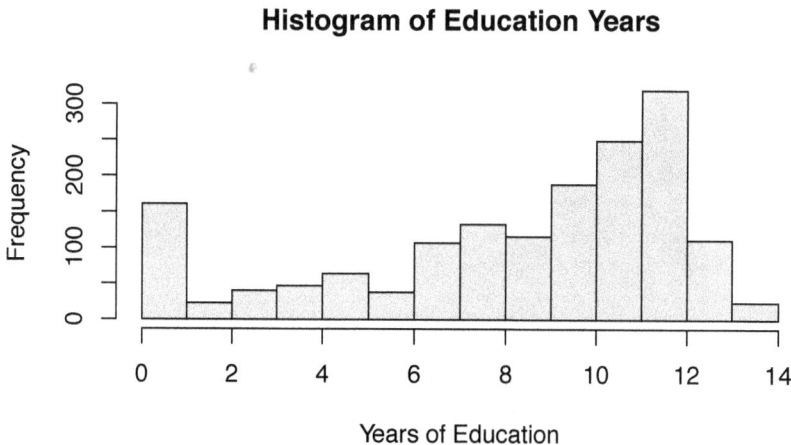

Histogram of Education Years

For our purposes, we want to represent education as whether a person has a high school education or less.

```r
# Categorize education to HS and above
tb_df$hs_less <- case_when(tb_df$education <= 12 ~ 1,
                           tb_df$education > 12 ~ 0,
                           TRUE ~ NA)
tb_df <- tb_df %>% select(-c(education))
```

There are several variables in the data related to how long a person has experienced symptoms. In the following code, we can see that the unit of the symptoms, recorded in `length_symp_unit_fac`, determines which other column is entered. For example, if `length_symp_unit_fac == 1`, then the only column without an NA value is `length_symp_days_fc`.

```
tb_df %>%
  group_by(length_symp_unit_fac) %>%
  summarize(missing_days = sum(is.na(length_symp_days_fac))/n(),
            missing_wks = sum(is.na(length_symp_wk_fac))/n(),
            missing_mnt = sum(is.na(length_symp_mnt_fac))/n(),
            missing_yr = sum(is.na(length_symp_yr_fac))/n())
#> # A tibble: 6 x 5
#>   length_symp_unit_fac missing_days missing_wks missing_mnt
↳   missing_yr
#>                  <int>        <dbl>       <dbl>       <dbl>      <dbl>
#> 1                    1            0           1           1          1
#> 2                    2            1           0           1          1
#> 3                    3            1           1           0          1
#> 4                    4            1           1           1          0
#> 5                   77            1           1           1          1
#> 6                   NA            1           1           1          1
```

Additionally, these measurements are positive integer values.

```
min(tb_df$length_symp_days_fac, na.rm = TRUE)
#> [1] 1
is.integer(tb_df$length_symp_days_fac)
#> [1] TRUE
```

This allows us to create a new variable that represents whether or not someone has had symptoms for more than two weeks. In our `case_when()` function call, we first check whether the duration is missing before checking for the cases when symptoms would be less than two weeks.

```
# Categorize number of weeks experiencing symptoms
tb_df <- tb_df %>%
  mutate(two_weeks = case_when((length_symp_unit_fac == 77 |
                 is.na(length_symp_unit_fac)) ~ NA,
               (length_symp_unit_fac == 1 &
                 length_symp_days_fac <= 14) ~ 0,
               (length_symp_unit_fac == 2 &
                 length_symp_wk_fac <= 2) ~ 0,
```

```
                    TRUE ~ 1))

tb_df <- tb_df %>%
  select(-c(length_symp_wk_fac, length_symp_days_fac,
            length_symp_mnt_fac, length_symp_yr_fac,
            length_symp_unit_fac))
```

Last, we update our symptom variables to have a summary column num_symptoms that represents the total number of classic TB symptoms rather than keeping track of individual symptoms. We also exclude anyone who does not have any TB symptoms.

```
# Count total number of symptoms
tb_df$num_symptoms <- tb_df$fever + tb_df$weight_loss + tb_df$cough +
  tb_df$night_sweats
tb_df$num_symptoms[tb_df$symptoms_missing == 1] <- NA
tb_df <- tb_df %>% select(-c(night_sweats, weight_loss, cough, fever,
                             symptoms_missing))

# Exclude observations with no TB symptoms
tb_df <- tb_df %>%
  filter(num_symptoms != 0)

table(tb_df$num_symptoms)
#>
#>   1   2   3   4
#> 600 344 265 196
```

Last, we convert all variables to factors.

```
# Convert all variables to factors
tb_df[] <- lapply(tb_df, function(x){return(as.factor(x))})
```

Our final data is summarized in the following table. The add_overall() function includes the overall summary statistics in addition to our stratified summaries. Our summary table looks similar to the one in the paper. However, it looks like we have a few more observations included. Additionally, our education variable shows a lower percentage of observations with post-high school education and positive HIV status.

```
tbl_summary(tb_df, by = "tb",
            label = list(
              tb= "Tuberculosis",
              age_group = "Age Group",
              hiv_pos = "HIV Positive",
              ever_smoke = "Ever Smoked",
              past_tb = "Past TB",
              male = "Male",
              hs_less = "High School or Less Educ.",
              two_weeks = "Two Weeks Symptoms",
              diabetes = "Diabetes",
              num_symptoms = "Number of Symptoms"
            )) %>%
  add_overall() %>%
  as_gt() %>%
  cols_width(everything() ~ "55pt")
```

Characteristic	Overall, N = 1,405[1]	TB Negative, N = 704[1]	TB Positive, N = 701[1]
Age Group			
[15,25)	205 (15%)	121 (17%)	84 (12%)
[25,35)	286 (20%)	120 (17%)	166 (24%)
[35,45)	338 (24%)	136 (19%)	202 (29%)
[45,55)	305 (22%)	158 (22%)	147 (21%)
[55,99)	271 (19%)	169 (24%)	102 (15%)
HIV Positive			
0	808 (59%)	503 (73%)	305 (45%)
1	556 (41%)	186 (27%)	370 (55%)
Unknown	41	15	26
Ever Smoked			
0	899 (64%)	483 (69%)	416 (60%)
1	496 (36%)	213 (31%)	283 (40%)
Unknown	10	8	2
Past TB			
0	1,186 (84%)	613 (87%)	573 (82%)
1	219 (16%)	91 (13%)	128 (18%)
Male			
0	669 (48%)	394 (56%)	275 (39%)
1	736 (52%)	310 (44%)	426 (61%)
Diabetes			

0	1,326 (97%)	658 (97%)	668 (96%)
1	47 (3.4%)	22 (3.2%)	25 (3.6%)
Unknown	32	24	8
High School or Less Educ.			
0	119 (8.5%)	73 (10%)	46 (6.6%)
1	1,276 (91%)	625 (90%)	651 (93%)
Unknown	10	6	4
Two Weeks Symptoms			
0	592 (44%)	386 (57%)	206 (31%)
1	760 (56%)	294 (43%)	466 (69%)
Unknown	53	24	29
Number of Symptoms			
1	600 (43%)	426 (61%)	174 (25%)
2	344 (24%)	181 (26%)	163 (23%)
3	265 (19%)	67 (9.5%)	198 (28%)
4	196 (14%)	30 (4.3%)	166 (24%)

[1]n (%)

7

Merging and Reshaping Data

In this chapter, we continue to look at some of the ways to manipulate data using the **tidyr** and **dplyr** packages, which are part of the **tidyverse** group of packages. In particular, we look at reshaping and merging data frames in order to get the data in the format we want. When reshaping data, we can convert between *wide form* (more columns, fewer rows) and *long form* (fewer columns, more rows). We can also use data pivots to put our data into what is called *tidy form*. Additionally, we look at combining information from multiple data frames into a single data frame. The key ideas when merging data are to think about what the common information is between the data frames and to consider which values we want to keep.

For this chapter, we use three datasets. The first dataset is covidcases, which contains the weekly COVID-19 case and death counts by county in the United States for 2020 (Guidotti and Ardia 2020; Guidotti 2022); the second dataset is mobility, which contains daily mobility estimates by state in 2020 (Warren and Skillman 2020); and the third dataset is lockdowndates, which contains the start and end dates for statewide stay-at-home orders (Raifman et al. 2022). Take a look at the first few rows of each data frame and read the documentation for the column descriptions.

```
library(tidyverse)
library(HDSinRdata)

data(covidcases)
data(lockdowndates)
data(mobility)
```

```
head(covidcases)
#> # A tibble: 6 x 5
#>    state       county  week weekly_cases weekly_deaths
#>    <chr>       <chr>   <dbl>      <int>          <int>
#> 1 California   Marin      9          1              0
#> 2 California   Orange     9          3              0
#> 3 Florida      Manatee    9          1              0
```

```
#> 4 California      Napa        9            1              0
#> 5 New Hampshire Grafton      9            2              0
#> 6 Washington     Spokane     9            4              0
```

```
head(mobility)
#> # A tibble: 6 x 5
#> # Groups:    state [1]
#>    state    date        samples   m50 m50_index
#>    <chr>    <chr>         <int> <dbl>     <dbl>
#> 1 Alabama 2020-03-01   267652  10.9      76.9
#> 2 Alabama 2020-03-02   287264  14.3      98.6
#> 3 Alabama 2020-03-03   292018  14.2      98.2
#> 4 Alabama 2020-03-04   298704  13.1      89.7
#> 5 Alabama 2020-03-05   288218  14.8      102.
#> 6 Alabama 2020-03-06   282982  17.9      126.
```

```
head(lockdowndates)
#> # A tibble: 6 x 3
#>    State       Lockdown_Start Lockdown_End
#>    <chr>       <chr>          <chr>
#> 1 Alabama     2020-04-04     2020-04-30
#> 2 Alaska      2020-03-28     2020-04-24
#> 3 Arizona     2020-03-31     2020-05-16
#> 4 Arkansas    None           None
#> 5 California  2020-03-19     2021-01-25
#> 6 Colorado    2020-03-26     2020-04-27
```

Both the mobility and lockdown data frames contain date columns. Right now, these columns in both datasets are of the class character, which we can see in the printed output. We can use the as.Date() function to tell R to treat these columns as dates instead of characters. When using this function, we need to specify the date format as an argument so that R knows how to parse this text to a date. Our format is given as %Y-%M-%D, where the %Y stands for the full four-digit year, %M is a two-digit month (e.g., January is coded "01" vs. "1"), and %D stands for the two-digit day (e.g., the third day is coded "03" vs. "3"). In the following code, we convert the classes of these columns to dates.

```
mobility$date <- as.Date(mobility$date, formula = "%Y-%M-%D")
lockdowndates$Lockdown_Start <- as.Date(lockdowndates$Lockdown_Start,
                                        formula = "%Y-%M-%D")
```

```
lockdowndates$Lockdown_End <- as.Date(lockdowndates$Lockdown_End,
                              formula = "%Y-%M-%D")
class(mobility$date)
#> [1] "Date"
class(lockdowndates$Lockdown_Start)
#> [1] "Date"
class(lockdowndates$Lockdown_End)
#> [1] "Date"
```

After coding these columns as dates, we can access information such as the day, month, year, or week from them. These functions are all available in the **lubridate** package (Spinu, Grolemund, and Wickham 2023), which is a package in the **tidyverse** that allows us to manipulate dates.

```
month(mobility$date[1])
#> [1] 3
week(mobility$date[1])
#> [1] 9
```

Next, we add a date column to `covidcases`. In this case, we need to use the week number to find the date. Luckily, we can add days, months, weeks, or years to dates using the **lubridate** package. January 1, 2020 was a Wednesday and is counted as the first week; so to find the corresponding Sunday for each week, we add the recorded week number minus 1 to December 29, 2019 (the last Sunday before 2020). We show a simple example of adding one week to this date before doing this conversion for the entire column.

```
as.Date("2019-12-29") + weeks(1)
#> [1] "2020-01-05"
```

```
covidcases$date <- as.Date("2019-12-29") + weeks(covidcases$week - 1)
head(covidcases)
#> # A tibble: 6 x 6
#>   state         county   week weekly_cases weekly_deaths date
#>   <chr>         <chr>    <dbl>        <int>         <int> <date>
#> 1 California    Marin       9            1             0 2020-02-23
#> 2 California    Orange      9            3             0 2020-02-23
#> 3 Florida       Manatee     9            1             0 2020-02-23
#> 4 California    Napa        9            1             0 2020-02-23
#> 5 New Hampshire Grafton     9            2             0 2020-02-23
#> 6 Washington    Spokane     9            4             0 2020-02-23
```

7.1 Tidy Data

The **tidyverse** is designed around interacting with **tidy data** with the premise that using data in a tidy format can streamline our analysis. Data is considered **tidy** if:

- Each variable is associated with a single column.

- Each observation is associated with a single row.

- Each value has its own cell.

Take a look at the sample data which stores information about the maternal mortality rate for five countries over time (Roser and Ritchie 2013). This data is *not* tidy because the variable for maternity mortality rate is associated with multiple columns. Every row should correspond to one class observation.

```
mat_mort1 <- data.frame(country = c("Turkey", "United States",
                                    "Sweden", "Japan"),
                        y2002 = c(64, 9.9, 4.17, 7.8),
                        y2007 = c(21.9, 12.7, 1.86, 3.6),
                        y2012 = c(15.2, 16, 5.4, 4.8))
head(mat_mort1)
#>          country y2002 y2007 y2012
#> 1          Turkey 64.00 21.90  15.2
#> 2 United States  9.90 12.70  16.0
#> 3          Sweden  4.17  1.86   5.4
#> 4           Japan  7.80  3.60   4.8
```

However, we can make this data tidy by creating separate columns for country, year, and maternity mortality rate as we demonstrate in the following code. Now every observation is associated with an individual row.

```
mat_mort2 <- data.frame(
    country = rep(c("Turkey", "United States", "Sweden", "Japan"), 3),
    year = c(rep(2002, 4), rep(2007, 4), rep(2012, 4)),
    mat_mort_rate = c(64.0, 9.9, 4.17, 7.8, 21.9, 12.7, 1.86, 3.6,
                      15.2, 16, 5.4, 4.8))
head(mat_mort2)
#>          country year mat_mort_rate
#> 1          Turkey 2002         64.00
#> 2 United States 2002          9.90
#> 3          Sweden 2002          4.17
```

```
#> 4          Japan 2002        7.80
#> 5         Turkey 2007       21.90
#> 6 United States 2007        12.70
```

7.2   Reshaping Data

The mobility and COVID-19 case data are both already in tidy form: each observation corresponds to a single row, and every column is a single variable. We might consider whether the lockdown dates should be re-formatted to be tidy. Another way to represent this data would be to have each observation be the start or end of a stay-at-home order.

To reshape our data, we use the `pivot_longer()` function to change the data from what is called **wide form** to what is called **long form**. This kind of pivot involves taking a subset of columns that we want to *gather* into a single column while increasing the number of rows in the dataset. Before pivoting, we have to think about which columns we are transforming. The image in Figure 7.1 shows a picture of some data on whether students have completed a physical, hearing, or eye exam. The data is presented in wide form on the left and long form on the right. To transform wide data to long data, we have identified a subset of columns `cols` that we want to transform (these `cols` are `phys`, `hear`, and `eye` in the left table). The long form contains a new column `names_to` that contains the exam type, and `values_to` that contains a binary variable indicating whether or not each exam was completed.

In our case, we want to take the lockdown start and end columns and create two new columns: one column will indicate whether or not a date represents the start or end of a lockdown, and the other will contain the date itself. These are called the *key* and *value* columns, respectively. The key column gets its values from the names of the columns we are transforming (or the keys), whereas the value column gets its values from the entries in those columns (or the values).

The `pivot_longer()` function takes in a data table, the columns `cols` that we are pivoting to longer form, the column name `names_to` that will store the data from the previous column names, and the column name `values_to` that will store the information from the columns gathered. In our case, we name the first column `Lockdown_Event`, since it will contain whether each date is the start or end of a lockdown, and we name the second column `Date`. Take a look at the result.

WIDE

name	sex	phys	hear	eye
Alex	F	1	0	0
May	F	1	1	1
Bo	M	1	0	1

LONG

name	sex	names_to	values_to
Alex	F	phys	1
May	F	phys	1
Bo	M	phys	1
Alex	F	hear	0
May	F	hear	1
Bo	M	hear	0
Alex	F	eye	0
May	F	eye	1
Bo	M	eye	1

Figure 7.1: Pivoting Longer.

```
lockdown_long <- lockdowndates %>%
   pivot_longer(cols = c("Lockdown_Start", "Lockdown_End"),
             names_to = "Lockdown_Event", values_to = "Date") %>%
   mutate(Date = as.Date(Date, formula ="%Y-%M-%D"),
         Lockdown_Event = ifelse(Lockdown_Event=="Lockdown_Start",
                             "Start", "End")) %>%
   na.omit()
head(lockdown_long)
#> # A tibble: 6 x 3
#>    State    Lockdown_Event Date
#>    <chr>    <chr>          <date>
#> 1 Alabama Start           2020-04-04
#> 2 Alabama End             2020-04-30
#> 3 Alaska   Start           2020-03-28
#> 4 Alaska   End             2020-04-24
#> 5 Arizona Start           2020-03-31
#> 6 Arizona End             2020-05-16
```

In R, we can also transform our data in the opposite direction (from long form to wide form instead of from wide form to long form) using the function pivot_wider(). This function again first takes in a data table, but now we specify the arguments names_from and values_from. The former indicates the column that R should get the new column names from, and the latter indicates where the row values should be taken from. For example, in order to pivot our lockdown data back to wide form in the following code, we specify that

names_from is the lockdown event and values_from is the date itself. Now we
are back to the same form as before!

```
lockdown_wide <- pivot_wider(lockdown_long,
                             names_from = Lockdown_Event,
                             values_from = Date)
head(lockdown_wide)
#> # A tibble: 6 x 3
#>   State       Start      End
#>   <chr>       <date>     <date>
#> 1 Alabama     2020-04-04 2020-04-30
#> 2 Alaska      2020-03-28 2020-04-24
#> 3 Arizona     2020-03-31 2020-05-16
#> 4 California  2020-03-19 2021-01-25
#> 5 Colorado    2020-03-26 2020-04-27
#> 6 Connecticut 2020-03-23 2020-05-20
```

Here's another example: suppose that I want to create a data frame where the
columns correspond to the number of cases for each state in New England,
and the rows correspond to the numbered months. First, I need to filter my
data to New England and then summarize my data to find the number of
cases per month. I use the month() function to be able to group by month and
state. Additionally, you can see that I add an ungroup() at the end. When
we summarize on data grouped by more than one variable, the summarized
output is still grouped. In this case, the warning message states that the data
is still grouped by state.

```
ne_cases <- covidcases %>%
  filter(state %in% c("Maine", "Vermont", "New Hampshire",
                      "Connecticut", "Rhode Island",
                      "Massachusetts")) %>%
  mutate(month = month(date)) %>%
  group_by(state, month) %>%
  summarize(total_cases = sum(weekly_cases)) %>%
  ungroup()
head(ne_cases)
#> # A tibble: 6 x 3
#>   state       month total_cases
#>   <chr>       <dbl>       <int>
#> 1 Connecticut     3        7489
#> 2 Connecticut     4       22764
#> 3 Connecticut     5       13640
#> 4 Connecticut     6        2913
```

```
#> 5 Connecticut      7       3062
#> 6 Connecticut      8       3031
```

Now, I need to convert this data to wide format with a column for each state, so my `names_from` argument is `state`. Further, I want each row to have the case values for each state, so my `values_from` argument is `total_cases`. The format of this data may not be tidy, but it allows me to quickly compare cases across states.

```
pivot_wider(ne_cases, names_from = state, values_from = total_cases)
#> # A tibble: 7 x 7
#>    month Connecticut Maine Massachusetts `New Hampshire` `Rhode
#> ↳  Island`
#>    <dbl>       <int> <int>         <int>           <int>   <int>
#> 1      3        7489   510         14971             744    1006
#> 2      4       22764   716         54704            1875    7513
#> 3      5       13640  1378         33913            2503    5558
#> 4      6        2913   831          6454             807    1426
#> 5      7        3062   540          8841             758    1741
#> # i 2 more rows
#> # i 1 more variable: Vermont <int>
```

7.2.1   Practice Question

Create a similar data frame as we did in the previous example but this time using the `mobility` dataset. In other words, create a data frame where the columns correspond to the average mobility for each state in New England, and the rows correspond to the numbered months. You should get a result that looks like in Figure 7.2.

```
# Insert your solution here:
```

The pivots seen so far were relatively simple in that there was only one set of values we were pivoting on (e.g., the lockdown date, COVID-19 cases). The **tidyr** package[1] provides examples of more complex pivots that you might want to apply to your data (Wickham, Vaughan, and Girlich 2023).

---

[1] https://tidyr.tidyverse.org/articles/pivot.html

A tibble: 7 × 7

month	Connecticut	Maine	Massachusetts	New Hampshire	Rhode Island	Vermont
<dbl>	<dbl>	<dbl>	<dbl>	<dbl>	<dbl>	<dbl>
3	4.3532330	3.815913	2.8208228	4.638525	3.5644032	3.6213499
4	0.9553716	1.048308	0.3332677	1.312718	0.6791034	0.4748011
5	2.5084593	4.013129	1.4697511	3.576088	2.1930056	2.6674897
6	4.5542111	5.788098	3.0946111	5.594582	3.9479722	4.5818615
7	5.2684875	6.173947	3.7516151	6.232202	4.4329086	5.0528288
8	4.9877706	6.016233	3.5173742	6.021194	3.9650753	4.6536179
9	5.3254444	6.295176	3.8391333	6.017727	4.3196667	4.9368462

Figure 7.2: Pivoting Mobility Data.

7.3 Merging Data with Joins

In the last section, we saw how to manipulate our current data into new formats. Now, we see how we can combine multiple data sources. Merging two data frames is called *joining*, and the functions we use to perform this joining depends on how we want to match values between the data frames. For example, we can join information about age and statin use from `table1` and `table2` matching by name.

```
table1 <- data.frame(age = c(14, 26, 32),
                     name = c("Alice", "Bob", "Alice"))
table2 <- data.frame(name = c("Carol", "Bob"),
                     statins = c(TRUE, FALSE))
full_join(table1, table2, by = "name")
#>   age  name statins
#> 1  14 Alice      NA
#> 2  26   Bob   FALSE
#> 3  32 Alice      NA
#> 4  NA Carol    TRUE
```

The following list gives an overview of the different possible joins. For each join type, we specify two tables, `table1` and `table2`, and the `by` argument, which specifies the columns used to match rows between tables.

Types of Joins:

- `left_join(table1, table2, by)`: Joins each row of table1 with all matches in table2.

- `right_join(table1, table2, by)`: Joins each row of table2 with all matches in table1 (the opposite of a left join)

- `inner_join(table1, table2, by)`: Looks for all matches between rows in table1 and table2. Rows that do not find a match are dropped.

- `full_join(table1, table2, by)`: Keeps all rows from both tables and joins those that match. Rows that do not find a match have NA values filled in.

- `semi_join(table1, table2, by)`: Keeps all rows in table1 that have a match in table2 but does not join to any information from table2.

- `anti_join(table1, table2, by)`: Keeps all rows in table1 that *do not* have a match in table2 but does not join to any information from table2. The opposite of a semi-join.

We first demonstrate a left-join using the `left_join()` function. This function takes in two data tables (table1 and table2) and the columns to match rows by. In a left-join, for every row of table1, we look for all matching rows in table2 and add any columns not used to do the matching. Thus, every row in table1 corresponds to at least one entry in the resulting table but possibly more if there are multiple matches. In the subsequent code chunk, we use a left-join to add the lockdown information to our `covidcases` data. In this case, the first table is `covidcases` and we match by `state`. Since the state column has a slightly different name in the two data frames ("state" in `covidcases` and "State" in `lockdowndates`), we specify that `state` is equivalent to `State` in the by argument.

```
covidcases_full <- left_join(covidcases, lockdowndates,
                       by = c("state" = "State"))
head(covidcases_full)
#> # A tibble: 6 x 8
#>   state          county   week weekly_cases weekly_deaths date
#>   <chr>          <chr>    <dbl>        <int>         <int> <date>
#> 1 California     Marin        9            1             0 2020-02-23
#> 2 California     Orange       9            3             0 2020-02-23
#> 3 Florida        Manatee      9            1             0 2020-02-23
#> 4 California     Napa         9            1             0 2020-02-23
#> 5 New Hampshire  Grafton      9            2             0 2020-02-23
```

```
#> 6 Washington    Spokane     9          4              0 2020-02-23
#> # i 2 more variables: Lockdown_Start <date>, Lockdown_End <date>
```

These two new columns allow us to determine whether the start of each recorded week was during a lockdown. We use the `between()` function to create a new column `lockdown` before dropping the two date columns. We can check that this column worked as expected by choosing a single county to look at.

```
covidcases_full <- covidcases_full %>%
  mutate(lockdown = between(date, Lockdown_Start, Lockdown_End)) %>%
  select(-c(Lockdown_Start, Lockdown_End))
covidcases_full %>%
  filter(state == "Alabama", county == "Jefferson",
         date <= as.Date("2020-05-10"))
#> # A tibble: 10 x 7
#>    state    county    week weekly_cases weekly_deaths date
#> ↵  lockdown
#>    <chr>    <chr>     <dbl>       <int>          <int> <date>       <lgl>
#> ↵
#> 1 Alabama Jefferson    11          21              0 2020-03-08
#> ↵  FALSE
#> 2 Alabama Jefferson    12          70              0 2020-03-15
#> ↵  FALSE
#> 3 Alabama Jefferson    13         191              0 2020-03-22
#> ↵  FALSE
#> 4 Alabama Jefferson    14         179             12 2020-03-29
#> ↵  FALSE
#> 5 Alabama Jefferson    15         159              4 2020-04-05 TRUE
#> ↵
#> # i 5 more rows
```

We now want to add in the mobility data. In the previous join, we wanted to keep any observation in `covidcases` regardless if it was in the `lockdowndates` data frame. Therefore, we used a left-join. In this case, we only want to keep observations that have mobility data for that state on each date. This indicates that we want to use an *inner-join*. The function `inner_join()` takes in two data tables (table1 and table2) and the columns to match rows by. The function only keeps rows in table1 that match to a row in table2. Again, those columns in table2 not used to match with table1 are added to the resulting outcome. In this case, we match by both state and date.

```
covidcases_full <- inner_join(covidcases_full, mobility,
                              by = c("state", "date")) %>%
  select(-c(samples, m50_index))
head(covidcases_full)
#> # A tibble: 6 x 8
#>    state        county  week weekly_cases weekly_deaths date
#>  ↳ lockdown
#>    <chr>        <chr>   <dbl>         <int>        <int> <date>      <lgl>
#>  ↳
#> 1 Florida      Okalo~    10             1            0 2020-03-01 FALSE
#>  ↳
#> 2 Georgia      Charl~    10             1            0 2020-03-01 FALSE
#>  ↳
#> 3 Massachus~   Essex     10             1            0 2020-03-01 FALSE
#>  ↳
#> 4 New York     Rockl~    10             6            0 2020-03-01 FALSE
#>  ↳
#> 5 Indiana      Hendr~    10             2            0 2020-03-01 FALSE
#>  ↳
#> 6 California   Marin     10             1            0 2020-03-01 FALSE
#>  ↳
#> # i 1 more variable: m50 <dbl>
```

7.3.1   Practice Question

Look at the two data frames, df_A and df_B, defined in the following code.
What kind of join would produce the data frame in Figure 7.3? Perform this
join yourself.

```
df_A <- data.frame(patient_id = c(12, 9, 12, 8, 14, 8),
                   visit_num = c(1, 1, 2, 1, 1, 2),
                   temp = c(97.5, 96, 98, 99, 102, 98.6),
                   systolic_bp = c(120, 138, 113, 182, 132, 146))
df_A
#>   patient_id visit_num  temp systolic_bp
#> 1         12         1  97.5         120
#> 2          9         1  96.0         138
#> 3         12         2  98.0         113
#> 4          8         1  99.0         182
#> 5         14         1 102.0         132
#> 6          8         2  98.6         146
df_B <- data.frame(patient_id = c(12, 12, 12, 8, 8, 8, 14, 14),
```

A data.frame: 5 × 5

patient_id	visit_num	temp	systolic_bp	digit_span
<dbl>	<dbl>	<dbl>	<dbl>	<dbl>
12	1	97.5	120	3
12	2	98.0	113	5
8	1	99.0	182	7
14	1	102.0	132	8
8	2	98.6	146	9

Figure 7.3: Joining Data.

```
                visit_num = c(1, 2, 3, 1, 2, 3, 1, 2),
                digit_span = c(3, 5, 7, 7, 9, 5, 8, 7))
df_B
#>   patient_id visit_num digit_span
#> 1         12         1          3
#> 2         12         2          5
#> 3         12         3          7
#> 4          8         1          7
#> 5          8         2          9
#> 6          8         3          5
#> 7         14         1          8
#> 8         14         2          7
```

```
# Insert your solution here:
```

7.4 Exercises

1. Take a look at the provided code. What is wrong with it? Hint: think about what causes the warning message.

```
visit_info <- data.frame(
  name.f = c("Phillip", "Phillip", "Phillip", "Jessica",
             "Jessica"),
  name.l = c("Johnson", "Johnson", "Richards", "Smith",
             "Abrams"),
  measure = c("height", "age", "age", "age", "height"),
  measurement = c(45, 186, 50, 37, 156)
)

contact_info <- data.frame(
first_name = c("Phillip", "Phillip", "Jessica", "Margaret"),
last_name = c("Richards", "Johnson", "Smith", "Reynolds"),
email = c("pr@aol.com", "phillipj@gmail.com",
          "jesssmith@brown.edu", "marg@hotmail.com")
)

left_join(visit_info, contact_info,
          by = c("name.f" = "first_name"))
#> Warning in left_join(visit_info, contact_info, by =
#>   c(name.f = "first_name")): Detected an unexpected
#>   many-to-many relationship between `x` and `y`.
#> i Row 1 of `x` matches multiple rows in `y`.
#> i Row 1 of `y` matches multiple rows in `x`.
#> i If a many-to-many relationship is expected, set
#>   `relationship =
#>   "many-to-many"` to silence this warning.
#>     name.f   name.l measure measurement last_name
#>   email
#> 1 Phillip  Johnson  height          45  Richards
#>   pr@aol.com
#> 2 Phillip  Johnson  height          45   Johnson
#>   phillipj@gmail.com
#> 3 Phillip  Johnson     age         186  Richards
#>   pr@aol.com
#> 4 Phillip  Johnson     age         186   Johnson
#>   phillipj@gmail.com
#> 5 Phillip Richards     age          50  Richards
#>   pr@aol.com
#> 6 Phillip Richards     age          50   Johnson
#>   phillipj@gmail.com
#> 7 Jessica    Smith     age          37     Smith
#>   jesssmith@brown.edu
#> 8 Jessica   Abrams  height         156     Smith
#>   jesssmith@brown.edu
```

2. First, use the covidcases data to create a new data frame called sub_cases containing the total number of cases by month for the states of California, Michigan, Connecticut, Rhode Island, Ohio, New York, and Massachusetts. Then, manipulate the mobility data to calculate the average m50 mobility measure for each month. Finally, merge these two datasets using an appropriate joining function.

3. Convert the sub_cases data frame from the previous exercise to wide format so that each row displays the cases in each state for a single month. Then, add on the average m50 overall for each month as an additional column using a join function.

8

Visualization with ggplot2

The package **ggplot2** (Wickham 2016) is another useful package in the **tidy-verse** that allows statisticians to use visualizations to communicate key findings and results in a compelling format. In this chapter, we learn about the three main components in a ggplot object and then expand on that format by learning more about the different layers we can use to create various plots. As with the **dplyr** functions, there are many functions to cover, and they build upon one another.

The three packages we use in this chapter are **tidyverse**, **HDSinRdata**, and **patchwork** (Pedersen 2022), the last of which is a nice package for combining multiple plots together into a single figure. We use the data from the Pittsburgh pain clinic (Alter et al. 2021) introduced in Chapter 3 to create our visuals. You can refresh your memory about this data by reading the data documentation. For the purposes of this chapter, we take a sample of 5,000 patients that are complete cases at baseline to reduce the computation time to display each plot. You can ignore how the code used to find this sample works.

```
library(tidyverse)
library(HDSinRdata)
library(patchwork)
data(pain)

# sampling data
set.seed(5)
pain_df_sub <- subset(pain,
                select = -c(PAIN_INTENSITY_AVERAGE.FOLLOW_UP))
pain_df <- pain[complete.cases(pain_df_sub), ]
pain_df <- pain_df[sample(1:nrow(pain_df), 5000, replace = FALSE),]
```

8.1   Intro to ggplot

We'll begin by demonstrating how to create a scatter plot in **ggplot2** to introduce the three key elements of a `ggplot2` object. Specifically, we create a scatter plot of a patient's depression vs. anxiety score. To start a graph, we can use the `ggplot()` function to create a `ggplot` object as shown in the following code. Note that this brings up a gray box; this is the base that we build up from.

```
ggplot()
```

Next, we can begin adding layers to our `ggplot` object. One type of layer is a **geom**, which creates a geometric object. In the next code chunk, we use the `geom_point()` function to add a scatter plot layer. For this function, we first need to specify which data we want to use, and then we need to tell R how to use that data to create the scatter plot using the `aes()` function, which creates an **aesthetic**. For a scatter plot, we need to at least specify the x-axis and y-axis in the aesthetic. Both the data and the aesthetic can either be specified in our initial `ggplot()` function, which passes this information to all future layers, or in the `geom_point()` function itself. In the following code, we specify the aesthetic in the geom function but also include two alternative ways to code the same image in the subsequent code chunk. The resulting plot shows a fairly linear relationship between anxiety and depression.

```
ggplot(pain_df) + geom_point(aes(x=PROMIS_ANXIETY,
                                 y = PROMIS_DEPRESSION))
```

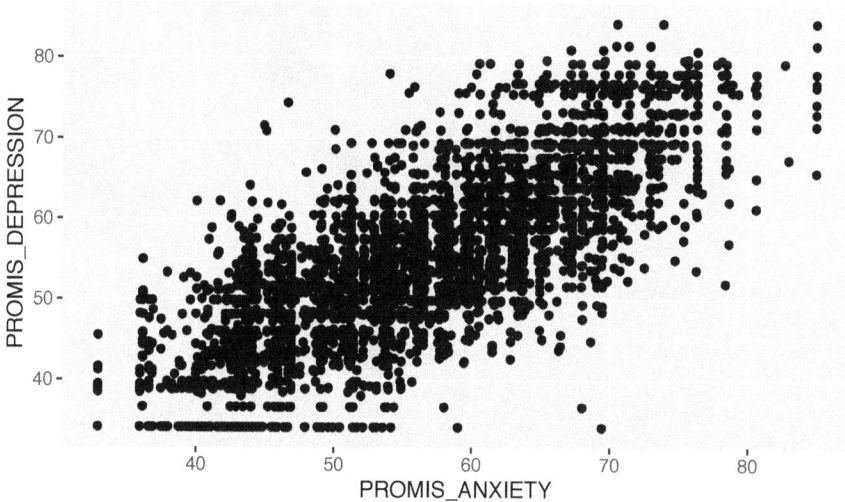

```
# Alternative 1:
ggplot(pain_df, aes(x = PROMIS_ANXIETY, y = PROMIS_DEPRESSION)) +
  geom_point()
# Alternative 2:
ggplot() +
  geom_point(data = pain_df, aes(x = PROMIS_ANXIETY,
                                 y = PROMIS_DEPRESSION))
```

If we want to improve our plot, we may want to add different labels and a title. To do so, we use the `labs()` function to add a layer in which we can specify all labels. Additionally, I have passed more information to the geometry layer by changing the color, size, and shape of the points. These things are specified outside of the `aes()` function since they do not come from the data; every point has the same color, size, and shape in this example.

```
ggplot(pain_df)+
  geom_point(aes(x = PROMIS_ANXIETY, y = PROMIS_DEPRESSION),
             color = "blue", size = 2, shape = 5) +
  labs(x = "PROMIS Anxiety Score", y = "PROMIS Depression Score",
       title = "Depression vs Anxiety Scores")
```

Depression vs Anxiety Scores

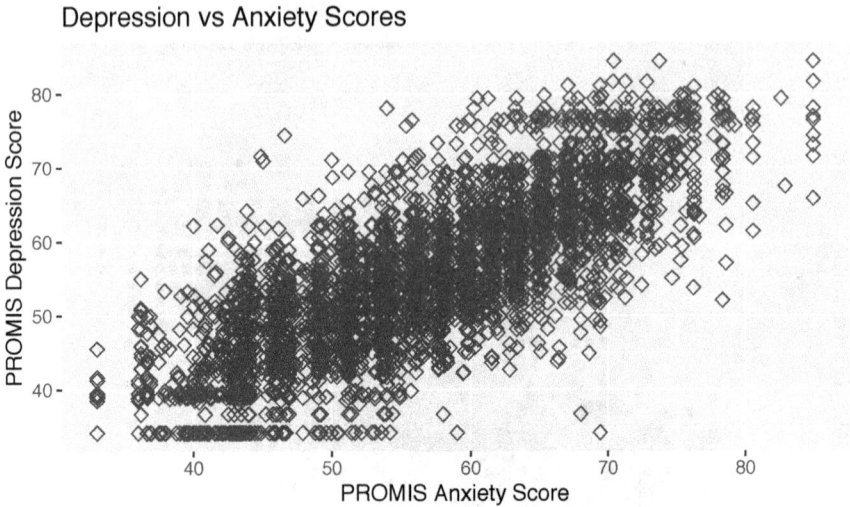

Let's create another example. This time, I create a histogram for initial recorded pain level. To find the corresponding geom for the type of plot we'd like to make, we can use the data visualization cheat sheet from Posit[1]. The first page lists all the geom options available along with what aesthetics we can set for each option. For example, here we are interested in plotting the distribution of one continuous variable, and under the `geom_histogram()` function we can see that we can specify `x` (the variable whose distribution we want to plot) as well as `binwidth`, `y`, `alpha`, `color`, `fill`, `linetype`, `size`, and `weight`. By default, the `y` value in a histogram is the count for each bin.

In the following code, you can see that we updated the color (`color`), fill (`fill`), and opacity (`alpha`) of our histogram bars and updated the number of bins to be 11 (to account for the possible values 0-10). Additionally, we used the `theme_minimal()` function to change the background colors used. You can find the available themes on the second page of the cheat sheet. Try changing the theme of the following plot to `theme_bw()`.

```
ggplot(pain_df)+
  geom_histogram(aes(x = PAIN_INTENSITY_AVERAGE), color = "violetred",
                 fill = "lightblue", alpha = 0.5, bins = 11) +
  labs(x = "Patient Reported Pain Intensity", y = "Count")+
  theme_minimal()
```

---

[1] https://posit.co/wp-content/uploads/2022/10/data-visualization-1.pdf

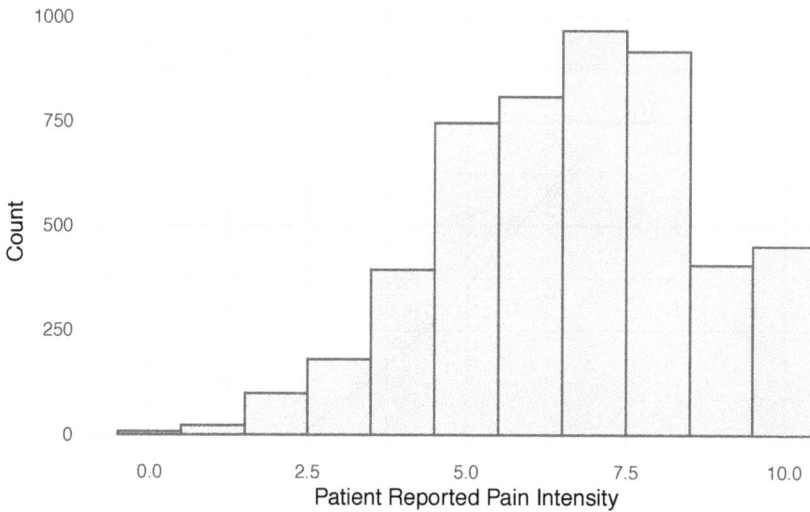

8.1.1   Practice Question

Recreate Figure 8.1.

```
# Insert your solution here:
```

8.2   Adjusting the Axes and Aesthetics

We can further control how each aesthetic element is displayed using *scale* functions. For example, suppose that I want to update the previous plot. In particular, I first want to update the x-axis to display all of the values 0 to 10 instead of 0, 2.5, 5, etc.. To update the x-axis, I need to find the corresponding scale function for x with continuous values. This function is `scale_x_continuous()`, which allows me to specify limits (`limits`), breaks (`breaks`), and labels (`labels`). The scale functions can be found on the second sheet of the cheat sheet. In this case, I just want to update the breaks to be all integer values from 0 to 10.

```
ggplot(pain_df)+
  geom_histogram(aes(x = PAIN_INTENSITY_AVERAGE), color = "violetred",
                 fill = "lightblue", alpha = 0.5, bins = 11) +
  labs(x = "Patient Reported Pain Intensity", y = "Count")+
  scale_x_continuous(breaks = 0:10)+
  theme_minimal()
```

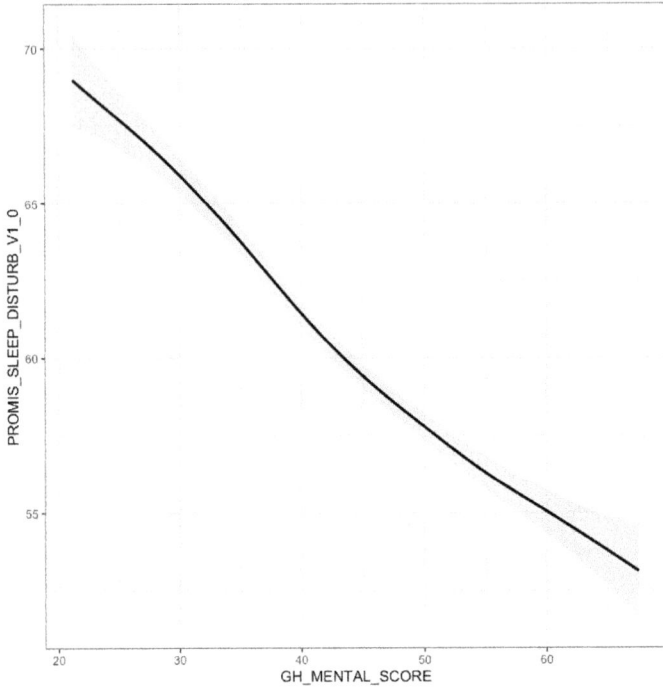

Figure 8.1: Line Plot.

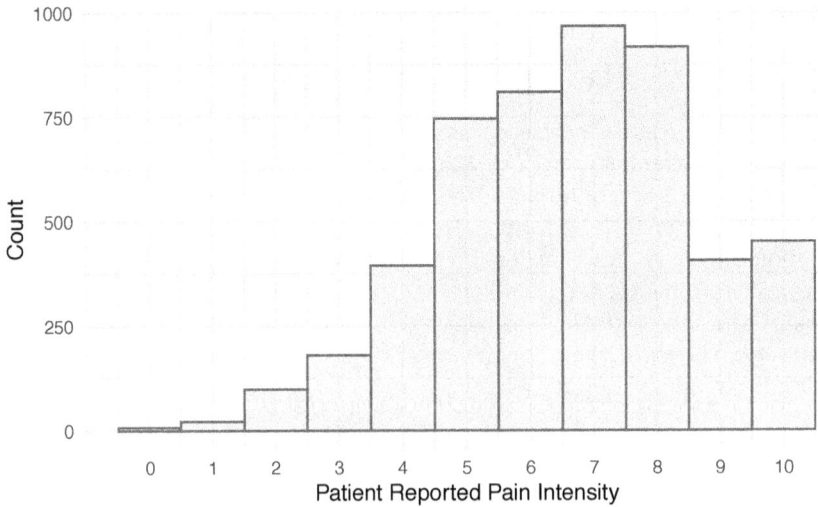

Now, let's take a more complex example. The following plot shows each patient's reported sleep disturbance vs. physical function and colors each point by their reported pain intensity. Since some points might overlap in values, we added `position="jitter"` to the `geom_point()` function to jitter the points, which corresponds to adding some random noise to each point's position. As presented, this plot is difficult to interpret. For example, the color of pain intensity makes it hard to see how pain changes, and the legend title needs to be simpler.

```
ggplot(pain_df)+
  geom_point(aes(x = PROMIS_PHYSICAL_FUNCTION,
                 y = PROMIS_SLEEP_DISTURB_V1_0,
                 color = PAIN_INTENSITY_AVERAGE), position="jitter")
```

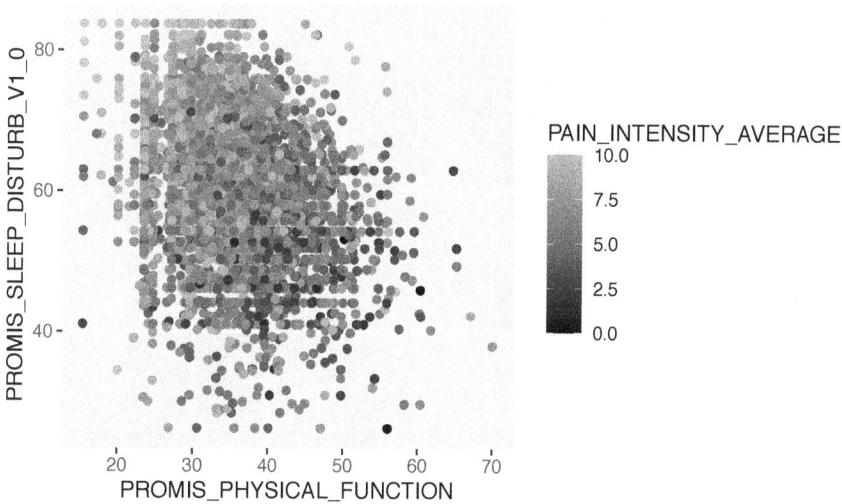

Suppose that we wanted to visualize the pain intensity and sleep disturbance for patients with below-average physical function. Note that both sleep disturbance and physical function are reported as T-Scores, meaning that the raw scores have been converted to a standardized score with mean 50 and standard deviation 10 within the population. We can use the scale functions to update our axes and labels to reflect this information. As before, we need to use the `scale_x_continuous()` function to update the x-axis for a continuous variable. In this case, we update the limits (to restrict to below-average physical function), breaks, and labels. We similarly update the y-axis.

Lastly, suppose we want to update the color aesthetic. As before, this aesthetic corresponds to a continuous variable. The cheat sheet provides several possible scale functions depending on how we want to specify the color gradient. We choose the `scale_color_gradient()` function, since this allows us to specify the low and high end colors. We can also specify the breaks for the legend values similar to how we specified the breaks for the x- and y-axes. The argument `name` also allows us to rename this legend. The palette then converts this to a continuous color gradient. Note that in contrast to the `scale_color_gradient()` function that we chose to use for this example, the functions `scale_color_gradient2()` and `scale_color_gradientn()` allow you to specify more color points in the gradient rather than just the two extreme colors.

We can observe that decreased physical function is associated with higher sleep disturbance, and that those with worse physical function and worse sleep disturbance tend to have higher reported pain. Note that this time we receive a warning message, which is because our axis limits have cut off some points. To avoid this message, we could use the function `coord_cartesian()` to specify our limits which clips the values rather than removing points outside the limits.

```
ggplot(pain_df)+
  geom_point(aes(x = PROMIS_PHYSICAL_FUNCTION,
                 y = PROMIS_SLEEP_DISTURB_V1_0,
                 color = PAIN_INTENSITY_AVERAGE),
             position = "jitter", alpha = 0.5) +
  scale_x_continuous(limits = c(15,50), breaks = c(20, 30, 40, 50),
                     labels = c("-3 SD", "-2 SD", "-1 SD",
                                "Pop Mean")) +
  scale_y_continuous(breaks = c(40, 50, 60, 70, 80),
                     labels = c("-1 SD", "Pop Mean", "+1 SD", "+2 SD",
                                "+3 SD")) +
  scale_color_gradient(breaks = seq(0,10,2), low = "green",
                       high = "red", "Reported Pain") +
  labs(x = "PROMIS Physical Function T-Score",
       y = "PROMIS Sleep Disturbance T-Score") +
  theme_minimal()
#> Warning: Removed 121 rows containing missing values or values
↳   outside the scale
#> range (`geom_point()`).
```

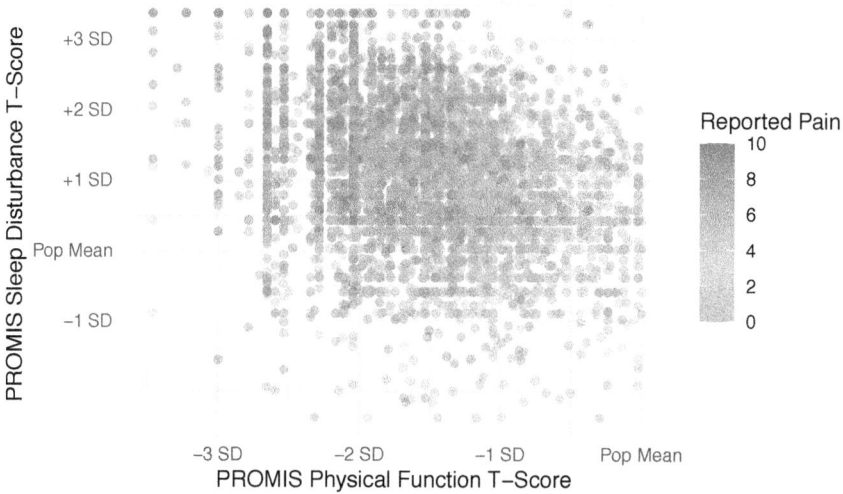

We now demonstrate these scale functions for discrete variables. In the subsequent example, we first create a new race variable that has only three categories since other groups have limited observations. We then create a boxplot for pain intensity by race. There are two discrete aesthetics here: color and the y-axis. This plot shows a higher median pain for black patients compared to other races.

```
pain_df$PAT_RACE_CAT <- ifelse(pain_df$PAT_RACE %in% c("BLACK",
                                                       "WHITE"),
                          pain_df$PAT_RACE, "OTHER")
pain_df$PAT_RACE_CAT <- as.factor(pain_df$PAT_RACE_CAT)


ggplot(pain_df)+
  geom_boxplot(aes(y = PAT_RACE_CAT, x = PAIN_INTENSITY_AVERAGE,
                   fill = PAT_RACE_CAT), alpha = 0.5) +
  theme_minimal()
```

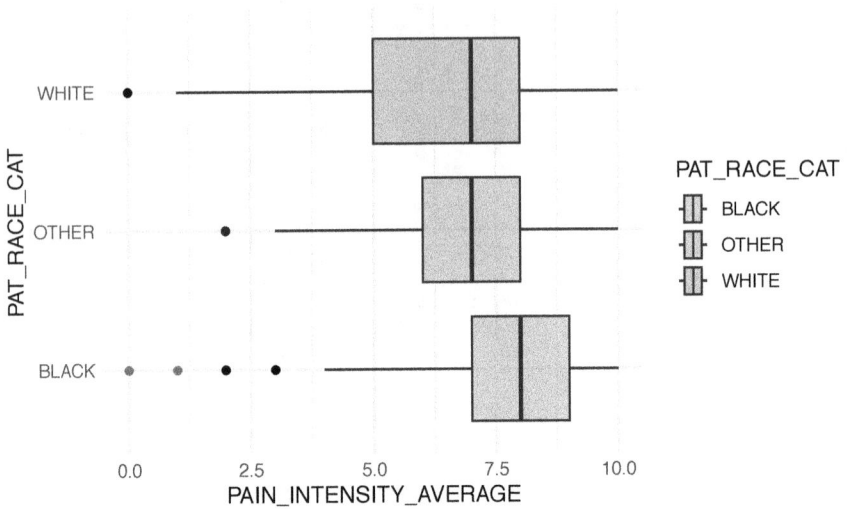

The function `scale_y_discrete()` is the scale function that corresponds to a discrete y-axis. In this case, we want to update the order and labels of this y-axis. To update the order, we can either re-factor the variable using `factor()` prior to plotting or update the `limits` argument of the scale function. The function `scale_fill_brewer()` is a scale function to control the color palette of a discrete variable used for the fill aesthetic. We use this function to specify the color palette (`palette`) and to specify that we do not want a legend (`guide`). Since we do not have a legend, we do not update the values and labels in this function.

```
ggplot(pain_df)+
  geom_boxplot(aes(y = PAT_RACE_CAT, x = PAIN_INTENSITY_AVERAGE,
                   fill = PAT_RACE_CAT), alpha = 0.5) +
  scale_x_continuous(breaks = c(0:10)) +
  scale_y_discrete(limits = c("OTHER", "WHITE", "BLACK"),
                   labels = c("Other", "White", "Black")) +
  scale_fill_brewer(palette = "Dark2", guide = "none") +
  labs(x = "Reported Pain Intensity", y = "Reported Race") +
  theme_minimal()
```

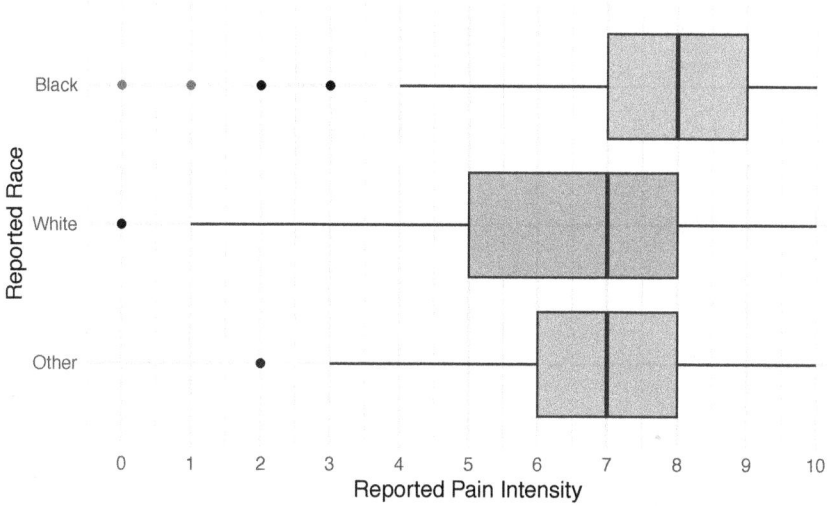

The **RColorBrewer** package (Neuwirth 2022) contains several default palettes to choose from, shown in the following output. You can also create your own palette using the `brewer.pal()` function from this package. To visualize a palette, you can use the available online tool[2].

```
library(RColorBrewer)
display.brewer.all()
```

[2]https://colorbrewer2.org/

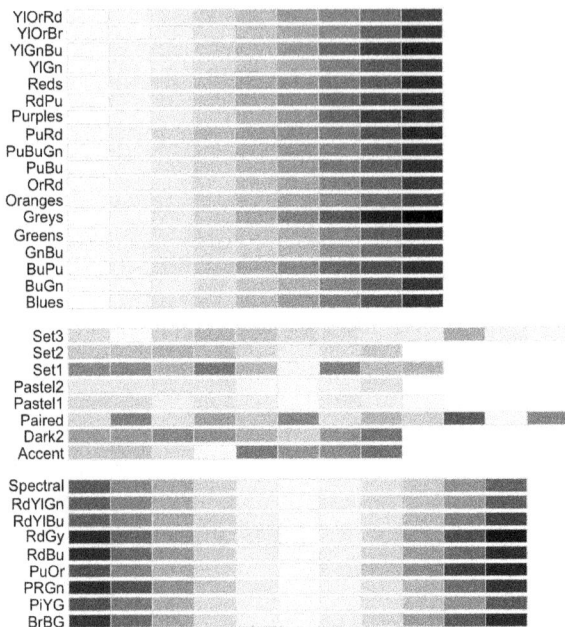

Figure 8.2: RColorBrewer Palettes.

Here is one more example of how you can use the scale functions; take a look at the next plot example. We used two `geom_histogram()` calls, or layers, to plot a histogram of pain at baseline and at follow-up. This allows us to visualize that pain at follow-up tends to be lower than at baseline.

We also specify the fill to be by "Baseline" and "Follow-up" within the aesthetic, even though this isn't a column in the data: this is a sort of manual way to color the bars. We use the `scale_fill_manual()` function to then specify the colors we want to use for these two categories using the `values` argument. We received three warnings when creating this plot! This is because we have many NA values for follow-up and because we did not specify the bin size for either histogram. C'est la vie.

```
ggplot(pain_df)+
  geom_histogram(aes(x = PAIN_INTENSITY_AVERAGE, fill = "Baseline")) +
  geom_histogram(aes(x = PAIN_INTENSITY_AVERAGE.FOLLOW_UP,
                     fill = "Follow-Up")) +
```

```
    scale_x_continuous(breaks = c(0:10)) +
    scale_fill_manual(values = c("violetred", "pink"),
                      name = "Measurement") +
    labs(x = "Reported Pain Intensity", y = "Count") +
    theme_minimal()
#> Warning: Removed 3604 rows containing non-finite outside the scale
↳   range
#> (`stat_bin()`).
```

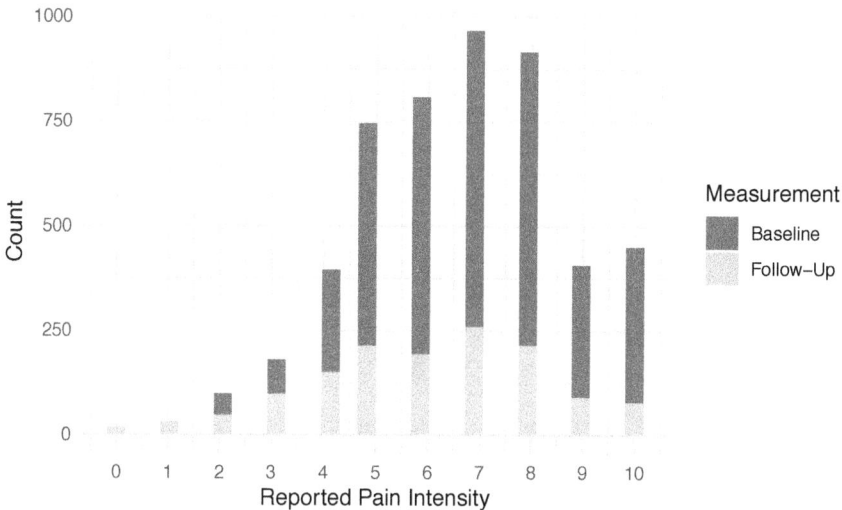

8.3 Adding Groups

In the previous example, we created two histograms using two calls to the geom_histogram() function. However, there is another way to create multiple layers like this when you want to separate the geom layer based on a variable. For example, suppose we want to visualize the distribution of physical function by whether someone has follow-up information. In the following code, we create the variable HAS_FOLLOW_UP before using it in our aesthetic for geom_density() as both the color and group. In fact, we do not have to add the group argument because as soon as we specify to **ggplot** that we want to color the density plots by this variable, it creates the grouping. Finally, we update the legend for this grouping using the scale_color_discrete() function, as the discrete variable HAS_FOLLOW_UP determines the color.

```
pain_df$HAS_FOLLOW_UP <-
  !is.na(pain_df$PAIN_INTENSITY_AVERAGE.FOLLOW_UP)
ggplot(pain_df) +
  geom_density(aes(x = PROMIS_PHYSICAL_FUNCTION,
                   group = HAS_FOLLOW_UP,
                   color= HAS_FOLLOW_UP)) +
  scale_x_continuous(breaks = c(0:10)) +
  scale_color_discrete(name = "Follow-Up", labels = c("No", "Yes")) +
  labs(x = "PROMIS Physical Function T-Score",
       y = "Estimated Density") +
  theme_minimal()
```

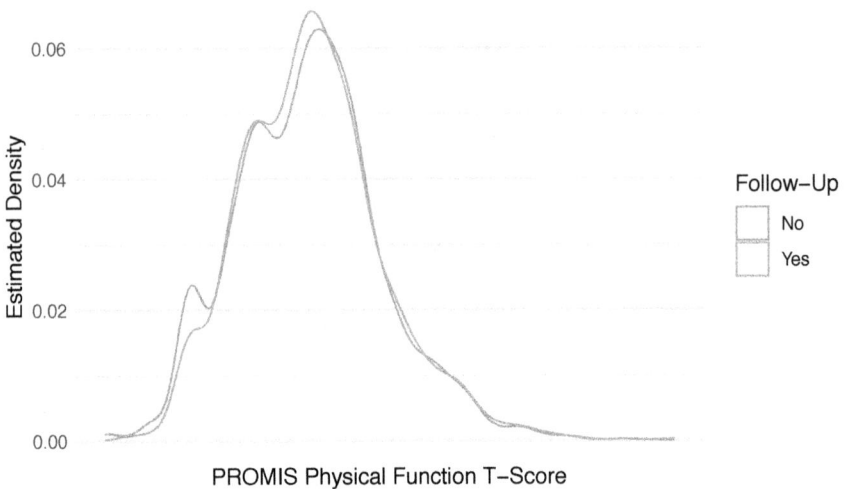

PROMIS Physical Function T-Score

Let's try another example. Suppose that we want to find the distribution of initial overall pain by those that do and do not have a follow-up. In this case, we want to plot the proportion of each pain score for each group rather than compare counts. We first need to find these proportions, which we do by grouping and summarizing over our data.

```
pain_df_grp <- pain_df %>%
  group_by(HAS_FOLLOW_UP, PAIN_INTENSITY_AVERAGE) %>%
  summarize(tot = n()) %>%
  mutate(prop = tot/sum(tot)) %>%
  ungroup()
head(pain_df_grp)
#> # A tibble: 6 x 4
```

```
#>   HAS_FOLLOW_UP PAIN_INTENSITY_AVERAGE    tot      prop
#>   <lgl>                           <dbl> <int>     <dbl>
#> 1 FALSE                               0     8   0.00222
#> 2 FALSE                               1    16   0.00444
#> 3 FALSE                               2    62   0.0172
#> 4 FALSE                               3   132   0.0366
#> 5 FALSE                               4   273   0.0757
#> 6 FALSE                               5   508   0.141
```

We can now use the `geom_col()` function to create a barplot of these proportions. By default, this function stacks the bars on top of each other when there is grouping. Try adding `position="dodge"` to the `geom_col()` function to place the bars side by side instead of on top of each other.

```
ggplot(pain_df_grp)+
  geom_col(aes(x = PAIN_INTENSITY_AVERAGE, y = prop,
               fill = HAS_FOLLOW_UP)) +
  scale_x_continuous(breaks = c(0:10)) +
  scale_fill_discrete(name = "Seen at Follow Up",
                      labels = c("No", "Yes")) +
  labs(x = "Reported Pain Intensity", y = "Proportion") +
  theme_minimal()
```

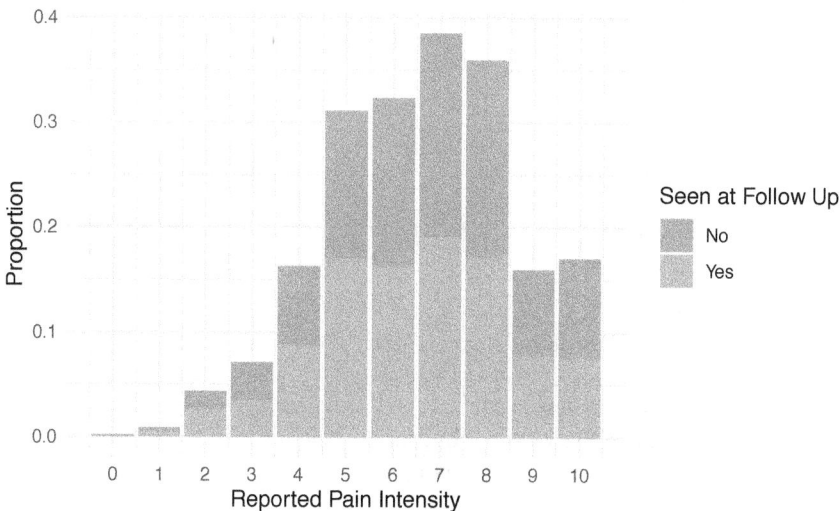

8.3.1   Practice Question

Recreate Figure 8.3.

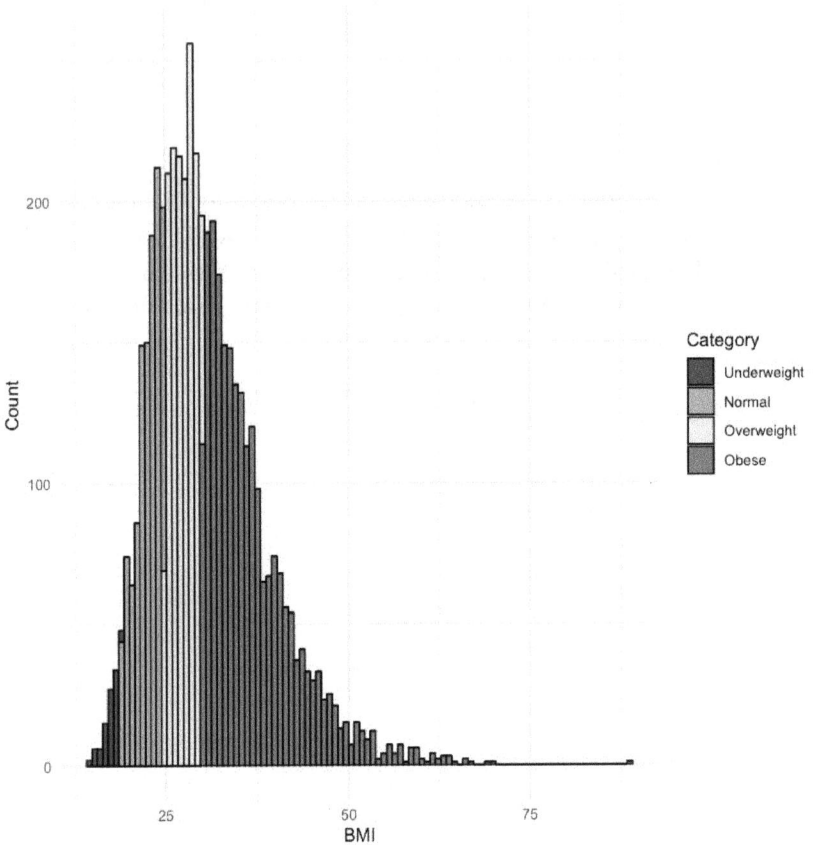

Figure 8.3: BMI Distribution.

```
# Insert your solution here:
```

Another way to visualize data by group is to add a facet wrap to your ggplot object. Facets divide a plot into subplots based on one or more discrete variable values. We can arrange these plots as a grid where the rows and/or columns correspond to the variables we are grouping by using facet_grid() and specifying the column and row variables using the col and row arguments respectively. Or we can wrap the plots into a rectangular format using facet_wrap() and specifying the columns using the facet argument. In the following code, we take one of our previous plots and add a facet grid where the columns of the grid are given by a racial group. If we had set row=vars(PAT_RACE_CAT), then this would stack the plots vertically. Note that we have to specify the variables inside the `vars()` function.

```
ggplot(pain_df)+
  geom_histogram(aes(x = PAIN_INTENSITY_AVERAGE, fill = "Baseline")) +
  geom_histogram(aes(x = PAIN_INTENSITY_AVERAGE.FOLLOW_UP,
                     fill = "Follow-Up")) +
  scale_x_continuous(breaks = c(0:10)) +
  scale_fill_manual(values = c("violetred", "pink"),
                    name = "Measurement") +
  labs(x= "Reported Pain Intensity", y = "Count") +
  facet_grid(row = vars(PAT_RACE_CAT))+
  theme_minimal()
#> Warning: Removed 3604 rows containing non-finite outside the scale
↪   range
#> (`stat_bin()`).
```

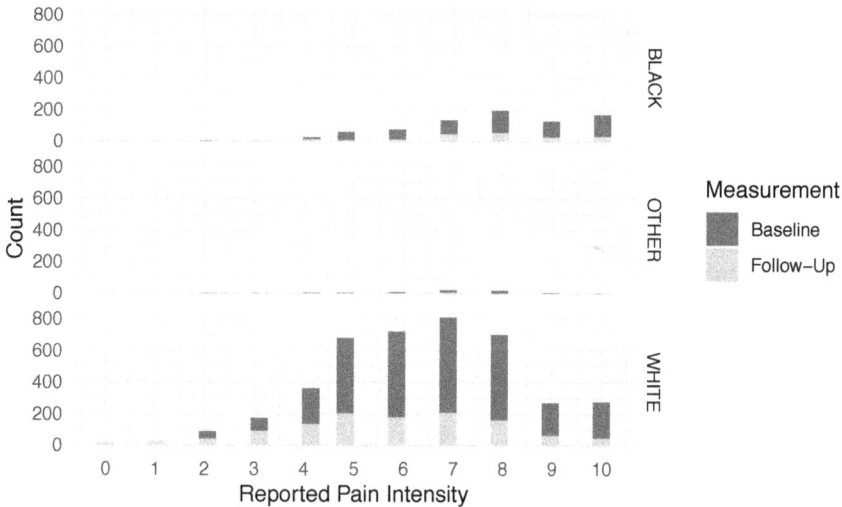

8.4 Extra Options

For our final plot, we will demonstrate additional features not yet covered in this chapter. To create this plot, we first find the number of participants who selected each body region as well as the average pain intensity for those patients. We also classify each body part region into larger groups.

```
pain_body_map <- data.frame(part = names(pain_df)[2:75])
pain_body_map$num_patients <- colSums(pain_df[, 2:75])
pain_body_map$perc_patients <- pain_body_map$num_patients /
                               nrow(pain_df)
pain_body_map$avg_pain <- colSums(pain_df[, 2:75] *
                          pain_df$PAIN_INTENSITY_AVERAGE) /
                          pain_body_map$num_patients
pain_body_map <- pain_body_map %>%
    mutate(region = case_when(
    part %in% c("X208", "X209", "X218", "X219", "X212",
               "X213") ~ "Back",
    part %in% c("X105", "X106", "X205", "X206") ~ "Neck",
    part %in% c("X107", "X110", "X207", "X210") ~ "Shoulders",
    part %in% c("X108", "X109", "X112", "X113") ~ "Chest/Abs",
    part %in% c("X126", "X127", "X228", "X229",
               "X131", "X132", "X233", "X234") ~ "Legs",
    part %in% c("X111", "X114", "X211", "X214", "X115", "X116",
               "X117", "X118", "X217", "X220") ~ "Arms",
    part %in% c("X119", "X124", "X221", "X226", "X125", "X128",
               "X227", "X230") ~ "Wrists/Hands",
    part %in% c("X215", "X216") ~ "Elbows",
    part %in% c("X135", "X136", "X237", "X238", "X133", "X134",
               "X235", "X236") ~ "Feet/Ankles",
    part %in% c("X129", "X130", "X231", "X232") ~ "Knees",
    part %in% c("X101", "X102", "X103", "X104", "X201", "X203",
               "X202", "X204") ~ "Head",
    part %in% c("X120", "X121", "X122", "X123", "X222", "X223",
               "X224", "X225") ~ "Hips"))

head(pain_body_map)
#>    part num_patients perc_patients avg_pain region
#> 1 X101          323        0.0646     6.69   Head
#> 2 X102          322        0.0644     6.82   Head
#> 3 X103          165        0.0330     6.86   Head
#> 4 X104          165        0.0330     6.95   Head
#> 5 X105          493        0.0986     6.90   Neck
#> 6 X106          507        0.1014     6.92   Neck
```

Within the theme we've chosen, we are able to update any of the theme options (see `?theme`). In the following code, we use the `theme()` function to update the legend position to the bottom and the grid lines to light pink. Additionally, we add a horizontal line using the `geom_hline()` function (`geom_vline()` and `geom_abline()` can add vertical or diagonal lines, respectively) and add a text annotation using the `annotate()` function. The resulting plot shows the average pain value for each body part as well as the proportion of patients who categorized it as being painful.

```
ggplot(pain_body_map) +
  geom_label(aes(x = perc_patients, y = avg_pain, label = part,
                 color = region)) +
  geom_hline(yintercept = mean(pain_body_map$avg_pain)) +
  annotate(geom = "text", label = "Average Pain Value",
           x = 0.35, y = 7.0) +
  labs(x = "Proportion Patients Selected Region",
       y = "Average Pain of Patients") +
  theme_minimal()+
  theme(legend.position="bottom",
        panel.grid.major = element_line(color = "lightpink"))
```

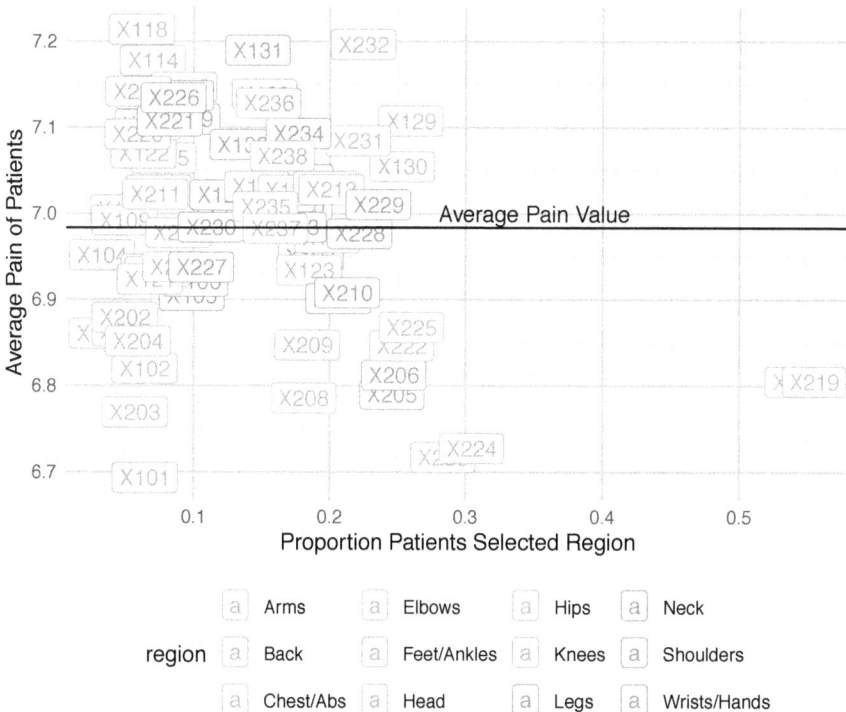

So far, we have not saved any of our figures as objects. In the next example, I create two plots and save them as objects named p1 and p2. If we want to save these plots, we can use the **ggsave()** function, which saves the last plot generated under the file name provided. Additionally, I can use the **patchwork**

package to incorporate multiple plots together. A + between plots adds them
together into a single figure, and then the `plot_layout()` function allows us to
specify the grid used to arrange our figures. We have added an extra element
using the `guide_area()` function to create a placeholder for the legends and
then used the `guide = "collect"` argument in the `plot_layout()` function to
specify that all guides should be put together.

```
p1 <- ggplot(pain_body_map) +
  geom_label(aes(x = perc_patients, y = avg_pain, label = part,
                 color = region)) +
  geom_hline(yintercept = mean(pain_body_map$avg_pain)) +
  annotate(geom = "text", label = "Average Pain Value",
           x = 0.35, y = 7.0) +
  labs(x = "Proportion of Patients Selecting Region",
       y = "Average Pain of Patients") +
  scale_color_discrete(name="Body Part")+
  theme_minimal()+
  theme(legend.position = "bottom",
        panel.grid.major = element_line(color = "lightpink"))

p2 <- ggplot(pain_body_map) +
  geom_histogram(aes(x = perc_patients), color = "violetred",
                 fill = "lightpink") +
  labs(x = "Proportion of Patients Selecting Region", y = "Count") +
  theme_minimal()+
  theme(panel.grid.major = element_line(color = "lightpink"))


p1 + p2 + guide_area() + plot_layout(ncol=1, guides = "collect",
                                     axes = "collect")
```

Body Part

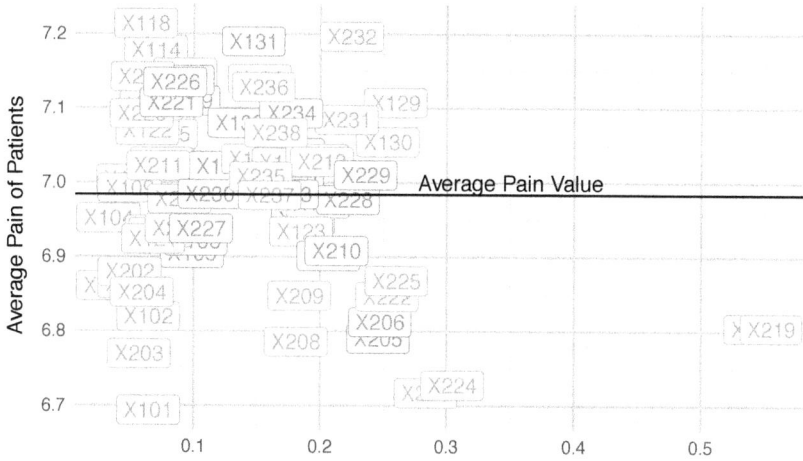

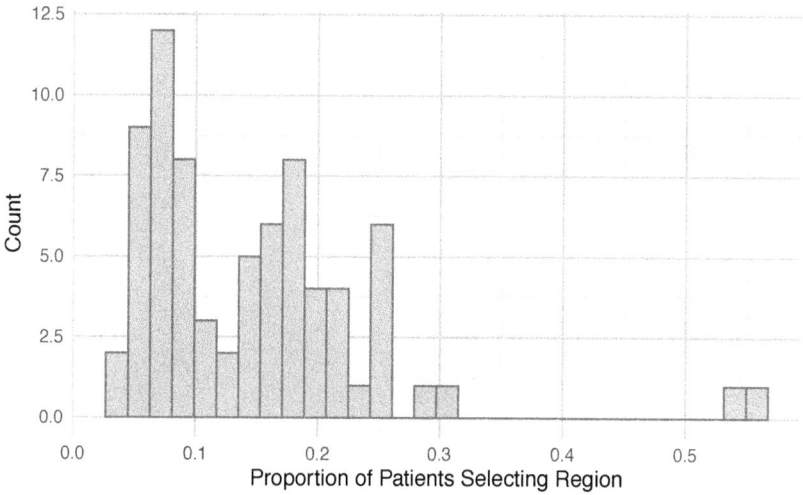

[a] Arms		[a] Elbows		[a] Hips		[a] Neck	
[a] Back		[a] Feet/Ankles		[a] Knees		[a] Shoulders	
[a] Chest/Abs		[a] Head		[a] Legs		[a] Wrists/Hands	

```
ggsave("images/visualization_ggplot/myplot.png", height=10)
```

8.5   Exercises

For this chapter's exercises, use the `covidcases` dataset that we first introduced in Chapter 5 to recreate some plots. These are complex plots, so try to build them up one step at a time and just try to get as close as possible to the given examples.

1. Replicate the following combined plot in Figure 8.4, which shows the weekly COVID-19 cases in the U.S. as well as the weekly cases by U.S. division. Hint: use the `scale_color_gradientn()` function to replicate the color scale.

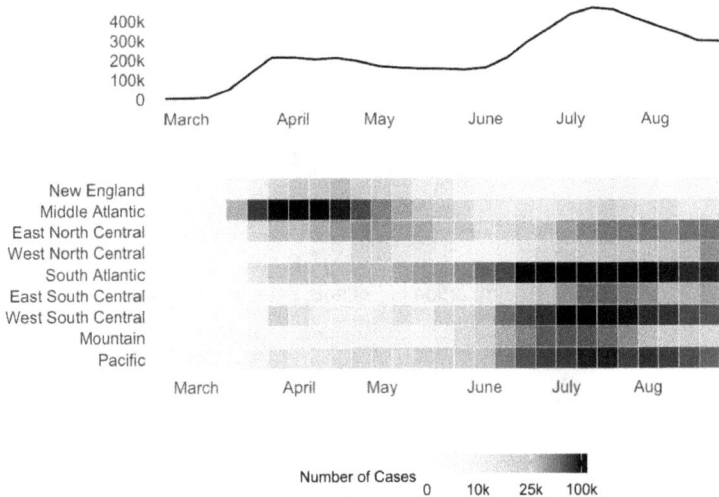

Figure 8.4: COVID-19 Cases Over Time by State.

2. Replicate the plot in Figure 8.5, which is a stacked area chart for the total deaths from COVID-19 in the states with the top ten total death counts overall.

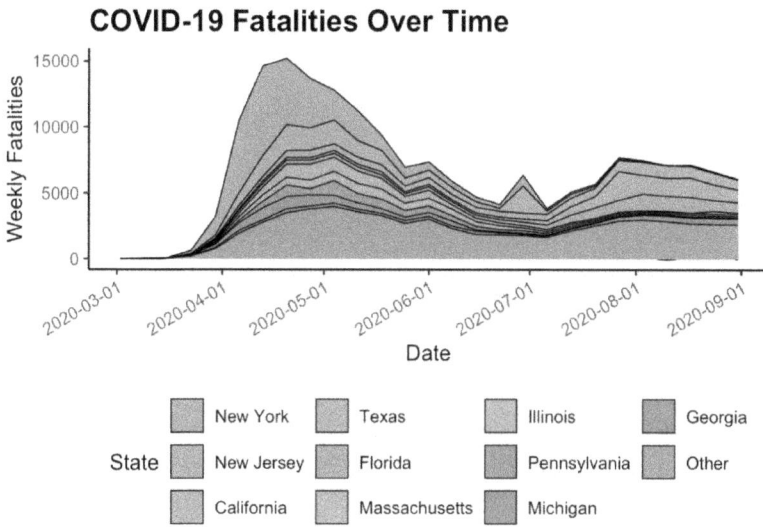

Figure 8.5: COVID-19 Cases Over Time by State.

9

Case Study: Exploring Early COVID-19 Data

In this chapter, we demonstrate a short exploratory analysis as a case study. This case study focuses on COVID-19 cases and deaths during 2020 using the covidcases and mobility datasets from the **HDSinRdata** package. A new package that is used in this case study is **usmap** package (Di Lorenzo 2024), which allows us to easily create spatial plots of the United States.

```
library(HDSinRdata)
library(tidyverse)
library(patchwork)
library(gt)
library(gtsummary)
library(usmap)
```

9.1 Pre-processing

We start by cleaning and merging our data. The covidcases data contains weekly confirmed COVID-19 cases and deaths at the state and county level in 2020. As the data description notes, some of these values may be negative due to data discrepancies in the cumulative counts data. The mobility data contains daily mobility statistics by state.

```
# Read in data
data(covidcases)
data(mobility)
```

First, we look at the columns in our data. We convert the date columns in the mobility data to be recognized as a date using the as.Date() function. The covidcases data has the week number of 2020. We create a similar column for the mobility data.

```
# Convert to date format and find week
mobility$date <- as.Date(mobility$date, formula = "%Y-%M-%D")
mobility$week <- week(mobility$date)
```

This allows us to summarize the mobility for a state across each week.

```
# Find average mobility for week
mobility_week <- mobility %>%
  group_by(state, week) %>%
  summarize(m50 = mean(m50, na.rm=TRUE), .groups = "drop")
head(mobility_week)
#> # A tibble: 6 x 3
#>   state     week   m50
#>   <chr>    <dbl> <dbl>
#> 1 Alabama      9 13.2
#> 2 Alabama     10 14.6
#> 3 Alabama     11 13.4
#> 4 Alabama     12  8.98
#> 5 Alabama     13  7.81
#> 6 Alabama     14  6.73
```

For both of our datasets, we want to check whether each state was observed across all dates and how the state's name is represented. For the mobility data, our data is at the state level, so we can use the `table()` function.

```
# Find number of dates recorded for each state
table(mobility_week$state)
#>
#>       Alabama        Alaska       Arizona      Arkansas
#>            27            27            27            27
#>    California      Colorado   Connecticut      Delaware
#>            27            27            27            27
#>       Florida       Georgia        Hawaii         Idaho
#>            27            27            27            27
#>      Illinois       Indiana          Iowa        Kansas
#>            27            27            27            27
#>      Kentucky     Louisiana         Maine      Maryland
#>            27            27            27            27
#> Massachusetts      Michigan     Minnesota   Mississippi
#>            27            27            27            27
#>      Missouri       Montana      Nebraska        Nevada
#>            27            27            27            27
```

```
#>    New Hampshire       New Jersey       New Mexico           New York
#>               27               27               27                 27
#>   North Carolina    North Dakota             Ohio           Oklahoma
#>               27               27               27                 27
#>           Oregon    Pennsylvania     Rhode Island     South Carolina
#>               27               27               27                 27
#>     South Dakota        Tennessee            Texas               Utah
#>               27               27               27                 27
#>          Vermont         Virginia       Washington  Washington, D.C.
#>               27               27               27                 27
#>    West Virginia        Wisconsin          Wyoming
#>               27               27               27
```

For the `covidcases` data, our data is at the county level. We need to summarize
the data instead. In this case, some states were observed for fewer weeks than
others.

```
# Find state names and number of weeks recorded for each state
unique(covidcases$state)
#>  [1] "California"        "Florida"
#>  [3] "New Hampshire"     "Washington"
#>  [5] "Massachusetts"     "Arizona"
#>  [7] "Texas"             "Georgia"
#>  [9] "New York"          "Wisconsin"
#> [11] "Oregon"            "North Carolina"
#> [13] "Nebraska"          "Illinois"
#> [15] "Utah"              "Indiana"
#> [17] "Tennessee"         "Pennsylvania"
#> [19] "Michigan"          "Oklahoma"
#> [21] "Kentucky"          "Connecticut"
#> [23] "Colorado"          "Virginia"
#> [25] "Nevada"            "South Dakota"
#> [27] "Minnesota"         "Ohio"
#> [29] "Vermont"           "New Jersey"
#> [31] "Maryland"          "Iowa"
#> [33] "Missouri"          "South Carolina"
#> [35] "Hawaii"            "District of Columbia"
#> [37] "Louisiana"         "Kansas"
#> [39] "Maine"             "Arkansas"
#> [41] "Idaho"             "Alabama"
#> [43] "Montana"           "Mississippi"
#> [45] "North Dakota"      "New Mexico"
#> [47] "Alaska"            "Wyoming"
```

```
#> [49] "Delaware"            "West Virginia"
#> [51] "Rhode Island"
num_wks <- covidcases %>%
  group_by(state) %>%
  summarize(num_weeks = n_distinct(week), .groups = "drop")
summary(num_wks)
#>     state            num_weeks
#>  Length:51        Min.   :23.0
#>  Class :character 1st Qu.:25.5
#>  Mode  :character Median :26.0
#>                   Mean   :26.0
#>                   3rd Qu.:27.0
#>                   Max.   :27.0
```

Note that D.C. is written differently for each data source. We update this name in the mobility data.

```
mobility_week$state[mobility_week$state == "Washington, D.C."] <-
  "District of Columbia"
```

After checking the formatting of the `state` and `week` columns, we can now merge our data together. In this case, we want to add the mobility data to the case data and use a `left_join()`.

```
# Join cases and mobility data
covid <- left_join(covidcases, mobility_week, by = c("state", "week"))
```

Next, we want to get some simple information about the continuous variables in our data. We observe two key points. First, we can see the negative values the data description warned us about, and second, there is no missing data.

```
summary(covid[, c("weekly_cases", "weekly_deaths", "m50")])
#>  weekly_cases    weekly_deaths       m50
#>  Min.   : -188  Min.   :-511   Min.   : 0.0
#>  1st Qu.:    2  1st Qu.:   0   1st Qu.: 5.0
#>  Median :    9  Median :   0   Median : 7.7
#>  Mean   :   87  Mean   :   3   Mean   : 7.7
#>  3rd Qu.:   39  3rd Qu.:   1   3rd Qu.: 9.9
#>  Max.   :35134  Max.   :5226   Max.   :49.4
```

These negative numbers are clear data discrepancies. When showing the dis-

tribution of cases in our exploratory analysis, we may choose to either code
these as 0 or NA. We decide to re-code these negative values as NA.

```r
# Set negative counts to NA
covid$weekly_cases <- replace(covid$weekly_cases,
                              which(covid$weekly_cases < 0),
                              NA)

covid$weekly_deaths <- replace(covid$weekly_deaths,
                               which(covid$weekly_deaths < 0),
                               NA)
```

As the last step in our pre-processing, we add in the state abbreviation and
region for each state using the `state.name` and `state.region` vectors available
in R. We code D.C. to be in the same region as Maryland and Virginia.

```r
# Add region and abbreviation and remove county
region_key <- data.frame(state = c(state.name,
                                   "District of Columbia"),
                         state_abb = c(state.abb, "DC"),
                         region = c(as.character(state.region),
                                   "South"))

covid <- covid %>%
  left_join(region_key, by = c("state"))

head(covid)
#> # A tibble: 6 x 8
#>    state   county  week weekly_cases weekly_deaths    m50 state_abb
#> ↳  region
#>    <chr>   <chr>   <dbl>        <int>         <int> <dbl> <chr>
#> ↳  <chr>
#> 1 Califo~ Marin       9            1             0  7.50 CA          West
#> 2 Califo~ Orange      9            3             0  7.50 CA          West
#> 3 Florida Manat~      9            1             0  9.68 FL          South
#> 4 Califo~ Napa        9            1             0  7.50 CA          West
#> 5 New Ha~ Graft~      9            2             0  7.67 NH          North~
#> 6 Washin~ Spoka~      9            4             0  4.01 WA          West
```

9.2 Mobility and Cases Over Time

Now that our data are merged and cleaned, we start exploring mobility and cases by region. The following summary table shows that these measures did differ by region overall.

```
covid %>%
  select(c("region", "m50", "weekly_cases", "weekly_deaths")) %>%
  tbl_summary(by = "region", missing = "no") %>%
  as_gt() %>%
  cols_width(everything() ~ "55pt")
```

Characteristic	North Central, N = 22,653[1]	Northeast, N = 5,165[1]	South, N = 32,276[1]	West, N = 9,436[1]
m50	7.4 (5.4, 8.8)	4.2 (1.6, 5.2)	9.7 (7.1, 11.3)	4.3 (2.9, 7.0)
weekly_cases	5 (1, 22)	15 (3, 91)	13 (3, 50)	5 (1, 38)
weekly_deaths	0 (0, 0)	0 (0, 4)	0 (0, 1)	0 (0, 1)

[1]Median (IQR)

We then plot mobility over time both for the whole country and by region. Across the country, we see a similar pattern in how mobility fluctuated, but certain regions had overall higher mobility than others.

```
# Average mobility in the US over time - overall
pmob1 <- covid %>%
  select(c(region, state, week, m50)) %>%
  distinct() %>%
  group_by(week) %>%
  summarize(avg_m50 = mean(m50, na.rm=TRUE), .groups="drop") %>%
  ggplot() +
  geom_line(aes(x = week, y = avg_m50)) +
  labs(x = "Week in 2020", y = "Average Mobility",
       title = "Average Mobility in the US") +
  theme_bw()

# Average mobility in the US over time - by region
pmob2 <- covid %>%
```

```
select(c(region, state, week, m50)) %>%
distinct() %>%
group_by(region, week) %>%
summarize(avg_m50 = mean(m50, na.rm=TRUE), .groups="drop") %>%
ggplot() +
geom_line(aes(x = week, y = avg_m50, color = region)) +
labs(x = "Week in 2020", y = "Average Mobility",
     title = "Average Mobility by Region in the US",
     color = "Region") +
theme_bw() +
theme(legend.position = "bottom")

pmob1+pmob2
```

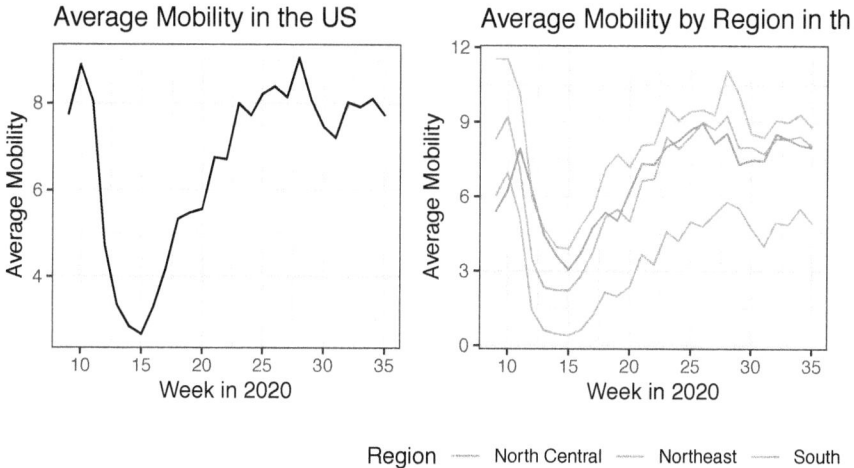

We then look at cases and deaths by region. A limitation of these data are that we do not have population counts which would allow us to standardize these numbers. However, a secondary y-axis using the sec_axis() function within scale_y_continuous() allows us to plot deaths and cases together. In this case, the secondary axis is scaled by 1/10th of the primary axis.

```
# Change in number cases over time, per region
covid %>%
  filter(!is.na(region)) %>%
  group_by(region, week) %>%
  summarize(weekly_cases = sum(weekly_cases, na.rm = TRUE),
```

```
                weekly_deaths = sum(weekly_deaths, na.rm = TRUE),
                .groups = "drop") %>%
ggplot() +
  geom_line(aes(x = week, y = weekly_cases, color = region,
              linetype = "Cases")) +
  geom_line(aes(x = week, y = weekly_deaths*10, color = region,
              linetype = "Deaths")) +
  scale_y_continuous(name = "Average Weekly Cases",
                  sec.axis = sec_axis(~./10,
                      name = "Average Weekly Deaths"))+
  scale_linetype(name = "Measure") +
  labs(x = "Week in 2020", color = "Region",
      title = "Weekly Cases Over Time by Region") +
  theme_bw()
```

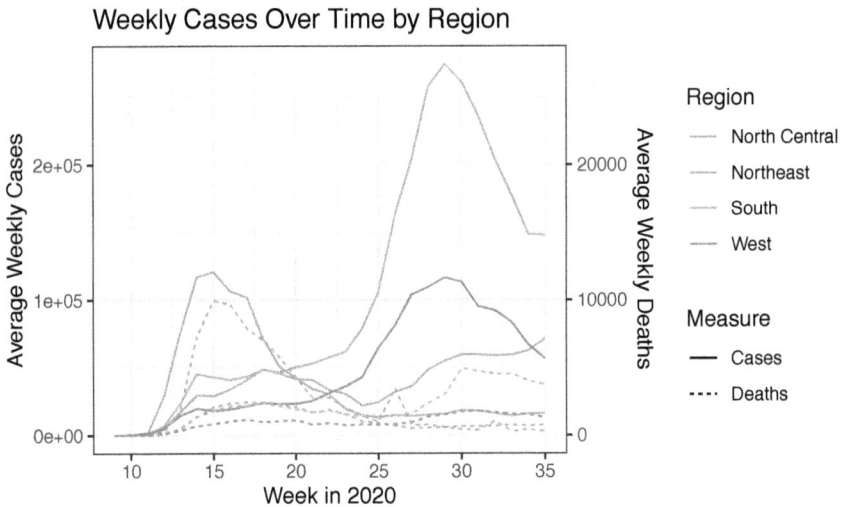

To examine how mobility and cases are related, we look at a scatter plot of mobility and cases in California.

```
covid_ca <- covid %>% filter(state == "California")
ggplot(covid_ca)+
  geom_point(aes(x = weekly_cases, y = m50), na.rm = TRUE) +
  labs(x = "Weekly Cases", y = "Average Mobility")
```

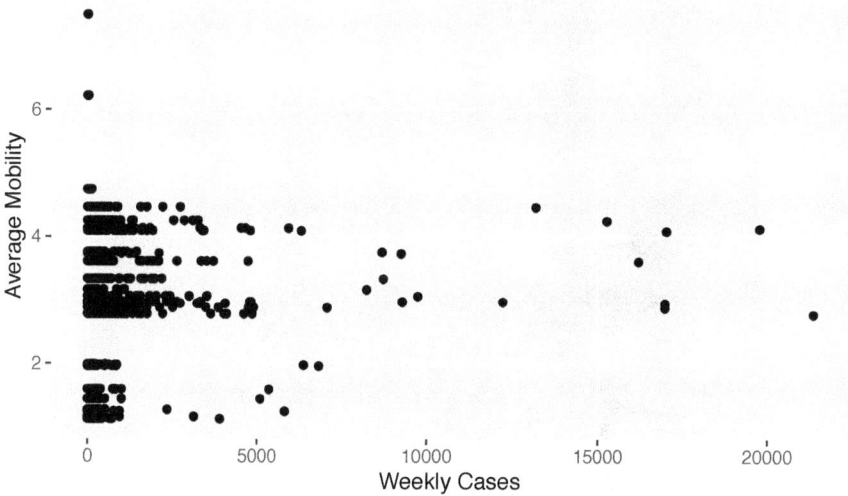

This motivates us to look at the correlation between these two columns by state. We plot this using the `plot_usmap()` function from the **usmap** package. Interestingly, we observe different relationships throughout the country, but none of the correlations are particularly strong.

```
# Calculate and plot correlation between cases and mobility, y state
covid_cor <- covid %>%
  group_by(state) %>%
  summarize(correlation = cor(weekly_cases, m50,
                               use = "complete.obs"))

plot_usmap(regions = "states", data = covid_cor,
           values = "correlation") +
  scale_fill_gradient2(low = "darkblue", high = "darkred",
                       mid="white", name = "Correlation") +
  labs(title = "Correlation Between Cases and Mobility") +
  theme(legend.position = "right")
```

Correlation Between Cases and Mobility

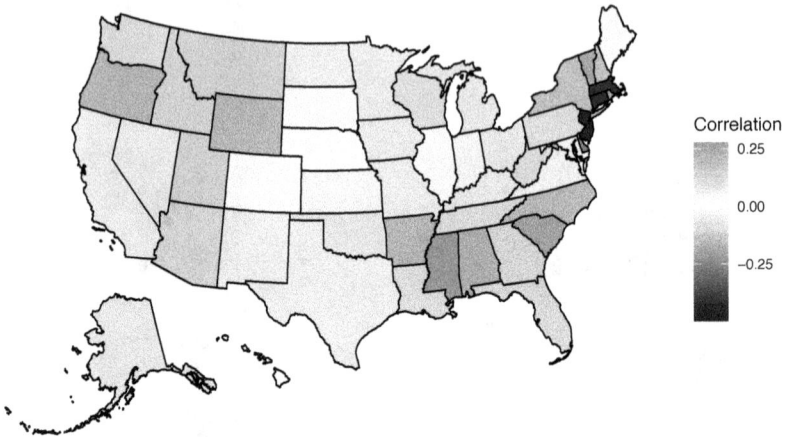

Last, we look at how the total cases and deaths are related to each other. This shows that the Northeast suffered more deaths per case overall, which may be related to the lower mobility and negative correlation between mobility and cases observed earlier.

```
# Relationship between cases and deaths summarized
covid %>%
  group_by(region, state_abb) %>%
  summarize(total_cases = sum(weekly_cases, na.rm = TRUE),
            total_deaths = sum(weekly_deaths, na.rm = TRUE),
            .groups = "drop") %>%
ggplot() +
  geom_label(aes(x = total_cases, y = total_deaths, color = region,
                 label = state_abb), size = 1.5) +
  labs(x = "Total Cases", y = "Total Deaths", color = "Region") +
  theme_bw()
```

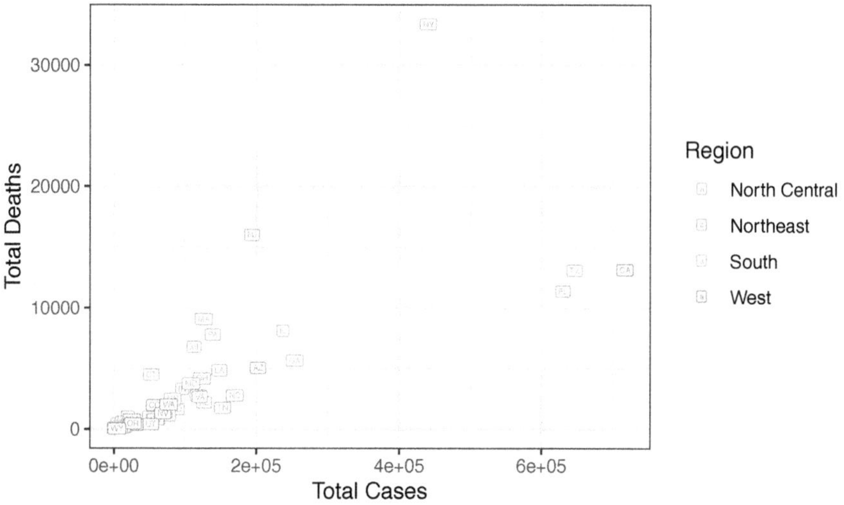
30000
20000
10000
0
Total Deaths
0e+00
2e+05
4e+05
6e+05
Total Cases
Region
North Central
Northeast
South
West

Part III

Distributions and Hypothesis Testing

10

Probability Distributions in R

In this chapter, we cover how to generate random samples in R from known probability distributions and empirical distributions. Base R provides a set of four functions for all common probability distributions. These can be used to generate random samples and to calculate the corresponding density, quantile, and cumulative functions that correspond to that distribution.

```
library(tidyverse)
library(HDSinRdata)

data(NHANESsample)
```

In the following code, we demonstrate an example of drawing random samples. Anytime we perform an operation in R in which the outcome has some randomness, we are using R's random number generator under the hood. This means that the results change every time we run our code. In order to make sure our code is replicable, we have to set a *random seed*, which makes the results the same every time. The `set.seed()` function takes in a numeric seed value. You can use any number as the seed. In the next code chunk, we first sample a random value from the numbers 1 to 10 without setting a seed. Note that every time you run this code chunk, the output can change. However, in the following code chunk we set a seed, which means that the result is always the same (in this case, it's equal to 2).

```
sample(1:10, 1)
#> [1] 1
```

```
set.seed(5)
sample(1:10, 1)
#> [1] 2
```

10.1   Probability Distribution Functions

All of the common discrete (e.g., Bernoulli, binomial) and continuous (e.g., normal, uniform, exponential, Poisson) probability distributions have corresponding functions in R. For each of these distributions, there are four available functions:

- `r[dist]()`: random sample function for the given distribution (e.g., `rnorm()`, `runif()`)
- `d[dist]()`: density function for the distribution (e.g., `dnorm()`, `dunif()`)
- `p[dist]()`: cumulative distribution function for the distribution (e.g., `pnorm()`, `punif()`)
- `q[dist]()`: quantile function for the distribution (e.g., `qnorm()`, `qunif()`)

Let's see how these work in practice, using the normal and binomial distributions as examples.

10.1.1   Random Samples

The following code generates a sample of 100 random numbers following a normal distribution with mean 5 and standard deviation 1. As you can see, the function takes in n (the number of observations), mean (the mean with default value 0), and sd (the standard deviation with default value 1). A histogram plot (using the built-in hist() function) shows that the generated values look roughly normally distributed.

```
x <- rnorm(n = 100, mean = 5, sd = 1)
hist(x)
```

Histogram of x

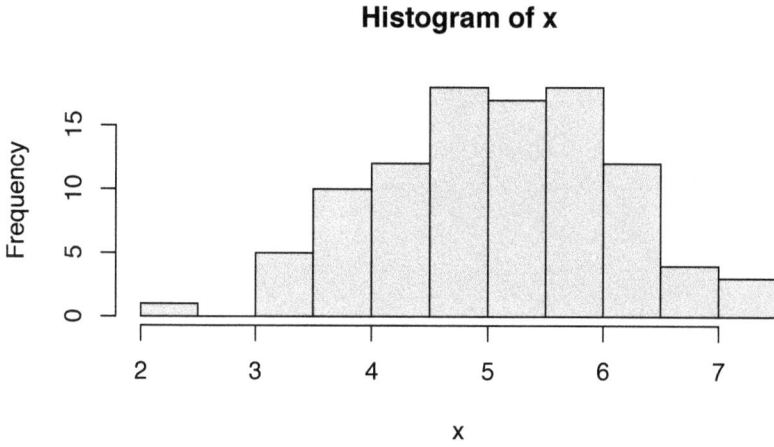

We can also input a vector instead of a single value for the mean or sd arguments if we want each sample to come from its own normal distribution. As an example, we generate 100 random numbers with the default standard deviation of 1 where half of the samples have a mean of 0, and the other half have a mean of 5.

```
x <- rnorm(n = 100, mean = rep(c(0,5), 50))
hist(x)
```

Histogram of x

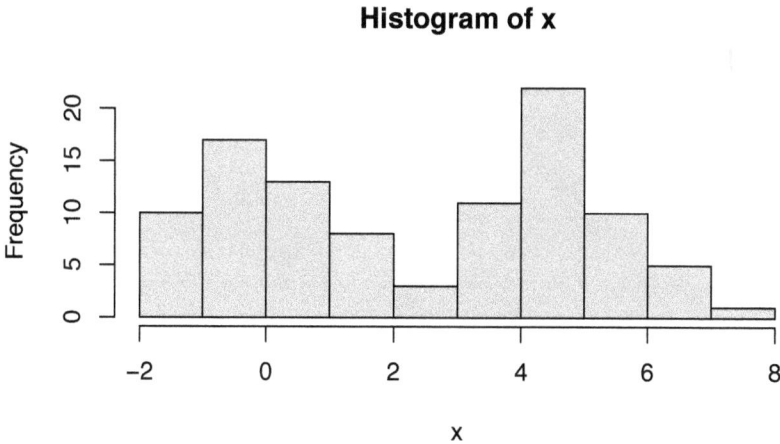

For the binomial distribution, the difference is that we need to specify a probability p and number of trials size (rather than mean and sd in the normal
case) to specify the distribution. In the following code, we generate 100 random numbers following a binomial distribution with 10 trials and a probability
0.5.

```
x <- rbinom(n = 100, p = 0.5, size = 10)
hist(x)
```

Histogram of x

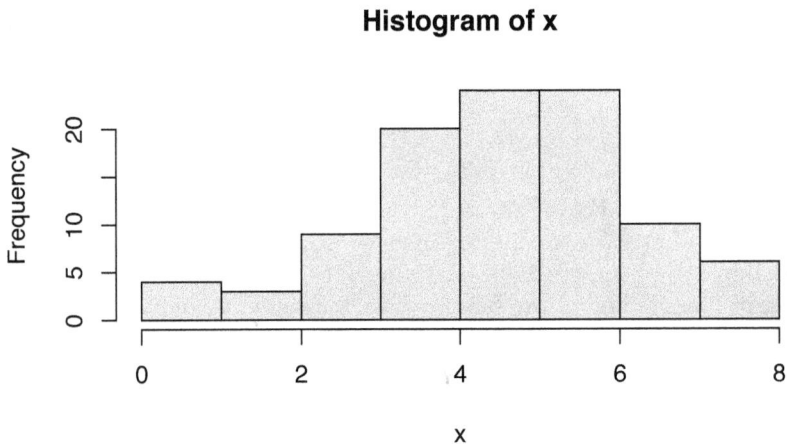

We can also specify a different size or probability of success for each sample.
We repeat our sample but this time let the probability of success be 0.25 for
half of the sample and 0.75 for the other half.

```
x <- rbinom(n = 100, p = rep(c(0.25, 0.75), 50), size = 10)
hist(x)
```

Histogram of x

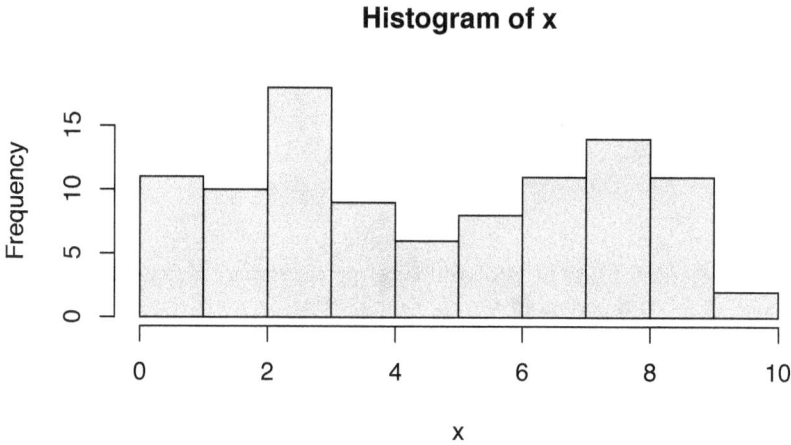

10.1.2 Density Function

Next, we look at the density function. Recall that the probability density function for a normal distribution with mean μ and standard deviation σ is given by the following formula.

$$f_X(x) = \frac{1}{\sigma\sqrt{2\pi}} \exp\left(-\frac{1}{2}\left(\frac{x-\mu}{\sigma}\right)^2\right)$$

Using the following code, we can compare some of the values from the dnorm() function to this equation and see that they are in fact equal. We could also specify the mean and standard deviation in this function but choose to use the default values (mean = 0 and sd = 1).

```
dnorm(0) == 1/sqrt(2*pi)
#> [1] TRUE
dnorm(1) == exp(-1/2)/sqrt(2*pi)
#> [1] TRUE
dnorm(2) == exp(-1/2*2^2)/sqrt(2*pi)
#> [1] TRUE
```

If we wanted to find the density function for several values, we can input a vector to this density function. In the following code, we find the values of the density function for a normal distribution with mean 1 and standard deviation 2 for values c(-1, 0, 1, 2, 3).

```
dnorm(c(-1, 0, 1, 2, 3), mean = 1, sd = 2)
#> [1] 0.121 0.176 0.199 0.176 0.121
```

For the binomial distribution, dbinom() returns the probability of a certain number of successes and corresponds to the probability density function.

$$P(X = x) = \binom{size}{x} p^x (1 - p)^{size - x}.$$

For example, we can find the probability of getting exactly 3 heads from 10 coin flips, each with a probability of 0.5 for heads.

```
dbinom(3, size = 10, p = 0.5)
#> [1] 0.117
```

While dnorm() allows us to specify any continuous values for x, dbinom() gives us a warning if x contains non-integer values, since the support of a binomial variable only includes integers.

```
dbinom(2.4, size = 10, p = 0.5)
#> Warning in dbinom(2.4, size = 10, p = 0.5): non-integer x = 2.400000
#> [1] 0
```

We can also specify a vector for a distribution's parameters to find the distribution function for different distributions. For example, I find the the probability density function for $X = 4$ for the distribution with $p = 0.25$ and $p = 0.5$.

```
dbinom(4, size = 10, p = c(0.25, 0.5))
#> [1] 0.146 0.205
```

10.1.3   Cumulative Distribution

Next, we take a look at the cumulative distribution function. For the normal distribution, the cumulative distribution is given by pnorm(), which takes in a value x, a mean, and a sd and returns the probability that a random variable following a $N(mean, sd)$ distribution is less than x. For example, for x equal to the mean, this returns a 50% probability because the normal distribution is symmetric with mean equal to the median. In the following code, we verify this for two different values of the mean.

```
pnorm(0)
#> [1] 0.5
pnorm(5, mean = 5, sd = 1)
#> [1] 0.5
```

Since the binomial distribution is discrete, it can only take on integer values from 0 to size. This means that, for example, the pbinom() function returns the same value for 3, 3.5, 3.6, all the way up to, but not including, 4. This is because $P(X \leq 3) = P(X \leq 3.2) = P(X \leq 3.5) = P(X \leq 3.6)$ and so on. Note that here we passed in a vector of values x.

```
pbinom(c(3, 3.5, 3.6, 4), size = 10, p = 0.5)
#> [1] 0.172 0.172 0.172 0.377
```

We can also vary the parameters for the distribution by passing a vector for size and/or p to the cumulative distribution function. In the subsequent code chunk, we find the probability that $X \leq 3$ and the probability that $X \leq 4$ with 12 trials and a probability 0.25 and with 10 trials and a probability 0.5.

```
pbinom(c(3, 3, 4, 4), size = c(12, 10, 12, 10),
       p=c(0.25, 0.5, 0.25, 0.5))
#> [1] 0.649 0.172 0.842 0.377
```

10.1.4 Quantile Distribution

Lastly, we have the quantile distribution function, which is the inverse of the cumulative distribution function. This function takes in a probability x, a mean, and a sd and returns the value for which the cumulative distribution function is equal to x. Thus, when x is equal to 0.5, the qnorm() function returns the median of the distribution, which is equal to the mean for the normal distribution.

```
qnorm(0.5)
#> [1] 0
qnorm(0.5, mean = 5, sd = 1)
#> [1] 5
```

For the discrete binomial distribution, the qbinom() function returns the largest integer value for which the probability of being less than or equal to that value is at most the inputted value x.

```
qbinom(c(0.2, 0.3), size = 10, p = 0.5)
#> [1] 2 3
```

10.1.5 Reference List for Probability Distributions

In the previous examples, we only used the normal and binomial distributions. The following list contains the other probability distributions available in R. For each distribution, we have given the arguments for the r[dist]() function. The other three functions have a similar format. Unless otherwise stated, the parameter n is the number of observations.

- **Beta**: rbeta(n, shape1, shape2, ncp = 0) with shape parameters shape1 and shape2 (and optional non-centrality parameter ncp).
- **Binomial**: rbinom(n, size, prob) with probability of success prob and number of trials size.
- **Cauchy**: rcauchy(n, location = 0, scale = 1) with location parameter location and scale parameter scale.
- **Chi-Square**: rchisq(n, df, ncp = 0) with df degrees of freedom and optional non-centrality parameter ncp.
- **Exponential**: rexp(n, rate = 1) with rate rate (i.e., mean = 1/rate).
- **F**: rf(n, df1, df2, ncp) with df1 and df2 degrees of freedom (and optional non-centrality parameter ncp).
- **Gamma**: rgamma(n, shape, rate = 1, scale = 1/rate) with parameters shape and scale (or alternatively specified by rate).
- **Geometric**: rgeom(n, prob) with probability parameter prob.
- **Hypergeometric**: rhyper(nn, m, n, k) with m white balls, n black balls, and k balls chosen.
- **Logistic**: rlogis(n, location = 0, scale = 1) with parameters location and scale.
- **Log Normal**: rlnorm(n, meanlog = 0, sdlog = 1) with mean meanlog and standard deviation sdlog on the log scale.
- **Negative Binomial**: rnbinom(n, size, prob, mu) with parameters size and prob.
- **Normal**: rnorm(n, mean = 0, sd = 1) with mean equal to mean and standard deviation equal to sd.
- **Poisson**: rpois(n, lambda) with parameter lambda.
- **Student t**: rt(n, df, ncp) with df degrees of freedom (and optional non-centrality parameter ncp).
- **Uniform**: runif(n, min = 0, max = 1) with minimum value min and maximum value max.
- **Weibull**: rweibull(n, shape, scale = 1) with parameters shape and scale.
- **Wilcoxon Rank Sum**: rwilcox(nn, m, n) with nn number of observations and sample sizes m and n.

- **Wilcoxon Signed Rank:** `rsignrank(nn, n)` with `nn` number of observations and sample size `n`.

10.1.6 Practice Question

Set the random seed to be `123`, and then generate 5 random numbers following a uniform distribution with min 1 and max 5. Then, find the 0.15 quantile for this same distribution (it should be equal to 1.6).

```
# Insert your solution here:
```

10.2 Empirical Distributions and Sampling Data

At the start of this chapter, we used the `sample()` function. This function can also be used to sample from an empirical distribution. The `sample(x, size, replace=FALSE, prob=NULL)` function takes in the values we want to sample from `x`, the number of observations we want to sample `size`, and whether we want to sample with replacement `replace`. If we don't want to sample such that each value has an equal probability of being chosen, we can also set a probability vector `prob`, which must have the same length as `x`. In the following code, we sample 500 rows without replacement from the `NHANESsample` data. To do so, we select 500 values from the indices 1 to the number of rows in the data. We then select rows of the data using these indices.

```
nhanes_sample_ids <- sample(1:nrow(NHANESsample), 500, replace =
  ↪   FALSE)
nhanes_sample <- NHANESsample[nhanes_sample_ids, ]
dim(nhanes_sample)
#> [1] 500   21
```

We now demonstrate sampling with replacement. By doing so, we create a new dataset that is sampled from the empirical distribution of the data and that is called a *bootstrap sample*.

```
nhanes_sample_ids <- sample(1:nrow(NHANESsample), nrow(NHANESsample),
                            replace = TRUE)
nhanes_sample <- NHANESsample[nhanes_sample_ids, ]
dim(nhanes_sample)
#> [1] 31265    21
```

Another way to sample from a data frame is to use the `slice_sample()` function from the **tidyverse**. In this function, we can either specify the number of observations to sample n or the proportion of observations to sample prop. Additionally, we can sample with or without replacement by setting the value of the argument `replace` (with default value FALSE). We use this function to randomly sample 20% of observations without replacement.

```
nhanes_sample <- NHANESsample %>%
  slice_sample(prop = 0.2, replace = FALSE)
dim(nhanes_sample)
#> [1] 6253    21
```

10.2.1   Practice Question

Set the random seed to 5 and then sample 50 observations with replacement from the set of integers from 1 to 100. Take the mean of those observations; it should be 56.7.

```
# Insert your solution here:
```

Beyond sampling, we can also find the empirical cumulative distribution. That is, we can use a given vector to infer a distribution. In the following case, we draw a random sample from a normal distribution vec and then find its empirical cumulative distribution using the `ecdf()` function. This function actually returns a function, which can then be used to find the sample cumulative distribution for different values similar to the `p[dist]()` functions. In our example, we find the sample probability that $X \leq 0$.

```
vec <- rnorm(100)
ecdf_vec <- ecdf(vec)
ecdf_vec(0)
#> [1] 0.63
```

We now plot this empirical distribution against the actual cdf using the `pnorm()` function. Note that in order to do so, we create a sequence of possible x values to pass to both `pnorm()` and `ecdf_vec()`.

```
df <- data.frame(x = seq(-3, 3, 0.05))
df$ecdf <- ecdf_vec(df$x)
df$distn = pnorm(df$x)
```

```
ggplot(df) +
  geom_line(aes(x = x, y = ecdf), color = "black") +
  geom_line(aes(x = x, y= distn), color = "red")
```

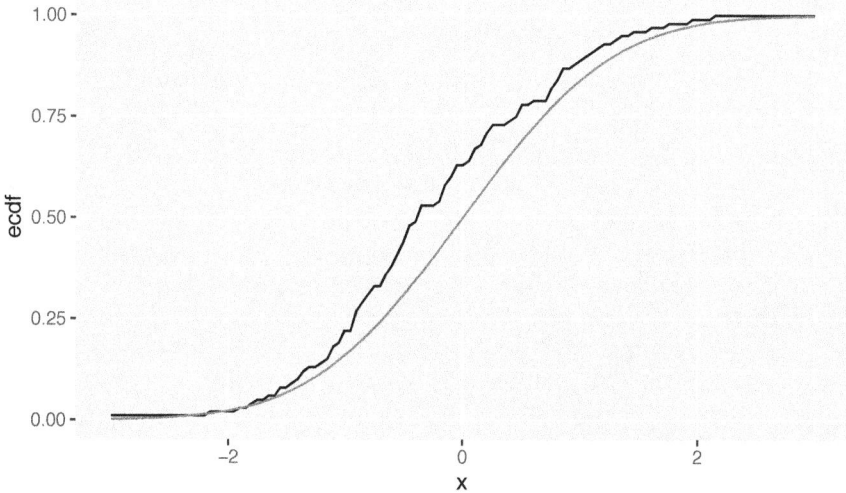

In practice, the empirical cumulative distribution might involve data from a given dataset that you want to use to represent the population's distribution. As an example, in the following code we find the empirical distribution of blood lead level from the NHANESsample data frame. A blood lead level of 5 μg/dL or above is considered elevated. We can see 96.4% of observations have a blood lead level below this threshold.

```
ecdf_lead <- ecdf(nhanes_sample$LEAD)
ecdf_lead(5)
#> [1] 0.961
```

10.3 Exercises

1. Assume the distribution of female heights is approximated by a normal distribution with a mean of 64 inches and a standard deviation of 2.2 inches. Using this distribution, answer the following questions.

- What is the probability that a randomly chosen female is 5 feet or shorter?

- What is the probability that a randomly chosen female is 6 feet or taller?

- Generate 500 random observations following this distribution and find the sample 0.15 quantile. Then, compare this to the 0.15 quantile using the qdist() function.

2. Compute the probability that the height of a randomly chosen female is within 1 SD from the average height.

3. Create a vector of 100 patient IDs, and then use the sample() function to assign half of them to a treatment group and the other half to a control group. Then, suppose those in the control group have a reduction in viral load distributed as $X \sim 100 * exp(mean = V)$, where V follows a uniform distribution between 1 and 2, whereas those who are in the treatment group have a reduction in viral load distributed as $X \sim 100 * exp(mean = 3)$. Plot distributions of reduction in viral load for both groups.

11

Hypothesis Testing

In this chapter, we look at hypothesis testing in R. We start with single sample distributions and tests, and then we look at hypothesis tests for comparing two samples. Examples include testing for positive correlations, performing two-sample paired t-tests, and testing for equal variance among groups. The data we use in this section comes from the Texas Health and Human Services Department and includes the reported number of induced terminations of pregnancy (ITOPs) from 2016 to 2021, stratified by both race and county (Texas Health & Human Services Commission 2016-2021). The data also contains the rate of abortions per 1000 females aged 15-49. Read the data documentation to see the full variable descriptions.

We use the **tidyverse**, **gt**, and **gtsummary** packages to help manipulate and summarize the data. The **car** package (Fox, Weisberg, and Price 2023) contains the function `leveneTest()` to implement a Levene's test for homogeneity of variance across groups, and all other hypothesis tests are available in base R.

```
library(tidyverse)
library(car)
library(HDSinRdata)
library(gt)
library(gtsummary)

data(tex_itop)
```

11.1 Univariate Distributions and One-Sample Tests

Let's begin by looking at a single outcome of interest - the number of induced terminations of pregnancy (referred to as ITOPs or abortions below) in 2021 per 1000 females ages 15-49 in each county. We use the number of females ages 15-49 as a proxy to scale the number of abortions by the population size,

though this is not truly reflective of the number of people who can give birth
in each county.

```
county_rates_2021 <- tex_itop$total_rate[tex_itop$year == 2021]
hist(county_rates_2021, breaks = 35)
```

Histogram of county_rates_2021

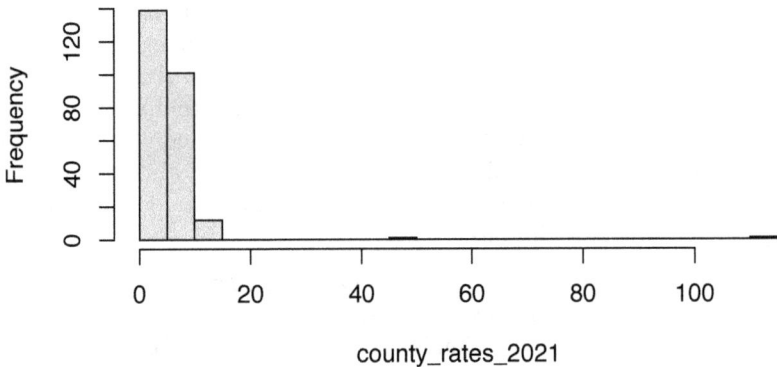

We can see in the figure that this is a heavy-tailed distribution. In the following
code, we find the ten counties with the highest rates and see that there are
some counties that have very few total abortions but that have some of the
highest abortion rates. This indicates a small population. On the other hand,
we also observe Harris county, which contains the city of Houston and has
both a high total abortion count and a high abortion rate.

```
tex_itop %>%
  filter(year == 2021) %>%
  slice_max(n = 10, total_rate) %>%
  dplyr::select(c(county, total_itop, total_rate))
#> # A tibble: 10 x 3
#>    county  total_itop total_rate
#>    <chr>        <dbl>      <dbl>
#> 1 Loving           1       111.
#> 2 Terrell          5        50
#> 3 Concho           4        13.9
#> 4 Harris       14122        13.5
```

```
#> 5 Irion              3          12.9
#> # i 5 more rows
```

Some of the counties are so small that we may want to consider dropping them from our analysis. In particular, among these small counties, the rates in Loving County and Terrell County are high enough that we might consider them to be outliers. For this one-sample analysis, however, we do not remove them. If we wanted to estimate the mean abortion rate among counties μ, we can do so by simply using the `mean()` function. For reference, the Centers for Disease Control estimated the national abortion rate in 2020 to be 11.2 abortions per 1,000 women aged 15–44 years (Kortsmit 2023).

```
mean(county_rates_2021, na.rm = TRUE)
#> [1] 5.17
```

Within R we can also calculate a confidence interval for this mean. Recall that a $(1 - \alpha)\%$ confidence interval for the mean is given by the equation $\hat{\mu} \pm z_{1-\alpha/2} \cdot \frac{\hat{\sigma}}{\sqrt{n}}$, where $\hat{\mu}$ is our sample mean, $\hat{\sigma}^2$ is the sample variance, and n is the number of observations.

In the subsequent code chunk, we use this formula to calculate a 95% confidence interval for the mean abortion rate among counties:

```
est_mean <- mean(county_rates_2021, na.rm = TRUE)
est_sd <- sd(county_rates_2021)
z_alpha <- dnorm(1 - 0.05 / 2)
n <- length(county_rates_2021)
c(est_mean - z_alpha * est_sd / sqrt(n),
  est_mean + z_alpha * est_sd / sqrt(n))
#> [1] 5.04 5.29
```

If we want to display this nicely, we can use the `round()` function, which allows us to specify a number of digits to be displayed, and the `paste()` function, which creates a single character string from multiple inputs.

```
lower <- round(est_mean - z_alpha*est_sd/sqrt(n), 3)
upper <- round(est_mean + z_alpha*est_sd/sqrt(n), 3)
paste("Confidence Interval: (", lower, ",", upper, ")")
#> [1] "Confidence Interval: ( 5.044 , 5.289 )"
```

Suppose that we wanted to run a hypothesis test to compare the mean to a pre-determined value. In particular, the Texas Heartbeat Act was introduced in 2021 and drastically reduced the number of eligible abortions. We could test whether there were significantly fewer abortions in 2021 compared to 2020 using a one-sided t-test. Our null hypothesis is that $\mu \geq 6.23$, the mean abortion rate in 2020. To run this hypothesis test, we use the `t.test()` function. For a one-sample t-test, we need to specify our sample `x`, the alternative hypothesis `alternative` (default is a two-sided test), the true value of the mean `mu` (default 0), and a confidence level `conf.level` (default 0.95). In the following code, we run this t-test, and we can see from the result that we reject the null hypothesis at the 0.05 level and observe a statistically significant decline in the abortion rate in 2021.

```
t.test(county_rates_2021, alternative = "less", mu = 6.23,
      conf.level=0.95)
#>
#>   One Sample t-test
#>
#> data:  county_rates_2021
#> t = -2, df = 253, p-value = 0.02
#> alternative hypothesis: true mean is less than 6.23
#> 95 percent confidence interval:
#>   -Inf 5.98
#> sample estimates:
#> mean of x
#>       5.17
```

The output for this test is printed. If we want to reference these values, we need to save the result. The object `t_test_res` is a list that contains information about the statistic, p-value, confidence interval, etc. The list of outputs is similar to other test objects, so it is useful to look at what is contained in each by reading the test documentation (`?t.test`). We find the p-value from `t_test_res`.

```
t_test_res <- t.test(county_rates_2021, alternative = "less",
                     mu = 6.23, conf.level = 0.95)
names(t_test_res)
#> [1] "statistic"    "parameter"    "p.value"     "conf.int"
#> [5] "estimate"     "null.value"   "stderr"      "alternative"
#> [9] "method"       "data.name"
```

```
t_test_res$p.value
#> [1] 0.0161
```

11.1.1 Practice Question

Test whether there were significantly more abortions in 2019 compared to 2020 using a one-sided t-test. Your test statistic should be -6.4736.

```
# Insert your solution here:
```

One thing to consider is that the `t.test()` function assumes that the sample x comes from a normal distribution. The one-sample Wilcoxon signed rank test is a non-parametric alternative to the one-sample t-test that can be used to compare the median value of a sample to a theoretical value without assuming that the data are normally distributed. This test can be performed using the `wilcox.test()` function and takes in the same arguments as the `t.test()` function. In the following output, we can see that we again reject the null hypothesis at the 0.05 level and conclude that the median abortion rate in 2021 was significantly lower than 5.14, which was the median rate in 2020.

```
wilcox_res <- wilcox.test(county_rates_2021, alternative = "less",
                    mu = 5.14, conf.level = 0.95)
wilcox_res
#>
#>  Wilcoxon signed rank test with continuity correction
#>
#> data:  county_rates_2021
#> V = 12807, p-value = 0.002
#> alternative hypothesis: true location is less than 5.14
wilcox_res$p.value
#> [1] 0.00193
```

11.2 Correlation and Covariance

We now look at two-sample tests. To start, we look at the 2020 and 2021 rates by county. We pivot our data into a wider format in order to create 2020 and 2021 rate columns, and, this time, we filter out the Loving and Terrell counties to remove outliers. We then create a scatter plot of 2021 vs. 2020 rates and observe a linear correlation between the two.

```
county_rates <- tex_itop %>%
  dplyr::select(c(county, total_rate, year)) %>%
  filter(!(county %in% c("Terrell", "Loving")),
```

```
        year %in% c(2020, 2021)) %>%
  pivot_wider(names_from = year, values_from = total_rate) %>%
  na.omit() %>%
  rename("y2020" = "2020", "y2021" = "2021")
head(county_rates)
#> # A tibble: 6 x 3
#>   county     y2020 y2021
#>   <chr>      <dbl> <dbl>
#> 1 Anderson    6.84 5.07
#> 2 Andrews     1.85 0.792
#> 3 Angelina    5.81 6.00
#> 4 Aransas     3.44 7.18
#> 5 Archer      1.47 0.733
#> 6 Armstrong   0    0
```

```
ggplot(county_rates) +
  geom_point(aes(x = y2020, y = y2021)) +
  labs(x = "2020 ITOP Rates", y ="2021 ITOP Rates")
```

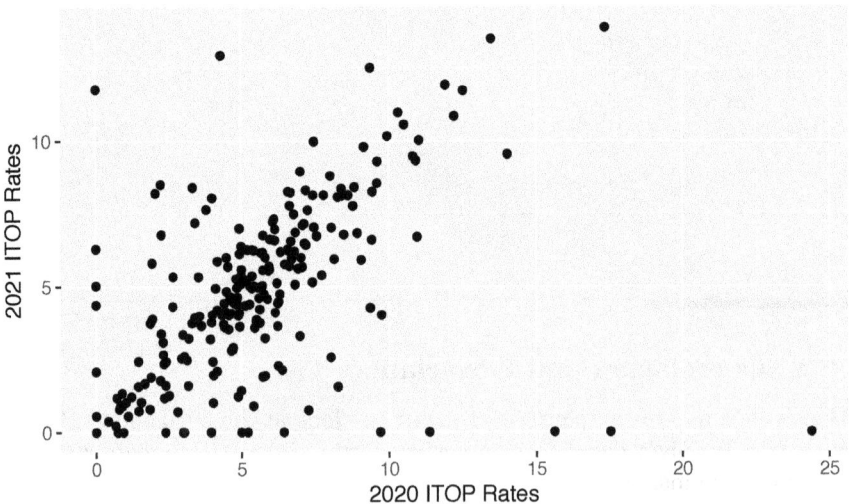

We have seen before how to calculate the correlation between two columns using the cor() function. We can also calculate the covariance using the cov() function. As suspected, there is a positive correlation. The estimated covariance is around 5.2.

```
cor(county_rates$y2020, county_rates$y2021)
#> [1] 0.5
cov(county_rates$y2020, county_rates$y2021)
#> [1] 5.2
```

Besides calculating the value of the correlation, we can also test whether this correlation is significantly different from zero. The function `cor.test()` tests for association between paired samples, using either Pearson's product moment correlation coefficient, Kendall's τ, or Spearman's ρ. Similar to the `t.test()` and `wilcox.test()` functions, we can also specify the `alternative` and `conf.level` arguments. In the following code, we test whether there is a non-zero correlation between the 2020 and 2021 county rates using Pearson's product-moment correlation. We can see from the resulting p-value that we can reject the null hypothesis that the correlation is zero and conclude that it is instead significantly different than zero. This time we also print the computed confidence interval for our estimate.

```
cor_test_res <- cor.test(county_rates$y2020,
                         county_rates$y2021,
                         method = "pearson")
cor_test_res
#>
#>   Pearson's product-moment correlation
#>
#> data:  county_rates$y2020 and county_rates$y2021
#> t = 9, df = 250, p-value <2e-16
#> alternative hypothesis: true correlation is not equal to 0
#> 95 percent confidence interval:
#>   0.401 0.587
#> sample estimates:
#> cor
#> 0.5


cor_test_res$conf.int
#> [1] 0.401 0.587
#> attr(,"conf.level")
#> [1] 0.95
```

11.3   Two-Sample Tests for Continuous Variables

If we wanted to directly compare the difference between 2020 and 2021 rates, we could use a two-sample test. In this case, because our samples are paired by county, we can use a two-sample paired t-test. Specifically, we use a two-sided test to test the null hypothesis that the rates are equal by specifying two different vectors x and y. Note that we used the default values of mu = 0 and alternative = "two.sided". Additionally, we used the default value var.equal = FALSE, which implies that the samples may have different variances. From the results, we reject the null hypothesis that the two county rates are equal at the 0.05 level. We also print a 95% confidence interval of the difference in means.

```
t_test_two_res <- t.test(x = county_rates$y2020,
                         y = county_rates$y2021)
t_test_two_res
#>
#>   Welch Two Sample t-test
#>
#> data:   county_rates$y2020 and county_rates$y2021
#> t = 2, df = 497, p-value = 0.01
#> alternative hypothesis: true difference in means is not equal to 0
#> 95 percent confidence interval:
#>   0.145 1.278
#> sample estimates:
#> mean of x mean of y
#>      5.28      4.57
t_test_two_res$conf.int
#> [1] 0.145 1.278
#> attr(,"conf.level")
#> [1] 0.95
```

In the tex_itop dataset, each county has also been categorized by whether it was urban or rural. Suppose we want to compare the change in abortion rates from 2020 to 2021 between rural and urban counties. First, we create a variable describing the rate change between these years using the following code. We choose to use the change in rate rather than percent change to avoid infinite or undefined values.

```
county_rates_type <- tex_itop %>%
  dplyr::select(c(county, urban, county_type, total_rate, year)) %>%
```

```
filter(total_rate < 15, year %in% c(2020, 2021)) %>%
pivot_wider(names_from = year, values_from = total_rate) %>%
na.omit() %>%
rename("y2020" = "2020", "y2021" = "2021") %>%
mutate(rate_change = (y2021 - y2020))
```

We again use a two-sample two-sided t-test, but this time the data are not
paired. In the following code, we show an alternative way to specify a t-test
using a formula lhs ~ rhs, where lhs is a numeric column and rhs is a factor
column with two levels. We must also specify the data in this case. From the
R output in this case, we would fail to reject the null hypothesis at the 0.05
level and conclude that the rate changes for urban and rural counties are not
significantly different. We also print the estimates used in the t-test using
estimate, which shows the estimated mean in both groups.

```
t_test_unpaired <- t.test(rate_change ~ urban,
                          data = county_rates_type)
t_test_unpaired
#>
#>  Welch Two Sample t-test
#>
#> data:  rate_change by urban
#> t = 0.1, df = 205, p-value = 0.9
#> alternative hypothesis: true difference in means between group
#>  Rural and group Urban is not equal to 0
#> 95 percent confidence interval:
#>  -0.495  0.563
#> sample estimates:
#> mean in group Rural mean in group Urban
#>               -0.469              -0.503
t_test_unpaired$estimate
#> mean in group Rural mean in group Urban
#>               -0.469              -0.503
```

Note that this yields the same results as if we had specified the data using
two vectors x and y.

```
x <- county_rates_type$rate_change[county_rates_type$urban == 'Urban']
y <- county_rates_type$rate_change[county_rates_type$urban == 'Rural']
t.test(x = x, y = y, paired = FALSE)
#>
#>  Welch Two Sample t-test
```

```
#>
#> data:  x and y
#> t = -0.1, df = 205, p-value = 0.9
#> alternative hypothesis: true difference in means is not equal to 0
#> 95 percent confidence interval:
#>  -0.563  0.495
#> sample estimates:
#> mean of x mean of y
#>    -0.503    -0.469
```

Besides a t-test, we can also use a two-sample Wilcoxon non-parametric test using the wilcox.test() function, which has the same arguments as the function t.test(). Both the t.test() and wilcox.test() can only compare two groups. When we want to compare two or more independent samples, we can use a Kruskal-Wallis rank sum test using the kruskal.test() function or a one-way analysis of variance (ANOVA) using the aov() function.

This time we use the column county_type, which is an indicator for whether the county is urban, suburban, or rural according to the RUCC (rural-urban continuum codes) from the U.S. Department of Agriculture. For the kruskal.test() function, we can either specify the arguments formula (rate_change ~ county_type) and data (county_rates_type) or we can specify two vectors: x, a numeric vector, and g, a factor representing the group. For the aov() function, we specify the test using a formula and the data. To see the p-value, we have to use the summary() function to print the result. Again, both tests suggest that we fail to reject the null hypothesis at the 0.05 level.

```
kruskal.test(county_rates_type$rate_change,
             county_rates_type$county_type)
#>
#>  Kruskal-Wallis rank sum test
#>
#> data:  county_rates_type$rate_change and
  ↪ county_rates_type$county_type
#> Kruskal-Wallis chi-squared = 2, df = 2, p-value = 0.3
```

```
aov_res <- aov(rate_change ~ county_type,
               data = county_rates_type)
summary(aov_res)
#>              Df Sum Sq Mean Sq F value Pr(>F)
#> county_type   2      7    3.36    0.53   0.59
#> Residuals   245   1547    6.31
```

11.3.1 Practice Question

Use an appropriate test to determine whether the ITOP rates in 2016 significantly differed by race. The test statistic should be 263.53 with associated p-value < 2.2e-16.

```
# Insert your solution here:
```

11.3.2 Two-Sample Variance Tests

We could also test whether the variance of a continuous variable is equal between groups. To start, we compare the variance in abortion rates in 2021 between urban and rural counties using an F-test. Our null hypothesis for this test is that the variance in both groups is equal. The function `var.test()` implements an F-test and has the same main arguments as the `t.test()` function: vectors x and y OR a `formula` and `data`, the alternative hypothesis `alternative`, and `conf.level`. Additionally, we can specify the hypothesized ratio of the variances through the argument `ratio` (default value 1). Note that this function assumes that the two samples come from normally distributed populations. We fail to reject the null hypothesis that the variances in rates are equal at the 0.05 level and print the estimate of the ratio of variances, which is around 1.11.

```
f_test <- var.test(y2021 ~ urban, county_rates_type)
f_test
#>
#>  F test to compare two variances
#>
#> data:  y2021 by urban
#> F = 1, num df = 187, denom df = 59, p-value = 0.6
#> alternative hypothesis: true ratio of variances is not equal to 1
#> 95 percent confidence interval:
#>   0.719 1.657
#> sample estimates:
#> ratio of variances
#>                1.12
f_test$estimate
#> ratio of variances
#>                1.12
```

Lastly, we implement a Levene's test to test whether group variances are equal when there are more than two groups. This test can be specified using a formula and dataset, as demonstrated, or by providing two vectors y, a

numeric vector, and **g**, a vector specifying the groups. This test is from the
car package and has slightly different output than other tests. In particular,
to access the p-value, we need to access the value named `'Pr(>F)'`. In this
case, we actually do reject the null hypothesis at the 0.05 level.

```
levene_test <- leveneTest(y2021 ~ as.factor(county_type),
                          county_rates_type)
print(levene_test)
#> Levene's Test for Homogeneity of Variance (center = median)
#>         Df F value Pr(>F)
#> group    2    3.41  0.034 *
#>        245
#> ---
#> Signif. codes:  0 '***' 0.001 '**' 0.01 '*' 0.05 '.' 0.1 ' ' 1
levene_test[['Pr(>F)']]
#> [1] 0.0345     NA
```

11.4   Two-Sample Tests for Categorical Variables

In the previous two-sample tests, we were comparing the distributions of continuous variables. We now look at comparing distributions of categorical variables. We first categorize counties by their abortion rate in 2020 being above
or below 11.2, which was the national average rate that year. We display the
distribution of this variable by the urban/rural grouping using a contingency
table below.

```
county_rates_type$below_nat_avg <-
   ifelse(county_rates_type$y2020 > 11.2, "Above Nat Avg",
          "Below Nat Avg")
table(county_rates_type$below_nat_avg, county_rates_type$urban)
#>
#>                 Rural Urban
#>   Above Nat Avg     3     4
#>   Below Nat Avg   185    56
```

We can use a Fisher's exact test to test whether the classifications of being
above and below the national average and being rural and urban are associated
with each other. In this case, the null hypothesis is that the odds of being
below the national average is equal between rural and urban counties. The
`fisher.test()` function can either take in a contingency table as a matrix or

can be specified by two factor vectors x and y, which is how we implement it in the following code. Additionally, there is the option to specify the `alternative` and `conf.level` arguments. We do not see a statistically significant difference between urban and rural counties at the 0.05 level with the estimated odds ratio being around 0.23.

```
fisher_test <- fisher.test(county_rates_type$urban,
                           county_rates_type$below_nat_avg)
fisher_test
#>
#>   Fisher's Exact Test for Count Data
#>
#> data:  county_rates_type$urban and county_rates_type$below_nat_avg
#> p-value = 0.06
#> alternative hypothesis: true odds ratio is not equal to 1
#> 95 percent confidence interval:
#>   0.0325 1.3955
#> sample estimates:
#> odds ratio
#>      0.229
fisher_test$estimate
#> odds ratio
#>      0.229
```

An alternative test is a Pearson's Chi-Squared test, which can be used for large sample sizes. The counts of rural and urban counties in the 'Above Nat Avg' category are very small, so we re-categorize our outcome to be at or above Texas's average to avoid this complication. The `chisq.test()` function also takes in a contingency table as a matrix or can be specified by two factor vectors x and y. Another useful argument is `correct` (default is TRUE) which indicates whether to apply a continuity correction. For this test, we observe a statistically significant difference in the proportion of counties above the national average between rural and urban counties and reject the null hypothesis at the 0.05 level.

```
tex_mean <- mean(county_rates_type$y2020)
county_rates_type$below_tex_avg <-
  ifelse(county_rates_type$y2020 > tex_mean, "Above Texas Ave",
         "Below Texas Ave")
table(county_rates_type$below_tex_avg, county_rates_type$urban)
#>
#>                   Rural Urban
```

```
#>   Above Texas Ave     84     39
#>   Below Texas Ave    104     21
```

```
chi_sq <- chisq.test(county_rates_type$below_tex_avg,
          county_rates_type$urban)
chi_sq
#>
#>   Pearson's Chi-squared test with Yates' continuity correction
#>
#> data:  county_rates_type$below_tex_avg and county_rates_type$urban
#> X-squared = 7, df = 1, p-value = 0.01
chi_sq$p.value
#> [1] 0.00953
```

11.4.1   Practice Question

Repeat the Chi-Squared test, but this time use the RUCC codes instead of the
urban column. You should get a p-value of 0.2799. Think about what could
explain the difference between these results.

```
# Insert your solution here:
```

11.5   Adding Hypothesis Tests to Summary Tables

In Chapter 4, we used the **gt** and **gtsummary** packages to create summary
tables of variables. When creating a stratified table (done by adding the by
argument), we can automatically add p-values for hypothesis tests comparing across populations using the add_p() function. By default, the add_p()
function uses a Kruskal-Wallis rank sum test for continuous variables (or a
Wilcoxon rank sum test when the by variable has two levels) and uses a Chi-
Squared Contingency Table Test for categorical variables (or a Fisher's Exact
Test for categorical variables with any expected cell count less than five). The
chosen tests are displayed as footnotes.

```
tbl_summary(tex_itop,
            by = "year",
            include = c(total_rate, white_rate, asian_rate,
```

```
                        hispanic_rate, black_rate,
                        native_american_rate),
            label = list(
              total_rate = "Overall",
              white_rate = "White",
              asian_rate = "Asian",
              hispanic_rate = "Hispanic",
              black_rate = "Black",
              native_american_rate = "Native American"),
            statistic = list(all_continuous() ~ "{mean} ({sd})")) %>%
  add_p() %>%
  modify_header(label = "**Variable**") %>%
  as_gt() %>%
  cols_width(label ~ "50pt",
             everything() ~ "30pt")
```

Variable	2016, N = 254[1]	2017, N = 254[1]	2018, N = 254[1]	2019, N = 254[1]	2020, N = 254[1]	2021, N = 254[1]	p-value[2]
Overall	4.8 (3.0)	4.9 (4.9)	5.3 (4.2)	4.9 (3.3)	6.2 (14.1)	5.2 (7.9)	0.2
White	4.7 (3.8)	5.1 (5.8)	5.4 (6.0)	5.1 (5.1)	6.8 (21.3)	5.5 (8.0)	0.3
Asian	7 (32)	12 (46)	8 (21)	7 (20)	14 (55)	7 (37)	0.066
Hispanic	3.9 (3.7)	4.7 (6.3)	4.6 (4.6)	4.6 (5.0)	4.6 (5.8)	4.4 (4.8)	0.7
Black	9 (21)	13 (65)	26 (153)	20 (80)	25 (111)	26 (121)	0.13
Native American	5.0 (24.0)	9.3 (65.0)	4.9 (17.8)	2.3 (12.4)	4.1 (21.1)	2.5 (10.1)	0.13

[1]Mean (SD)
[2]Kruskal-Wallis rank sum test

We observe that a Kruskal-Wallis rank sum test was used to compare abortion rates across year for each racial group. All of the reported p-values are above 0.05, so overall it indicates that there were not statistically significant changes across years in the abortion rate.

11.6 Exercises

For the following exercises, we use the `pain` data from the **HDSinRdata** package.

```
data(pain)
```

1. Determine whether the presence or absence of follow-up information is significantly associated with the initial average pain intensity. What do the results suggest?

2. First, plot `PROMIS_PAIN_BEHAVIOR` grouped by race (you can use the `PAT_RACE_CAT` variable that we defined in Chapter 8). What do you observe? Next, choose an appropriate test to determine whether this variable differs significantly by race.

3. Examine the association between `CCI_BIN` and `MEDICAID_BIN`. Are these variables significantly related to each other? How would you describe their relationship?

4. Recreate the summary table in Figure 11.1. Then, recreate the p-values for `PROMIS_DEPRESSION`, `PROMIS_ANXIETY`, and `MEDICAID_BIN` using the appropriate tests.

Characteristic	BLACK, N = 1,379[1]	OTHER, N = 145[1]	WHITE, N = 7,271[1]	p-value[2]
PAIN_INTENSITY_AVERAGE	8.00 (7.00, 9.00)	7.00 (6.00, 8.00)	6.00 (5.00, 8.00)	<0.001
PROMIS_PHYSICAL_FUNCTION	35 (30, 38)	35 (31, 41)	35 (30, 39)	<0.001
PROMIS_PAIN_BEHAVIOR	62.6 (60.9, 64.3)	62.3 (59.8, 63.4)	61.6 (59.0, 63.4)	<0.001
PROMIS_DEPRESSION	57 (50, 64)	55 (48, 64)	55 (48, 62)	0.004
PROMIS_ANXIETY	60 (51, 65)	58 (51, 65)	56 (50, 63)	<0.001
PROMIS_SLEEP_DISTURB_V1_0	63 (56, 68)	61 (54, 68)	60 (54, 65)	<0.001
PROMIS_PAIN_INTERFERENCE	68 (64, 72)	68 (64, 72)	67 (63, 72)	<0.001
GH_MENTAL_SCORE	41 (36, 48)	44 (34, 51)	44 (36, 51)	<0.001
GH_PHYSICAL_SCORE	32 (30, 37)	35 (30, 40)	35 (30, 40)	<0.001
AGE_AT_CONTACT	53 (43, 61)	48 (37, 58)	57 (46, 67)	<0.001
BMI	32 (27, 37)	27 (23, 33)	29 (25, 34)	<0.001
PAT_SEX				<0.001
female	930 (67%)	92 (63%)	4,220 (58%)	
male	449 (33%)	53 (37%)	3,051 (42%)	
MEDICAID_BIN	573 (42%)	52 (36%)	1,536 (21%)	<0.001

[1] Median (IQR); n (%)

[2] Kruskal-Wallis rank sum test; Pearson's Chi-squared test

Figure 11.1: Stratified Summary Table.

12

Case Study: Analyzing Blood Lead Level and Hypertension

For this chapter, we use the `NHANESsample` dataset seen in Chapter 4. The sample contains lead, blood pressure, BMI, smoking status, alcohol use, and demographic variables from NHANES 1999-2018. Variable selection and feature engineering were conducted to replicate the pre-processing conducted by Huang (2022). We further replicate the regression analysis by Huang (2022) in Chapter 13. Use the help operator `?NHANESsample` to read the variable descriptions. Note that we ignore survey weights for this analysis.

```
library(HDSinRdata)
library(tidyverse)
library(gt)
library(gtsummary)

data("NHANESsample")
```

Our analysis focuses on using hypothesis testing to look at the association between hypertension and blood lead levels by sex. We first select some demographic and clinical variables that we believe may be relevant, including age, sex, race, body mass index, and smoking status. We do a complete case analysis and drop any observations with missing data.

```
NHANESsample <- NHANESsample %>%
  select("AGE", "SEX", "RACE", "SMOKE", "LEAD", "BMI_CAT",
         "HYP", "ALC") %>%
  na.omit()
```

We begin with a summary table stratified by hypertension status. As expected, we see statistically significant differences between the two groups across all included variables. We also observe higher blood lead levels and a higher proportion of male participants for those with hypertension.

```
tbl_summary(NHANESsample, by = c("HYP"),
            label = list(SMOKE ~ "SMOKING STATUS",
                         BMI_CAT ~ "BMI",
                         ALC ~ "ALCOHOL USE")) %>%
  add_p() %>%
  add_overall() %>%
  modify_spanning_header(c("stat_1", "stat_2") ~
                          "**Hypertension Status**") %>%
  as_gt() %>%
  cols_width(everything() ~ "55pt")
```

		Hypertension Status		
Characteristic	**Overall**, N = 30,425[1]	**0**, N = 13,735[1]	**1**, N = 16,690[1]	**p-value**[2]
AGE	48 (34, 63)	37 (28, 50)	57 (44, 69)	<0.001
SEX				<0.001
Male	16,031 (53%)	6,410 (47%)	9,621 (58%)	
Female	14,394 (47%)	7,325 (53%)	7,069 (42%)	
RACE				<0.001
Mexican American	5,184 (17%)	2,725 (20%)	2,459 (15%)	
Other Hispanic	2,207 (7.3%)	1,145 (8.3%)	1,062 (6.4%)	
Non-Hispanic White	15,108 (50%)	6,750 (49%)	8,358 (50%)	
Non-Hispanic Black	5,853 (19%)	2,077 (15%)	3,776 (23%)	
Other Race	2,073 (6.8%)	1,038 (7.6%)	1,035 (6.2%)	
SMOKING STATUS				<0.001
NeverSmoke	14,682 (48%)	7,210 (52%)	7,472 (45%)	
QuitSmoke	8,566 (28%)	2,990 (22%)	5,576 (33%)	
StillSmoke	7,177 (24%)	3,535 (26%)	3,642 (22%)	
LEAD	1.39 (0.85, 2.20)	1.14 (0.71, 1.85)	1.59 (1.00, 2.48)	<0.001
BMI				<0.001
BMI<=25	9,007 (30%)	5,313 (39%)	3,694 (22%)	

25<BMI<30	10,456 (34%)	4,718 (34%)	5,738 (34%)	
BMI>=30	10,962 (36%)	3,704 (27%)	7,258 (43%)	
ALCOHOL USE	24,174 (79%)	11,624 (85%)	12,550 (75%)	<0.001

[1]Median (IQR); n (%)
[2]Wilcoxon rank sum test; Pearson's Chi-squared test

We also plot the distribution of blood lead levels (on a log scale) by sex and hypertension status. We can visually see that male observations tend to have higher blood lead levels and that having hypertension is associated with higher blood lead levels.

```
ggplot(NHANESsample) +
  geom_boxplot(aes(x=LEAD,
                   y = interaction(HYP,SEX),
                   color = interaction(HYP,SEX))) +
  scale_x_continuous(trans = "log", breaks = c(0.1, 1, 10, 50)) +
  scale_y_discrete(labels = c("Male : 0", "Male : 1",
                              "Female : 0", "Female : 1")) +
  guides(color = "none") +
  labs(x="Blood Lead Level",
       y = "Sex : Hypertension Status")
```

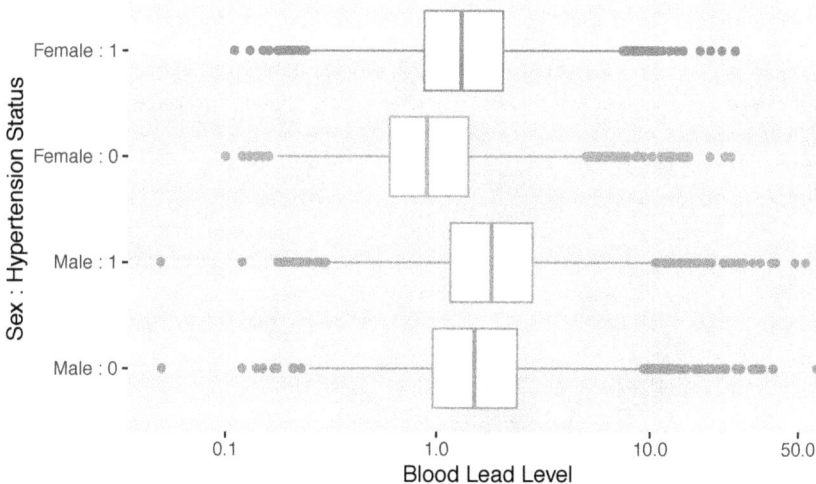

In Chapter 10, we explored that log blood lead levels could be approximated by a normal distribution. To test our hypothesis that there is a difference in mean log blood lead level between those with and without hypertension, we use a two-sample unpaired t-test. This shows a statistically significant difference between the two groups at the 0.05 level.

```
t.test(log(LEAD) ~ HYP, data = NHANESsample)
#>
#>  Welch Two Sample t-test
#>
#> data:  log(LEAD) by HYP
#> t = -37, df = 28853, p-value <2e-16
#> alternative hypothesis: true difference in means between group 0
  ↵  and group 1 is not equal to 0
#> 95 percent confidence interval:
#>   -0.314 -0.282
#> sample estimates:
#> mean in group 0 mean in group 1
#>           0.161           0.459
```

Finally, we repeat this test for a stratified analysis and present the results in a concise table. For both groups, we find a statistically significant difference at the 0.05 level.

```
# stratify the data
nhanes_male <- NHANESsample[NHANESsample$SEX == "Male",]
nhanes_female <- NHANESsample[NHANESsample$SEX == "Female",]

# t-test for each
test_male <- t.test(log(LEAD) ~ HYP, data = nhanes_male)
test_female <- t.test(log(LEAD) ~ HYP, data = nhanes_female)

# create data frame
res_df <- data.frame(group = c("Male", "Female"),
                  statistic = signif(c(test_male$statistic,
                                  test_female$statistic), 3),
                  p.value = signif(c(test_male$p.value,
                                  test_female$p.value), 3))
res_df
#>     group statistic   p.value
#> 1    Male     -14.7  1.84e-48
#> 2  Female     -32.3 4.35e-221
```

In Chapter 13, we use linear regression to further explore the association between blood lead level and hypertension adjusting for other potential confounders.

Part IV

Regression

13

Linear Regression

This chapter introduces you to linear regression analysis in R. We cover how to fit linear regression models, check model assumptions using diagnostic plots, change model formulas by adding transformations and interactions, calculate performance metrics, and perform variable selection using stepwise selection.

For this chapter, we use the `NHANESsample` dataset seen in Chapter 4. The sample contains lead, blood pressure, BMI, smoking status, alcohol use, and demographic variables from NHANES 1999-2018. Variable selection and feature engineering were conducted in an effort to replicate the regression analyses conducted by Huang (2022). Use the help operator `?NHANESsample` to read the variable descriptions. Note that we ignore survey weights for this analysis.

We use the **broom** package (Robinson, Hayes, and Couch 2023) to present the estimated coefficients for our regression models and the **car** package to compute variance inflation factors.

```
library(HDSinRdata)
library(tidyverse)
library(broom)
library(car)

data(NHANESsample)
```

13.1 Simple Linear Regression

In Chapter 4, we presented some initial exploratory analysis for this data. In this chapter, we use linear regression to understand the association between blood lead levels and systolic blood pressure, adjusting for possible confounders. Replicating the analysis of Huang (2022), we create summary columns for systolic and diastolic blood pressure. If an observation has one blood pressure reading, then we use that value. If there is more than one blood pressure reading, then we drop the first observation and average the rest. We do a complete case analysis by dropping any observation with NA values. This leaves us with 30,405 observations.

```
NHANESsample$SBP <- apply(NHANESsample[,c("SBP1", "SBP2", "SBP3",
                                          "SBP4")], 1,
    function(x) case_when(sum(!is.na(x)) == 0 ~ NA,
                          sum(!is.na(x)) == 1 ~ sum(x, na.rm = TRUE),
                          sum(!is.na(x)) > 1 ~ mean(x[-1],
                                                    na.rm = TRUE)))
NHANESsample$DBP <- apply(NHANESsample[,c("DBP1", "DBP2", "DBP3",
                                          "DBP4")], 1,
    function(x) case_when(sum(!is.na(x)) == 0 ~ NA,
                          sum(!is.na(x)) == 1 ~ sum(x, na.rm = TRUE),
                          sum(!is.na(x)) > 1 ~ mean(x[-1],
                                                    na.rm = TRUE)))
nhanes_df <- na.omit(subset(NHANESsample,
                     select= -c(SBP1, SBP2, SBP3, SBP4, DBP1,
                                DBP2, DBP3, DBP4)))
dim(nhanes_df)
#> [1] 30405    15
```

Next, we make sure any categorical variables are coded as factors.

```
nhanes_df$SEX <- as.factor(nhanes_df$SEX)
nhanes_df$RACE <- as.factor(nhanes_df$RACE)
nhanes_df$EDUCATION <- as.factor(nhanes_df$EDUCATION)
nhanes_df$BMI_CAT <- as.factor(nhanes_df$BMI_CAT)
nhanes_df$LEAD_QUANTILE <- as.factor(nhanes_df$LEAD_QUANTILE)
```

We start with simple linear regression. In the following code, we plot the relationship between blood lead level and systolic blood pressure. For a simple linear regression scenario with a single continuous independent variable, a scatter plot allows us to easily visualize whether we meet the assumptions underlying linear regression. The survey sampling for the NHANES survey allows us to assume that each observation is independent. If we meet the assumptions of linear regression, we also expect the plot to show that the average systolic blood pressure increases linearly with blood lead level and that the observations look normally distributed with equal variance along that line. We do not observe that to be the case. We come back to this in the section on transformations and interactions.

```
plot(nhanes_df$LEAD, nhanes_df$SBP,
```

```
xlab = "Blood Lead Level", ylab = "Systolic Blood Pressure",
pch = 16)
```

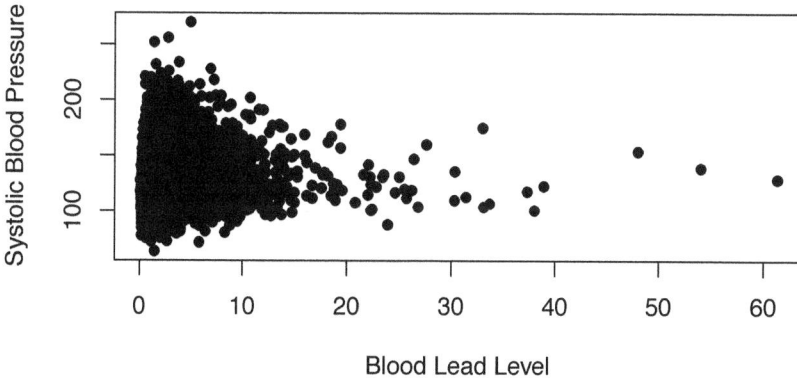

Despite our observations, we continue by fitting a simple linear regression model to explain the association between SBP and LEAD. The function lm(formula = y ~ x, data) fits a linear model in R. The first argument is the formula of the linear model: on the left-hand side of the ~ we put the outcome variable, and on the right-hand side we put the independent variable. When we have multiple independent variables, we separate them with a + (e.g., y~x1+x2). The output of this function is an lm object.

We can call the summary() function on this object to print a summary of the model, which includes the estimated coefficients, information about the residuals, the R-squared and adjusted R-squared values, and the F-statistic. Recall, that we previously used the summary() function to get summary statistics about a vector. This is an example of how multiple functions can have the same name. R figures out which summary() function to use by identifying that the argument we passed in is a lm object.

```
simp_model <- lm(formula = SBP ~ LEAD, data = nhanes_df)
summary(simp_model)
#>
#> Call:
#> lm(formula = SBP ~ LEAD, data = nhanes_df)
#>
```

```
#> Residuals:
#>    Min      1Q Median      3Q     Max
#> -96.36 -12.52   -2.79    9.36 140.88
#>
#> Coefficients:
#>               Estimate Std. Error t value Pr(>|t|)
#> (Intercept)  120.665      0.149    807.1   <2e-16 ***
#> LEAD           1.708      0.058     29.4   <2e-16 ***
#> ---
#> Signif. codes:  0 '***' 0.001 '**' 0.01 '*' 0.05 '.' 0.1 ' ' 1
#>
#> Residual standard error: 18.5 on 30403 degrees of freedom
#> Multiple R-squared:  0.0277, Adjusted R-squared:  0.0277
#> F-statistic:  867 on 1 and 30403 DF,  p-value: <2e-16
```

To visualize this model, we can add the estimated regression line to our scatter plot. In `ggplot2`, this can be done with the `geom_smooth()` function. In base R, we use the `abline()` function, which can take in a regression model as an input. We can see that the estimated regression line does not fit our data very well.

```
plot(nhanes_df$LEAD, nhanes_df$SBP,
     ylab = c("Systolic Blood Pressure"),
     xlab = c("Blood Lead Level"), pch = 16)
abline(simp_model, col = 2, lwd = 2)
```

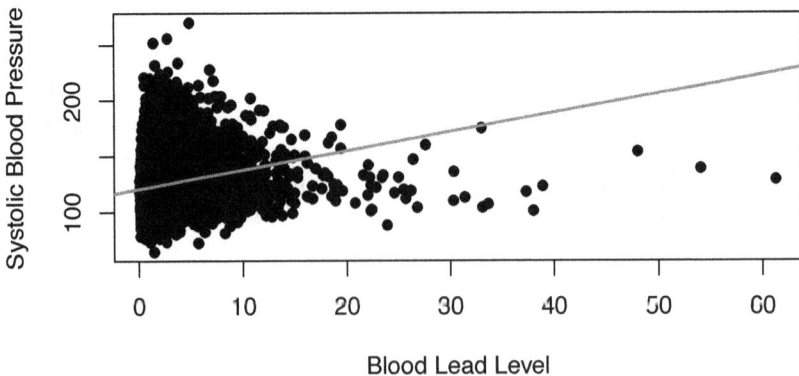

13.1.1 Practice Question

Fit a simple linear regression model with SBP as the outcome and AGE as the independent variable. The estimated coefficient for AGE should be 0.47693. Then, plot these two variables against each other and add the estimated regression line to the plot, as we did previously. You should see that this regression has a better fit than the previous one.

```
# Insert your solution here:
```

13.2 Multiple Linear Regression

We now create a model that is similar to the previous one except that it also adjusts for age and sex. To add these variables into the model, we have to specify a new formula. In the following code chunk, we fit this model and then print a summary, again using the summary() function.

```
adj_model <- lm(SBP ~ LEAD + AGE + SEX, data = nhanes_df)
summary(adj_model)
#>
#> Call:
#> lm(formula = SBP ~ LEAD + AGE + SEX, data = nhanes_df)
#>
#> Residuals:
#>    Min     1Q Median     3Q    Max
#> -65.62 -10.59  -1.55   8.55 131.60
#>
#> Coefficients:
#>              Estimate Std. Error t value Pr(>|t|)
#> (Intercept) 101.78541    0.30353  335.34  < 2e-16 ***
#> LEAD          0.40007    0.05525    7.24 4.5e-13 ***
#> AGE           0.46193    0.00557   82.97  < 2e-16 ***
#> SEXFemale    -2.77774    0.19567  -14.20  < 2e-16 ***
#> ---
#> Signif. codes:  0 '***' 0.001 '**' 0.01 '*' 0.05 '.' 0.1 ' ' 1
#>
#> Residual standard error: 16.6 on 30401 degrees of freedom
#> Multiple R-squared:  0.212,  Adjusted R-squared:  0.212
#> F-statistic: 2.72e+03 on 3 and 30401 DF,  p-value: <2e-16
```

We can also extract the estimated regression coefficients from the model using the `coef()` function or by using the `tidy()` function from the **broom** package. This function puts the coefficient estimates, standard errors, statistics, and p-values in a data frame. We can also add a confidence interval by specifying `conf.int = TRUE`. In our example, we add a 95% confidence interval (which is the default value for `conf.level`).

```
coef(adj_model)
#> (Intercept)         LEAD        AGE    SEXFemale
#>      101.785        0.400      0.462       -2.778
```

```
tidy(adj_model, conf.int = TRUE, conf.level = 0.95)
#> # A tibble: 4 x 7
#>   term           estimate std.error statistic  p.value conf.low
#>   ↳ conf.high
#>   <chr>             <dbl>     <dbl>     <dbl>    <dbl>    <dbl>    <dbl>
#> 1 (Intercept)      102.     0.304      335.    0        101.     102.
#> 2 LEAD             0.400    0.0552      7.24  4.54e-13   0.292    0.508
#> 3 AGE              0.462    0.00557    83.0    0         0.451    0.473
#> 4 SEXFemale       -2.78     0.196     -14.2   1.36e-45  -3.16    -2.39
```

Some other useful summary functions are `resid()`, which returns the residual values for the model, and `fitted()`, which returns the fitted values or estimated y values. We can also predict on new data using the `predict()` function. In the following plot, we look at the distribution of the residual values and then plot the fitted vs. true values. We observe some extreme residual values as well as the fact that the absolute residual values increase with increased blood pressure values.

```
summary(resid(adj_model))
#>    Min. 1st Qu.  Median    Mean 3rd Qu.    Max.
#>   -65.6   -10.6    -1.6     0.0     8.5   131.6
```

```
plot(nhanes_df$SBP, fitted(adj_model),
     xlab = "True Systolic Blood Pressure",
     ylab = "Predicted Systolic Blood Pressure", pch = 16)
abline(a = 0, b = 1, col = "red", lwd = 2)
```

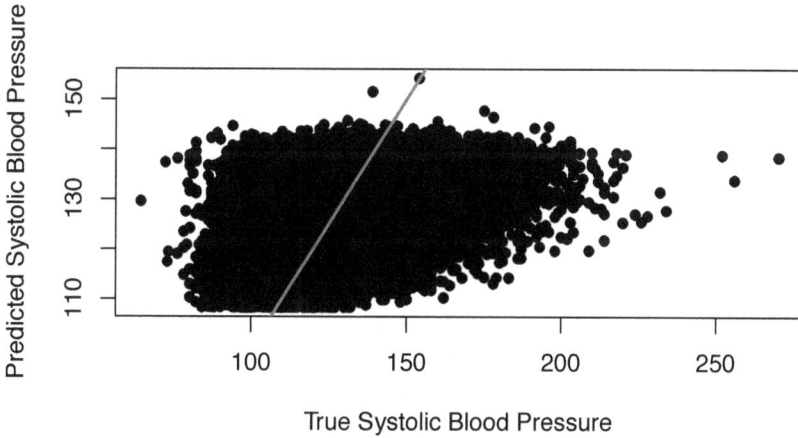

We can next perform a nested hypothesis test between our simple linear regression model and our adjusted model using the `anova()` function. We pass both models to this function along with the argument `test="F"` to indicate that we are performing an F-test. The `print()` function shows the two tested models along with the associated p-value, which indicates a significantly better fit for the adjusted model.

```
print(anova(simp_model, adj_model, test= "F"))
#> Analysis of Variance Table
#>
#> Model 1: SBP ~ LEAD
#> Model 2: SBP ~ LEAD + AGE + SEX
#>   Res.Df      RSS Df Sum of Sq      F Pr(>F)
#> 1  30403 10375769
#> 2  30401  8413303  2   1962467 3546 <2e-16 ***
#> ---
#> Signif. codes:  0 '***' 0.001 '**' 0.01 '*' 0.05 '.' 0.1 ' ' 1
```

The model summary for the adjusted model displays the estimated coefficient for sex as `SEXFemale`, which indicates that the reference level for sex is male. If we want to change our reference level, we can reorder the factor variable either by using the `factor()` function and specifying `Female` as the first level or by using the `relevel()` function. The `ref` argument in the `relevel()` function specifies the new reference level. Now, when we run the model, we can see that the estimated coefficient for sex is labeled as `SEXMale`.

```
nhanes_df$SEX <- relevel(nhanes_df$SEX, ref = "Female")
adj_model2 <- lm(SBP ~ LEAD + AGE + SEX, data = nhanes_df)
tidy(adj_model2)
#> # A tibble: 4 x 5
#>   term         estimate std.error statistic   p.value
#>   <chr>           <dbl>     <dbl>     <dbl>     <dbl>
#> 1 (Intercept)    99.0      0.293     338.    0
#> 2 LEAD            0.400    0.0552      7.24  4.54e-13
#> 3 AGE             0.462    0.00557    83.0   0
#> 4 SEXMale         2.78     0.196      14.2   1.36e-45
```

The formula passed to the lm() function also allows us to use the . to indicate
that we would like to include all remaining columns as independent variables
or the - to exclude variables. In the following code chunk, we show how we
could use these to fit a model with LEAD, AGE, and SEX as included covariates
by excluding all other variables instead of by specifying these three variables
themselves.

```
lm(SBP ~ . - ID - RACE - EDUCATION - INCOME - SMOKE - YEAR - BMI_CAT -
   LEAD_QUANTILE - DBP - ALC - HYP - RACE, data = nhanes_df)
#>
#> Call:
#> lm(formula = SBP ~ . - ID - RACE - EDUCATION - INCOME - SMOKE -
#>     YEAR - BMI_CAT - LEAD_QUANTILE - DBP - ALC - HYP - RACE,
#>     data = nhanes_df)
#>
#> Coefficients:
#> (Intercept)          AGE      SEXMale          LEAD
#>      99.008        0.462        2.778         0.400
```

13.3   Diagnostic Plots and Measures

We can tell from the previous plot that our model doesn't have a great fit.
We use some further diagnostic plots and measures to learn more. R has some
built-in plots available for linear regression models, which can be displayed
using the plot() function. Similar the summary() function, this function acts
differently when passed an lm object. The four plots include (a) Residuals
vs. Fitted, (b) a QQ-plot for the residuals, (c) Standardized residuals (sqrt)
vs. Fitted, and (d) Standardized Residuals vs. Leverage. In the last plot, you

may observe that there is a dashed line. Any points outside of these lines have
a Cook's distance of greater than 0.5. Additionally, points with labels correspond to the points with the largest residuals, so this last plot summarizes the
outliers, leverage, and influential points. The plots show that our residuals do
not look normally distributed and that we have may have some high leverage
points.

```
par(mfrow = c(2, 2)) # plots all four plots together
plot(adj_model)
```

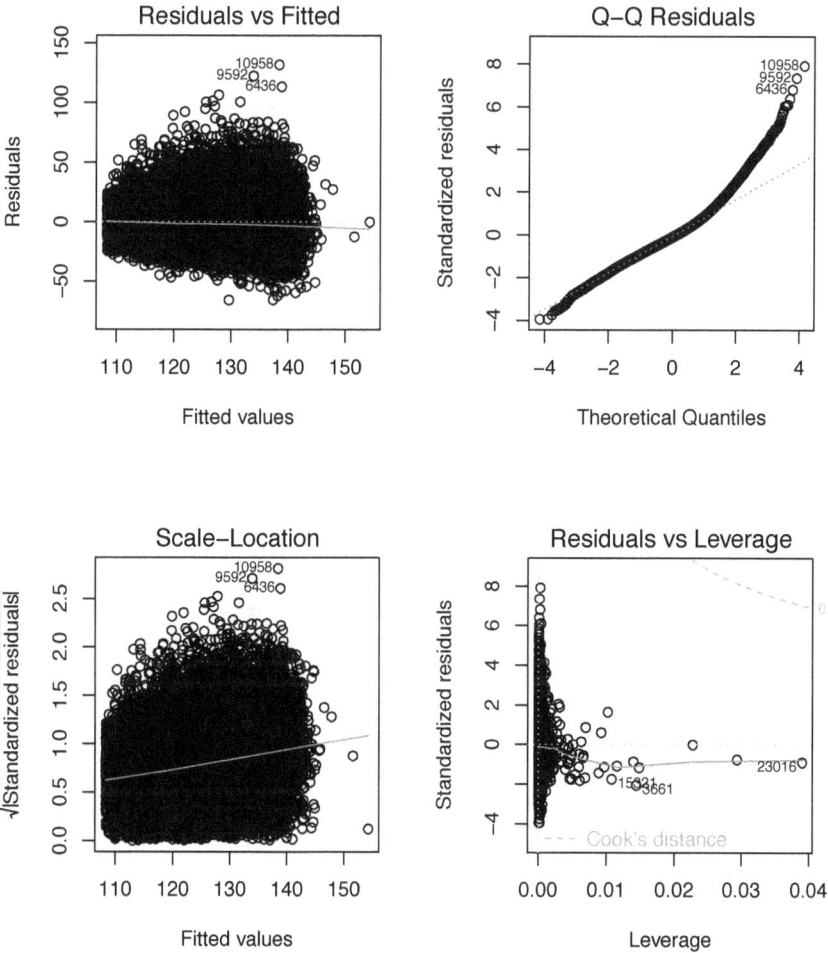

13.3.1   Normality

Beyond the default plots, we can also plot a histogram of the residuals and a
qq-plot. The qqnorm() and qqline() functions can take in the residuals from
our model as an argument. The latter adds the theoretical red line for reference.
As both the histogram and qq-plot show, the residuals are positively skewed,
and thus the assumption of normality is not satisfied for our residuals. Later
in this chapter, we discuss how we might transform this dataset and/or model
to satisfy this assumption.

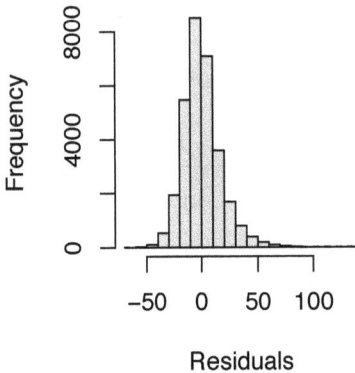

```
par(mfrow = c(1, 2)) # plot next to each other
hist(resid(adj_model), xlab = "Residuals",
    main = "Histogram of Residuals")
qqnorm(resid(adj_model))
qqline(resid(adj_model), col = "red")
```

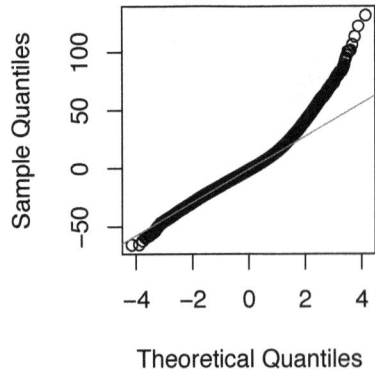

Instead of using the direct residuals, we can also find the standardized residuals with the function rstandard(). The standardized residuals are the raw
residuals divided by an estimate of the standard deviation for the residual,
which is different for each observation.

```
par(mfrow = c(1, 2))
hist(rstandard(adj_model), xlab = "Standardized Residuals",
    main = "Histogram of Standardized Residuals",
    cex.main = 0.65)
qqnorm(rstandard(adj_model), cex.main = 0.65)
qqline(rstandard(adj_model), col = "red")
```

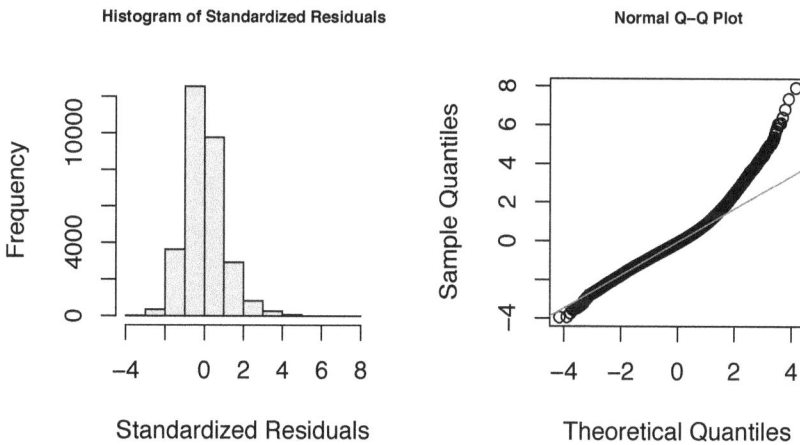

Histogram of Standardized Residuals   Normal Q–Q Plot

13.3.2 Homoscedasticity, Linearity, and Collinearity

We can also create a residual vs. fitted plot or plot the residuals against included covariates. In the following code, we plot the blood lead level against the residuals. In both plots, we are looking for the points to be spread roughly evenly around 0 with no discerning pattern. However, both plots show a funnel shape, indicating a growing and shrinking variance of residuals by level, respectively. This indicates that we are violating the homoscedasticity assumption.

```
par(mfrow = c(1, 2))
plot(fitted(adj_model), resid(adj_model),
     xlab = "Fitted Values", ylab = "Residuals")
plot(nhanes_df$LEAD, resid(adj_model),
     xlab = "Blood Lead Level", ylab = "Residuals")
```

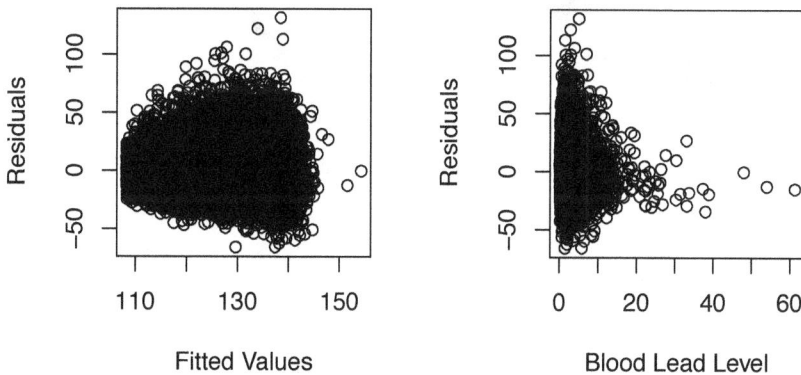

Fitted Values   Blood Lead Level

To quantify any collinearity between the included covariates, we can calculate the variance inflation factors. The `vif()` function in the **car** package allows us to calculate the variance inflation factors or generalized variance inflation factors for all covariates. In our case, all the VIF values are around 1, indicating low levels of collinearity.

```
vif(adj_model)
#> LEAD  AGE  SEX
#> 1.12 1.07 1.05
```

13.3.3 Practice Question

Fit a linear regression model with SBP as the outcome and with INCOME, RACE, EDUCATION, and ALC as independent variables. Then, plot the residuals vs. the fitted values as well and make a QQ-plot for the standardized residuals from this model. They should look like Figure 13.1.

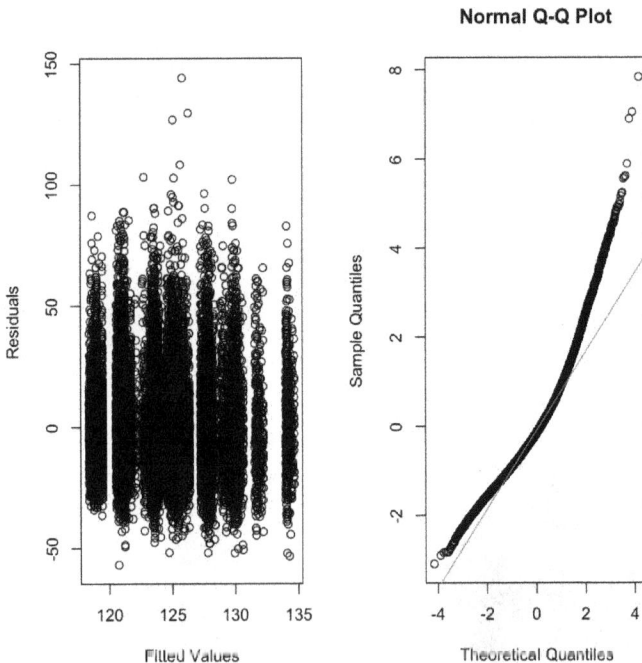

Figure 13.1: Residual Plots.

```
# Insert your solution here:
```

13.3.4   Leverage and Influence

We may also be interested in how each observation is influencing the model. Leverage values measure how much an individual observation's y value influences its own predicted value and indicate whether observations have extreme predictor values compared to the rest of the data. Leverage values range from 0 to 1 and sum to the number of estimated coefficients. Observations with high leverage have the potential to significantly impact the estimated regression coefficients and the overall fit of the model. Therefore, examining leverage values helps identify observations that may be influential or outliers. In the following code chunk, we find the ten highest leverage values and then find those observations in the data.

```
sort(hatvalues(adj_model), decreasing = TRUE)[1:10]
#>    23016    2511    3091   21891    3661     511   21892   15321
#>     6511
#> 0.03899 0.02936 0.02270 0.01484 0.01443 0.01399 0.01159 0.01080
#>   0.01022
#>     3452
#> 0.00968
nhanes_df[order(hatvalues(adj_model), decreasing = TRUE),] %>%
  select(c(SBP, LEAD, AGE, SEX)) %>%
  head(10)
#>         SBP LEAD AGE   SEX
#> 23016 129 61.3  38 Male
#> 2511  139 54.0  61 Male
#> 3091  154 48.0  72 Male
#> 21891 123 38.9  54 Male
#> 3661  101 38.0  39 Male
#> 511   118 37.3  34 Male
#> 21892 107 33.7  21 Male
#> 15321 104 33.1  39 Male
#> 6511  175 33.0  71 Male
#> 3452  113 31.4  38 Male
```

Some other measures of influence are the DFBETAs and Cook's distance, which measure how much each observation influences the estimated coefficients and the estimated y values, respectively. The influence.measures() function provides a set of measures that quantify the influence of each observation on a linear regression model: these include the DFBETAS for each model variable,

DFFITS, covariance ratios, Cook's distances, and the leverage values. The
output returns the values in a matrix called `infmat`, which we convert to a
data frame.

```
inf_mat <- influence.measures(adj_model)[['infmat']]
as.data.frame(inf_mat) %>% head()
#>       dfb.1_   dfb.LEAD    dfb.AGE   dfb.SEXF    dffit cov.r   cook.d
#> 1  0.013880 -0.017564 -1.68e-02  0.008319 -0.03427 1.000 2.93e-04
#> 2 -0.000732  0.000348 -3.92e-05  0.001051 -0.00150 1.000 5.59e-07
#> 3  0.022137  0.005749 -1.45e-02 -0.016843  0.02964 0.999 2.19e-04
#> 4  0.000499  0.001043 -2.07e-03  0.001631 -0.00312 1.000 2.43e-06
#> 5  0.002259 -0.002725 -2.50e-03  0.000973 -0.00498 1.000 6.20e-06
#> 6 -0.001283 -0.000559  1.65e-03 -0.002929 -0.00441 1.000 4.87e-06
#>        hat
#> 1 1.90e-04
#> 2 6.61e-05
#> 3 8.28e-05
#> 4 1.18e-04
#> 5 2.35e-04
#> 6 8.09e-05
```

13.4   Interactions and Transformations

We now try to improve our model. To start, we look at potential transformations for our outcome variable. We consider a log transformation for both
our outcome, systolic blood pressure, and our predictor of interest, blood lead
level. Both of these variables have a fairly skewed distribution and may benefit from such a transformation. In the following code, you can see that the
transformed variables have distributions that are more symmetrical.

```
par(mfrow=c(2,2))
hist(nhanes_df$SBP, xlab = "Systolic Blood Pressure",
     main = "")
hist(log(nhanes_df$SBP), xlab = "Log Systolic Blood Pressure",
     main = "")
hist(nhanes_df$LEAD, xlab = "Blood Lead Level",
     main = "")
hist(log(nhanes_df$LEAD), xlab = "Log Blood Lead Level",
     main = "")
```

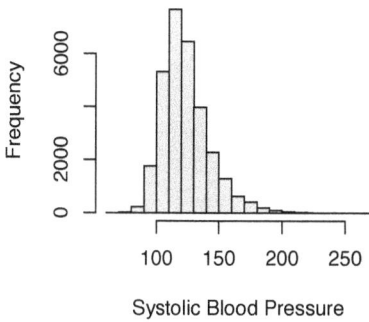

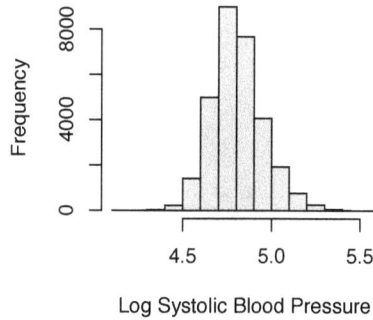

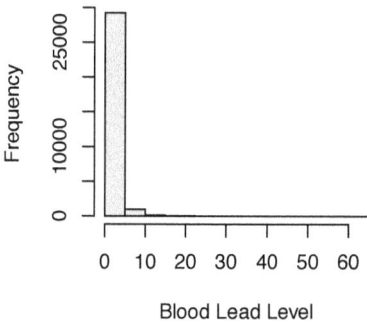

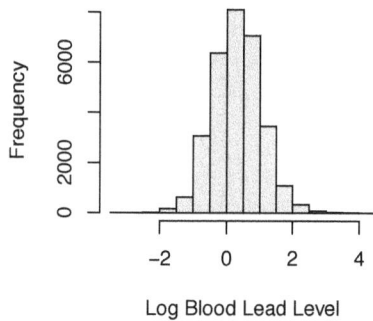

To add a transformation to a model, we can simply apply the transformation in the formula for lm(). We find the adjusted R-squared for each potential model to compare their fits in addition to plotting the four qq-plots. Both indicate that the model with the log-log transformation (that is, with a log transformation applied to both the SBP and the LEAD variables) is the best fit, though the model with just a log transformation for SBP has a similar qq-plot.

```
model_nlog_nlog <- lm(SBP ~ LEAD + AGE + SEX, data = nhanes_df)
model_log_nlog <- lm(log(SBP) ~ LEAD + AGE + SEX, data = nhanes_df)
model_nlog_log <- lm(SBP ~ log(LEAD) + AGE + SEX, data = nhanes_df)
model_log_log <- lm(log(SBP) ~ log(LEAD) + AGE + SEX,
                    data = nhanes_df)
```

```
summary(model_nlog_nlog)$adj.r.squared
#> [1] 0.212
summary(model_log_nlog)$adj.r.squared
#> [1] 0.215
summary(model_nlog_log)$adj.r.squared
#> [1] 0.212
summary(model_log_log)$adj.r.squared
#> [1] 0.215


par(mfrow=c(2,2))
qqnorm(rstandard(model_nlog_nlog), main = "Original Model")
qqline(rstandard(model_nlog_nlog), col = "red")
qqnorm(rstandard(model_log_nlog), main = "Log SBP")
qqline(rstandard(model_log_nlog), col = "red")
qqnorm(rstandard(model_nlog_log), main = "Log Lead")
qqline(rstandard(model_nlog_log), col = "red")
qqnorm(rstandard(model_log_log), main = "Log SBP, Log Lead")
qqline(rstandard(model_log_log), col = "red")
```

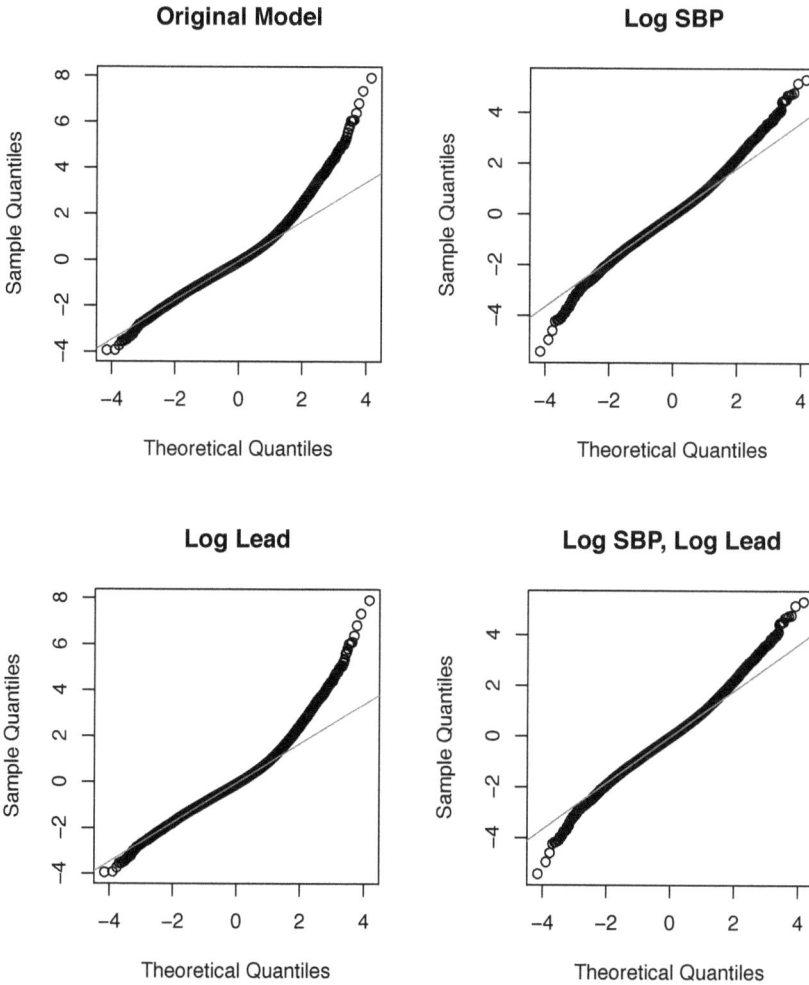

13.4.1 Practice Question

Instead of adding in a log transformation for LEAD like we did previously, try a square root transformation sqrt(LEAD) and an inverse transformation 1/LEAD while keeping the log transformation for the outcome log(SBP). Which model fits better according to the adjusted R-squared? The resulting QQ-plots should look like Figure 13.2.

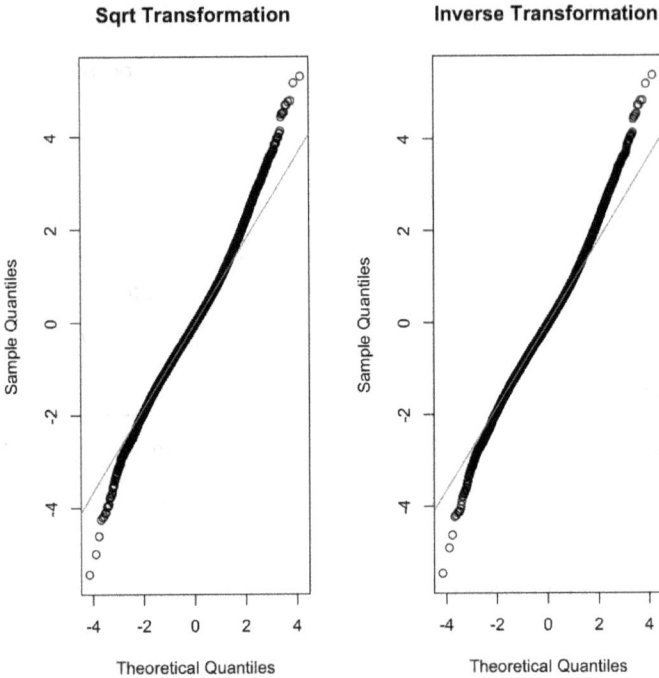

Figure 13.2: QQ-Plots for Possible Transformations.

```
# Insert your solution here:
```

Additionally, we might consider polynomial transformations. The poly(x, de-gree=1) function allows us to specify a polynomial transformation where we might have higher degree terms. We do not pursue this approach for this particular example, but we show some example code for creating such a transformation (in this case, a cubic transformation for blood lead level).

```
model_poly <- lm(SBP ~ poly(LEAD, 3) + AGE + SEX, data = nhanes_df)
```

We can summarize the outcome for our log-log model using the tidy() function again. We observe small p-values for each estimated coefficient.

```
tidy(model_log_log)
#> # A tibble: 4 x 5
#>   term         estimate std.error statistic  p.value
#>   <chr>           <dbl>     <dbl>     <dbl>    <dbl>
```

```
#> 1 (Intercept)  4.62    0.00239     1932.  0
#> 2 log(LEAD)    0.00891 0.00118      7.53 5.34e-14
#> 3 AGE          0.00349 0.0000457   76.4  0
#> 4 SEXMale      0.0254  0.00155     16.4  2.06e-60
```

Another component that we may want to add to our model is an interaction term. For example, we may consider an interaction between sex and blood lead level. We add an interaction to the formula using a : between the two variables. The output shows that the coefficient for this interaction is indeed significant.

```
model_interaction <- lm(log(SBP) ~ log(LEAD) + AGE + SEX +
                        SEX:log(LEAD), data=nhanes_df)
summary(model_interaction)
#>
#> Call:
#> lm(formula = log(SBP) ~ log(LEAD) + AGE + SEX + SEX:log(LEAD),
#>     data = nhanes_df)
#>
#> Residuals:
#>     Min      1Q  Median      3Q     Max
#> -0.6981 -0.0816 -0.0049  0.0752  0.6599
#>
#> Coefficients:
#>                    Estimate Std. Error t value Pr(>|t|)
#> (Intercept)        4.62e+00   2.39e-03  1936.2   <2e-16 ***
#> log(LEAD)          2.36e-02   1.68e-03    14.1   <2e-16 ***
#> AGE                3.45e-03   4.58e-05    75.3   <2e-16 ***
#> SEXMale            3.32e-02   1.67e-03    19.9   <2e-16 ***
#> log(LEAD):SEXMale -2.66e-02   2.16e-03   -12.3   <2e-16 ***
#> ---
#> Signif. codes:  0 '***' 0.001 '**' 0.01 '*' 0.05 '.' 0.1 ' ' 1
#>
#> Residual standard error: 0.128 on 30400 degrees of freedom
#> Multiple R-squared:  0.219,  Adjusted R-squared:  0.219
#> F-statistic: 2.13e+03 on 4 and 30400 DF,  p-value: <2e-16
```

13.5   Evaluation Metrics

In addition to adjusted R-squared, there are a few other metrics that can help us to understand how well our model fits the data and can also help with model selection. The AIC() and BIC() functions find the Akaike information criterion (AIC) and Bayesian information criterion (BIC) values, respectively. Both AIC and BIC balance the trade-off between model complexity and goodness of fit. AIC takes into account both the goodness of fit (captured by the likelihood of the model) and the complexity of the model (captured by the number of parameters used). Lower AIC values are preferable. BIC is similar to AIC but has a stronger penalty for model complexity compared to AIC. Both measures indicate a preference for keeping the interaction term.

```
AIC(model_log_log)
#> [1] -38610
AIC(model_interaction)
#> [1] -38760
```

```
BIC(model_log_log)
#> [1] -38569
BIC(model_interaction)
#> [1] -38710
```

The predict() function allows us to calculate the predicted y values. When called on a model with no data specified, it returns the predicted values for the training data. We could also specify new data using the newdata argument. The new data provided must contain the columns given in the model formula. We use the predict() function to find the predicted values from our model and then calculate the mean absolute error (MAE) and mean squared error (MSE) for our model. MAE is less sensitive to outliers compared to MSE. The MAE indicates that our model has fairly high residuals on average. While this model may be helpful for understanding the relationship between blood lead level and systolic blood pressure, it would not be very useful as a tool to predict the latter.

```
pred_y <- predict(model_interaction)
```

```
mae <- mean(abs(nhanes_df$SBP - pred_y))
```

```
mae
#> [1] 119
```

```
mse <- mean((nhanes_df$SBP - pred_y)^2)
mse
#> [1] 14502
```

13.6   Stepwise Selection

So far we have ignored the other variables in the data frame. When performing variable selection, there are multiple methods to use. We conclude this chapter by demonstrating how to implement one such method, **stepwise selection**, in R. Chapter 15 expands upon this model selection technique by showing how to implement regularized models in R.

The `step()` function takes in an initial model along with a `direction` ("forward", "backward", or "both"), and a `scope`. The scope specifies the lower and upper model formulas to consider. In the following example, we use forward selection so the lower formula is the formula for our current model, and the upper formula contains the other covariates we are considering adding in. These two formulas must be nested, that is, all terms in the lower formula must be contained in the upper formula.

By default, the `step()` function prints each step in the process and uses AIC to guide its decisions. We can set `trace=0` to avoid the print behavior and update the argument `k` to `log(n)` to use BIC, where `n` is the number of observations. In the output, we see that the algorithm first adds in race, then BMI, then income, then education, and then smoking status. In fact, all variables were added to the model! The final output is an `lm` object that we can use just like the ones earlier in this chapter. We get the summary of the final model and see that the adjusted R-squared has improved to 0.2479.

```
lower_formula <- "log(SBP) ~ log(LEAD) + AGE + SEX:log(LEAD)"
upper_formula <- "log(SBP) ~ log(LEAD) + AGE + SEX:log(LEAD) + SEX +
  RACE + EDUCATION + SMOKE + INCOME + BMI_CAT"
mod_step <- step(model_interaction, direction = 'forward',
                scope = list(lower = lower_formula,
                             upper = upper_formula))
#> Start:  AIC=-125048
```

```
#> log(SBP) ~ log(LEAD) + AGE + SEX + SEX:log(LEAD)
#>
#>             Df Sum of Sq RSS     AIC
#> + RACE       4      9.16 488 -125605
#> + BMI_CAT    2      8.97 488 -125597
#> + INCOME     1      2.87 494 -125222
#> + EDUCATION  2      1.90 495 -125160
#> + SMOKE      2      0.35 497 -125065
#> <none>                  497 -125048
#>
#> Step:  AIC=-125605
#> log(SBP) ~ log(LEAD) + AGE + SEX + RACE + log(LEAD):SEX
#>
#>             Df Sum of Sq RSS     AIC
#> + BMI_CAT    2      7.16 481 -126050
#> + INCOME     1      1.80 486 -125715
#> + EDUCATION  2      1.34 487 -125684
#> + SMOKE      2      0.13 488 -125609
#> <none>                  488 -125605
#>
#> Step:  AIC=-126050
#> log(SBP) ~ log(LEAD) + AGE + SEX + RACE + BMI_CAT + log(LEAD):SEX
#>
#>             Df Sum of Sq RSS     AIC
#> + INCOME     1     1.617 479 -126151
#> + EDUCATION  2     1.112 480 -126117
#> + SMOKE      2     0.261 481 -126063
#> <none>                  481 -126050
#>
#> Step:  AIC=-126151
#> log(SBP) ~ log(LEAD) + AGE + SEX + RACE + BMI_CAT + INCOME +
#>     log(LEAD):SEX
#>
#>             Df Sum of Sq RSS     AIC
#> + EDUCATION  2     0.418 479 -126173
#> + SMOKE      2     0.258 479 -126163
#> <none>                  479 -126151
#>
#> Step:  AIC=-126173
#> log(SBP) ~ log(LEAD) + AGE + SEX + RACE + BMI_CAT + INCOME +
#>     EDUCATION + log(LEAD):SEX
#>
#>             Df Sum of Sq RSS     AIC
```

```
#> + SMOKE   2       0.286 479 -126187
#> <none>                  479 -126173
#>
#> Step:  AIC=-126187
#> log(SBP) ~ log(LEAD) + AGE + SEX + RACE + BMI_CAT + INCOME +
#>     EDUCATION + SMOKE + log(LEAD):SEX


summary(mod_step)
#>
#> Call:
#> lm(formula = log(SBP) ~ log(LEAD) + AGE + SEX + RACE + BMI_CAT +
#>     INCOME + EDUCATION + SMOKE + log(LEAD):SEX, data = nhanes_df)
#>
#> Residuals:
#>     Min      1Q  Median      3Q     Max
#> -0.6713 -0.0799 -0.0039  0.0738  0.6797
#>
#> Coefficients:
#>                         Estimate Std. Error t value Pr(>|t|)
#> (Intercept)             4.61e+00   3.32e-03 1391.51  < 2e-16 ***
#> log(LEAD)               2.28e-02   1.69e-03   13.47  < 2e-16 ***
#> AGE                     3.48e-03   4.85e-05   71.87  < 2e-16 ***
#> SEXMale                 3.47e-02   1.65e-03   20.94  < 2e-16 ***
#> RACEOther Hispanic     -7.11e-03   3.22e-03   -2.20    0.027 *
#> RACENon-Hispanic White -4.45e-03   2.20e-03   -2.02    0.043 *
#> RACENon-Hispanic Black  3.37e-02   2.47e-03   13.66  < 2e-16 ***
#> RACEOther Race          6.27e-03   3.39e-03    1.85    0.064 .
#> BMI_CAT25<BMI<30        1.51e-02   1.84e-03    8.23  < 2e-16 ***
#> BMI_CATBMI>=30          3.78e-02   1.83e-03   20.62  < 2e-16 ***
#> INCOME                 -3.89e-03   5.00e-04   -7.78  7.6e-15 ***
#> EDUCATIONHS            -1.94e-05   2.19e-03   -0.01    0.993
#> EDUCATIONMoreThanHS    -8.69e-03   2.07e-03   -4.20  2.6e-05 ***
#> SMOKEQuitSmoke         -7.56e-03   1.80e-03   -4.21  2.6e-05 ***
#> SMOKEStillSmoke        -4.04e-03   1.94e-03   -2.08    0.038 *
#> log(LEAD):SEXMale      -2.61e-02   2.12e-03  -12.28  < 2e-16 ***
#> ---
#> Signif. codes:  0 '***' 0.001 '**' 0.01 '*' 0.05 '.' 0.1 ' ' 1
#>
#> Residual standard error: 0.126 on 30389 degrees of freedom
#> Multiple R-squared:  0.248,  Adjusted R-squared:  0.248
#> F-statistic:  669 on 15 and 30389 DF,  p-value: <2e-16
```

13.7 Exercises

For these exercises, we continue using the nhanes_df data.

1. Construct a linear model using DBP as the output and LEAD, AGE, and EVER_SMOKE as features, and print the output.

2. Use forward stepwise selection to add possible interactions to the linear model from the previous question.

3. Draw a QQ-plot for the model in Question 2, and describe the distribution that you observe.

4. Report the MAE and MSE of the model developed in Question 2. Then, find the row numbers of the observations with the top 5 Cook's Distance values for this model.

5. Look at some diagnostic plots for the model and use what you observe from these plots to choose a transformation that improves the fit of this model. Then, fit and summarize this new model with the transformation included. How do the MSE and MAE of the new model compare to the previous one? Note that your predictions will be on the transformed scale, so you'll need to convert them to the correct scale.

14

Logistic Regression

This chapter builds on the previous chapter and continues with regression analysis in R. Specifically, we cover binary logistic regression using the `glm()` function, which can be used to fit generalized linear models. Many of the functions learned in the last chapter can also be used with a `glm` object. For example, the `glm()` function expects a formula in the same way as the `lm()` function. We also cover diagnostic plots and model evaluation specific to a binary outcome.

The data used in this chapter is from the 2021 National Youth Tobacco Survey (NYTS) (Centers for Disease Control and Prevention (CDC) 2021). This dataset contains 20,413 participants and a set of variables relating to demographic information, frequency of tobacco use, and methods of obtaining said tobacco as reported by students on the 2021 NYTS. We use logistic regression to examine whether survey setting is associated with youth reporting of current tobacco use, similar to the analysis presented in Park-Lee et al. (2023). Note that we ignore survey weights for this analysis.

We use the **broom** package again to present the estimated coefficients, the **tidyverse** package to create a calibration plot, the **lmtest** (Hothorn et al. 2022) package to perform likelihood ratio tests, and the **pROC** package (Robin et al. 2023) to create receiver operating characteristic curves.

```
library(broom)
library(tidyverse)
library(pROC)
library(lmtest)
library(HDSinRdata)

data(nyts)
```

14.1   Generalized Linear Models in R

The glm(formula, data, family) function in R is used to fit generalized linear models. The three main arguments we must specify to the function are:

- formula - the relationship between the independent variables and the outcome of interest,

- data - the dataset used to train the model, and

- family - a description of the error distribution and link function to be used in the model.

In binary logistic regression, we assume a binomial outcome and use the logit link function. We can specify this by setting family = binomial. By default, this assumes the link function is the logit function. Note that we can even use the glm() function to implement linear regression by setting family = gaussian. Using our example from Chapter 13, running glm(SBP ~ LEAD, data = nhanes_df, family = gaussian) would be equivalent to lm(SBP ~ LEAD, data = nhanes_df).

Our outcome of interest is current e-cigarette use, e_cig_use, so we need to create this variable from the variables that are currently in the data. We set e_cig_use to 0 if the respondent answered that they have not used e-cigarettes in the last 30 days and 1 otherwise. We can see that there are only 1,435 respondents who reported e-cigarette use. This is a low percentage of the overall sample, which will likely impact our results.

```
nyts$e_cig_use <- as.factor(ifelse(nyts$num_e_cigs == 0, "0", "1"))
table(nyts$e_cig_use)
#>
#>      0     1
#> 18683  1435
```

Looking at the covariate of interest, survey setting, we can see that there are 85 respondents who took the survey in "Some other place". Since we are interested in the impact of taking the survey at school compared to other settings, we simplify this variable to have two levels: "school" and "home/other".

```
table(nyts$location)
#>
#>        At home (virtual learning) In a school building/classroom
#>                              8738                          10737
```

```
#>               Some other place
#>                        85
nyts$location <- ifelse(nyts$location ==
                  "In a school building/classroom",
                "school", "home/other")
nyts$location <- as.factor(nyts$location)
```

To start, we create a model to predict e-cigarette use from school setting adjusting for the covariates sex, school level, race, and ethnicity. Note that we specify our formula and data as with the lm() function. We then use the summary() function again to print a summary of this fitted model. The output is slightly different from an lm object. We can see the null and residual deviances are reported along with the AIC. Adding transformations and interactions is equivalent to that in the lm() function and is not demonstrated in this chapter.

```
mod_start <- glm(e_cig_use ~ grade + sex + race_and_ethnicity +
                location, data = nyts, family = binomial)
summary(mod_start)
#>
#> Call:
#> glm(formula = e_cig_use ~ grade + sex + race_and_ethnicity +
#>     location, family = binomial, data = nyts)
#>
#> Coefficients:
#>
#>                                    Estimate Std. Error z value
#> (Intercept)                        -4.6017     0.1539  -29.91
#> grade7th                            0.4461     0.1753    2.54
#> grade8th                            0.9677     0.1607    6.02
#> grade9th                            1.3830     0.1549    8.93
#> grade10th                           1.9183     0.1513   12.68
#> grade11th                           2.1385     0.1491   14.34
#> grade12th                           2.4286     0.1492   16.28
#> gradeUngraded or Other Grade        2.5213     0.4487    5.62
#> sexFemale                           0.1922     0.0580    3.32
#> race_and_ethnicitynon-Hispanic Black   -0.6614  0.1121   -5.90
#> race_and_ethnicitynon-Hispanic other race -0.1021 0.1515
#>   ↳  -0.67
#> race_and_ethnicitynon-Hispanic White    0.1983   0.0739   2.68
#> locationschool                      0.7223     0.0648   11.14
#>                                    Pr(>|z|)
#> (Intercept)                         < 2e-16 ***
#> grade7th                            0.01095 *
#> grade8th                            1.7e-09 ***
```

```
#> grade9th                                      < 2e-16 ***
#> grade10th                                     < 2e-16 ***
#> grade11th                                     < 2e-16 ***
#> grade12th                                     < 2e-16 ***
#> gradeUngraded or Other Grade                  1.9e-08 ***
#> sexFemale                                     0.00091 ***
#> race_and_ethnicitynon-Hispanic Black          3.6e-09 ***
#> race_and_ethnicitynon-Hispanic other race     0.50061
#> race_and_ethnicitynon-Hispanic White          0.00726 **
#> locationschool                                < 2e-16 ***
#> ---
#> Signif. codes:  0 '***' 0.001 '**' 0.01 '*' 0.05 '.' 0.1 ' ' 1
#>
#> (Dispersion parameter for binomial family taken to be 1)
#>
#>     Null deviance: 9754.9  on 18746  degrees of freedom
#> Residual deviance: 8886.8  on 18734  degrees of freedom
#>   (1666 observations deleted due to missingness)
#> AIC: 8913
#>
#> Number of Fisher Scoring iterations: 6
```

We can use the `tidy()` function from the **broom** package to display the estimated coefficients from the previous model. This time we add the `exponen-
tiate = TRUE` argument to exponentiate our coefficients so we can interpret
them as estimated change in odds rather than log odds. For example, we can
see that those who answered the survey at school have double the estimated
odds of reporting e-cigarette use compared to those who took the survey at
home/other, adjusting for grade, sex, race, and ethnicity.

```
tidy(mod_start, exponentiate = TRUE)
#> # A tibble: 13 x 5
#>    term          estimate std.error statistic   p.value
#>    <chr>            <dbl>     <dbl>     <dbl>     <dbl>
#> 1 (Intercept)     0.0100     0.154     -29.9 1.68e-196
#> 2 grade7th          1.56     0.175      2.54 1.10e-  2
#> 3 grade8th          2.63     0.161      6.02 1.73e-  9
#> 4 grade9th          3.99     0.155      8.93 4.41e- 19
#> 5 grade10th         6.81     0.151      12.7 7.94e- 37
#> # i 8 more rows
```

14.1.1 Practice Question

Fit a logistic regression model with cigarette use as the outcome and age, race_and_ethnicity, LGBT, and family_affluence as well as an interaction between family_affluence and race_and_ethnicity as independent variables. Your AIC should be 2430.8.

```
# Insert your solution here:
```

14.2 Residuals, Discrimination, and Calibration

Next, we look at the distribution of the residuals. The `resid()` function can be used to find the residuals again, but this time we might want to specify the Pearson and deviance residuals by specifying the `type` argument. We plot histograms for both of these residual types using the following code. In both plots, we can observe a multi-modal distribution, which reflects the binary nature of our outcome.

```
par(mfrow=c(1,2))
hist(resid(mod_start, type = "pearson"), main = "Pearson Residuals")
hist(resid(mod_start, type = "deviance"), main = "Deviance Residuals")
```

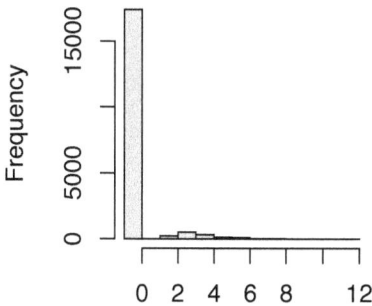

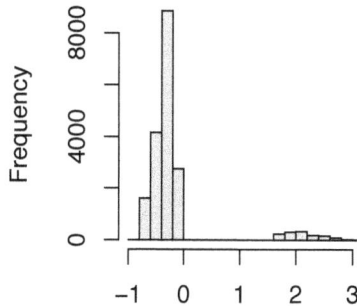

To further evaluate the fit of our model, we may want to observe the predicted probabilities. The `predict()` function by default returns the predicted value on the scale of the linear predictors. In this case, that is the predicted log odds. If we want to find the predicted probabilities, we can update the argument by specifying `type="response"`. Additionally, we can predict on data not used to train the model by using the argument `newdata`. Note that there are only 18,747 predicted probabilities despite our training data having more observations. This is because the `glm()` function (and `lm()` function) drop any observations with NA values when training. In the last chapter, we omitted incomplete cases prior to analysis so that the predicted probabilities corresponded directly to the rows in our data.

```
pred_probs <- predict(mod_start, type = "response")
length(pred_probs)
#> [1] 18747
```

If we want to find the class for each observation used in fitting the model, we can use the model's output, which stores the model matrix x and the outcome vector y. We plot the distribution of estimated probabilities for each class. Note that all the predicted probabilities are below 0.5, the typical cut-off for prediction. This is in part due to the fact that we have such an imbalanced outcome.

```
ggplot() +
  geom_histogram(aes(x = pred_probs, fill = as.factor(mod_start$y)),
                 bins = 30) +
  scale_fill_discrete(name = "E-Cig Use") +
  labs(x = "Predicted Probabilities", y = "Count")
```

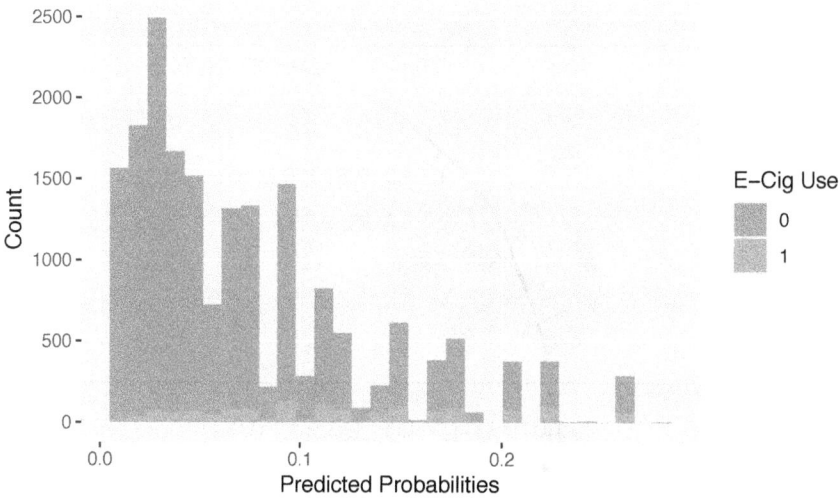

14.2.1 Receiver Operating Characteristic Curve

We now plot the receiver operating characteristic (ROC) curve and compute the area under the curve (AUC). The `roc()` function from the **pROC** package builds a ROC curve. The function has several ways to specify a response and predictor. For example, we can specify the response vector `response` and predictor vector `predictor`. By default, with a 0/1 outcome, the `roc()` function assumes class 0 is controls and class 1 is cases. We can also specify this in the `levels` argument to set the value of the response for controls and cases, respectively. Additionally, the function assumes the predictor vector specifies predicted probabilities for the class 1. We can change the argument `direction = ">"` if the opposite is true. We can plot the ROC curve by calling the `plot()` function. We can add some extra information by adding the AUC (`print.auc = TRUE`) and the threshold that maximizes sensitivity + specificity (`print.thres = TRUE`).

```
roc_mod <- roc(predictor = pred_probs,
               response = as.factor(mod_start$y),
               levels = c(0,1), direction = "<")
plot(roc_mod, print.auc = TRUE, print.thres = TRUE)
```

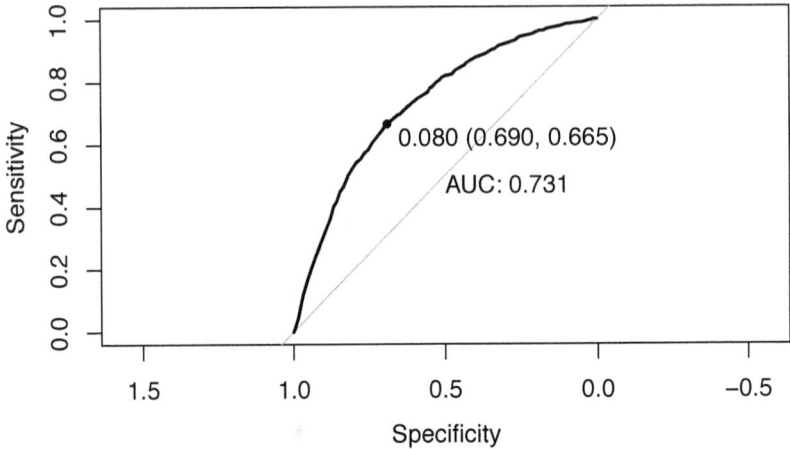

If we want to understand more about the curve, we can use the `coords()` function to find the coordinates for each threshold used to create the curve. The argument `x= "all"` specifies that we want to find all thresholds, but we could also specify only to return local maxima.

```
roc_vals <- coords(roc = roc_mod, x = "all")
head(roc_vals)
#>    threshold specificity sensitivity
#> 1       -Inf     0.00000       1.000
#> 2    0.00569     0.00523       1.000
#> 3    0.00713     0.01070       1.000
#> 4    0.00850     0.01547       0.999
#> 5    0.00934     0.01835       0.998
#> 6    0.00982     0.02404       0.996
```

For example, we could use this information to find the highest threshold with a corresponding sensitivity above 0.75. This returns a threshold of 0.062. If we were to predict class 1 for all observations with a predicted probability above 0.062, then we would achieve a sensitivity of 0.77 and specificity of 0.56 on the training data.

```
roc_vals[roc_vals$sensitivity > 0.75, ] %>% tail(n = 1)
#>     threshold specificity sensitivity
#> 63      0.062       0.555       0.768
```

We use the threshold of 0.080 indicated on our ROC curve to create predicted classes for our response. By comparing the result to our outcome using the `table()` function, we can directly calculate measures like sensitivity, specificity, positive and negative predictive values, and overall accuracy.

```
pred_ys <- ifelse(pred_probs > 0.08, 1, 0)
tab_outcome <- table(mod_start$y, pred_ys)
tab_outcome
#>      pred_ys
#>           0     1
#>   0  11992  5395
#>   1    455   905
```

```
sens <- tab_outcome[2, 2]/(tab_outcome[2, 1]+tab_outcome[2, 2])
spec <- tab_outcome[1, 1]/(tab_outcome[1, 1]+tab_outcome[1, 2])
ppv <- tab_outcome[2, 2]/(tab_outcome[1, 2]+tab_outcome[2, 2])
npv <- tab_outcome[1, 1]/(tab_outcome[1, 1]+tab_outcome[2, 1])
acc <- (tab_outcome[1, 1]+tab_outcome[2, 2])/sum(tab_outcome)
```

```
data.frame(Measures = c("Sens", "Spec", "PPV", "NPV", "Acc"),
           Values = round(c(sens, spec, ppv, npv, acc),3))
#>   Measures Values
#> 1     Sens  0.665
#> 2     Spec  0.690
#> 3      PPV  0.144
#> 4      NPV  0.963
#> 5      Acc  0.688
```

14.2.2 Calibration Plot

Another useful plot is a calibration plot. This type of plot groups the data by the estimated probabilities and compares the mean probability with the observed proportion of observations in class 1. It visualizes how close our estimated distribution and true distribution are to each other. There are several packages that can create calibration plots, but we demonstrate how to do this using the **ggplot2** package. First, we create a data frame with the predicted probabilities and the outcome variable. Additionally, we group this data into `num_cuts` groups based on the predicted probabilities using the `cut()` function. Within each group, we find the model's predicted mean along with the observed proportion and estimated standard errors.

```
num_cuts <- 10
calib_data <-  data.frame(prob = pred_probs,
                          bin = cut(pred_probs, breaks = num_cuts),
                          class = mod_start$y)
calib_data <- calib_data %>%
              group_by(bin) %>%
              summarize(observed = sum(class)/n(),
                        expected = sum(prob)/n(),
                        se = sqrt(observed * (1-observed) / n()))
calib_data
#> # A tibble: 10 x 4
#>   bin                observed expected      se
#>   <fct>                 <dbl>    <dbl>   <dbl>
#> 1 (0.00488,0.0322]     0.0212   0.0203 0.00188
#> 2 (0.0322,0.0592]      0.0440   0.0441 0.00328
#> 3 (0.0592,0.0862]      0.0621   0.0708 0.00451
#> 4 (0.0862,0.113]       0.0986   0.0988 0.00587
#> 5 (0.113,0.14]         0.131    0.123  0.0131
#> # i 5 more rows
```

Next, we plot the observed vs. expected proportions. We also used the estimated standard error to create corresponding 95% confidence intervals. The red line indicates a perfect fit where our estimated and true distributions match. Overall, the plot shows that our model could be better calibrated.

```
ggplot(calib_data) +
  geom_abline(intercept = 0, slope = 1, color = "red") +
  geom_errorbar(aes(x = expected, ymin = observed - 1.96 * se,
                    ymax = observed + 1.96 * se),
                colour="black", width=.01)+
  geom_point(aes(x = expected, y = observed)) +
  labs(x = "Expected Proportion", y = "Observed Proportion") +
  theme_minimal()
```

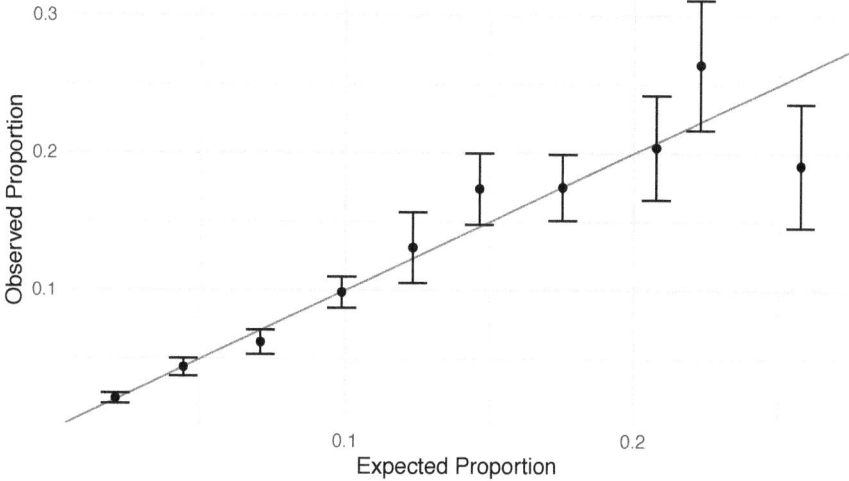

14.2.3   Practice Question

Create a calibration plot with five cuts for your model from the previous practice question (recall that this model should have cigarette use as the outcome and age, race_and_ethnicity, LGBT, and family_affluence as well as an interaction between family_affluence and race_and_ethnicity as independent variables). It should look like Figure 14.1.

```
# Insert your solution here:
```

14.3   Variable Selection and Likelihood Ratio Tests

In the last chapter, we introduced the step() function to implement stepwise variable selection. This function also works with glm objects. In this case, we use this function to implement backward selection from a larger set of covariates. We first remove any observations with NA values to ensure that our training data does not change size as the formula changes.

```
nyts_sub <- nyts %>%
  dplyr::select(location, sex, grade, otherlang, grades_in_past_year,
            perceived_e_cig_use, race_and_ethnicity, LGBT,
```

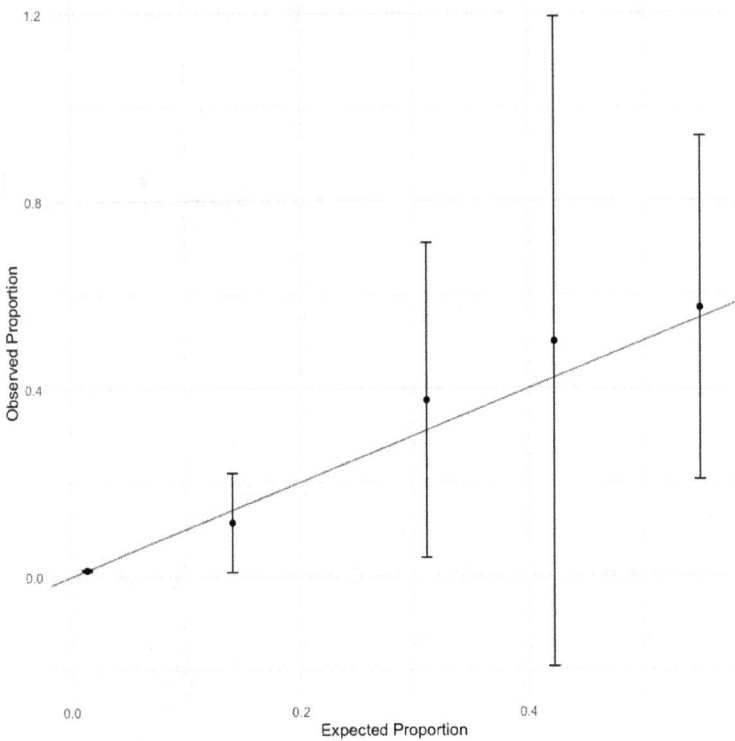

Figure 14.1: Calibration Plot.

```
                    psych_distress, family_affluence, e_cig_use) %>%
  na.omit()
head(nyts_sub)
#> # A tibble: 6 x 11
#>   location sex   grade otherlang grades_in_past_year
↳ perceived_e_cig_use
#>   <fct>    <fct> <fct> <fct>     <fct>                              <dbl>
#> 1 school   Male  6th   No        Mostly A's                             0
#> 2 school   Fema~ 6th   No        Mostly A's                             0
#> 3 school   Fema~ 6th   No        Mostly C's                             0
#> 4 school   Fema~ 6th   No        Mostly A's                             0
#> 5 school   Fema~ 6th   No        Mostly B's                             0
#> 6 school   Male  6th   No        Not Sure                               0
#> # i 5 more variables: race_and_ethnicity <chr>, LGBT <chr>,
#> #   psych_distress <chr>, family_affluence <chr>, e_cig_use <fct>
```

To implement backward selection, we first create a model with all the covariates included. The period . in the formula indicates that we want to include all variables. Next, we use the `step()` function. Since we are using backward selection, we only need to specify the lower formula in the scope.

```
model_full <- glm(e_cig_use ~ ., data = nyts_sub, family = binomial)
mod_step <- step(model_full, direction = 'backward',
                 scope = list(lower = "e_cig_use ~ sex + grade +
                 race_and_ethnicity + location"))
#> Start:  AIC=6093
#> e_cig_use ~ location + sex + grade + otherlang +
  ↵  grades_in_past_year +
#>       perceived_e_cig_use + race_and_ethnicity + LGBT +
  ↵  psych_distress +
#>       family_affluence
#>
#>                          Df Deviance  AIC
#> - family_affluence        2     6038 6090
#> <none>                          6037 6093
#> - otherlang               1     6042 6096
#> - LGBT                    2     6051 6103
#> - psych_distress          3     6106 6156
#> - grades_in_past_year     6     6126 6170
#> - perceived_e_cig_use     1     6416 6470
#>
#> Step:  AIC=6090
#> e_cig_use ~ location + sex + grade + otherlang +
  ↵  grades_in_past_year +
#>       perceived_e_cig_use + race_and_ethnicity + LGBT + psych_distress
#>
#>                          Df Deviance  AIC
#> <none>                          6038 6090
#> - otherlang               1     6043 6093
#> - LGBT                    2     6052 6100
#> - psych_distress          3     6106 6152
#> - grades_in_past_year     6     6128 6168
#> - perceived_e_cig_use     1     6418 6468
```

Stepwise selection keeps most variables in the model and only drops family affluence. In the following output, we can see the AUC for this model has improved to 0.818.

```
roc_mod_step <- roc(predictor = predict(mod_step, type = "response"),
                    response = as.factor(mod_step$y),
                    levels = c(0, 1), direction = "<")
plot(roc_mod_step, print.auc = TRUE, print.thres = TRUE)
```

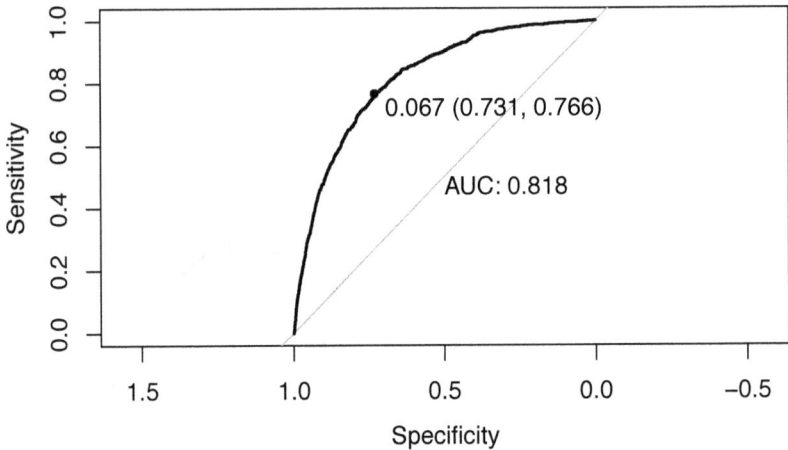

If we want to compare this model to our previous one, we could use a likelihood ratio test since the two models are nested. The lrtest() function from the **lmtest** package allows us to input two nested glm models and performs a corresponding Chi-squared likelihood ratio test. First, we need to ensure that our initial model is fit on the same data used in the stepwise selection. The output indicates a statistically significant improvement in the model likelihood with the inclusion of the other variables.

```
mod_start2 <- glm(e_cig_use ~ grade + sex + race_and_ethnicity +
                    location, data = nyts_sub, family = binomial)
```

```
print(lrtest(mod_start2, mod_step))
#> Likelihood ratio test
#>
#> Model 1: e_cig_use ~ grade + sex + race_and_ethnicity + location
#> Model 2: e_cig_use ~ location + sex + grade + otherlang +
  ↪ grades_in_past_year +
#>     perceived_e_cig_use + race_and_ethnicity + LGBT + psych_distress
#>   #Df LogLik Df Chisq Pr(>Chisq)
```

```
#> 1   13   -3369
#> 2   26   -3019 13    701      <2e-16 ***
#> ---
#> Signif. codes:   0 '***' 0.001 '**' 0.01 '*' 0.05 '.' 0.1 ' ' 1
```

14.4   Extending Beyond Binary Outcomes

The glm() function can be used to fit models for other possible families and
non-binary outcomes. For example, we can fit models where the outcome might
follow a Poisson distribution or negative binomial distribution by updating the
family argument. In the following code, we fit a Poisson model to model the
number of e-cigarettes used in the last 30 days by setting family = poisson.
However, despite our outcome being a count value, this model does not appear
to be a good fit for our data.

```r
mod_poisson <- glm(num_e_cigs ~ grade + sex + race_and_ethnicity +
                   location, data = nyts, family = poisson)
```

```r
par(mfrow=c(1,2))
hist(predict(mod_poisson, type = "response"), main = "Model",
     xlab = "Predicted Values")
hist(nyts$num_e_cigs, main = "Observed", xlab = "Number E-Cigs")
```

Model   **Observed**

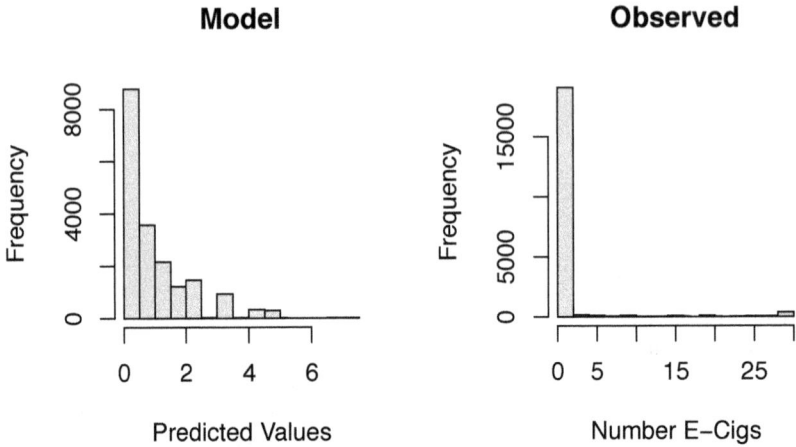

14.5   Exercises

1. Create a new variable `tobacco_use` representing any tobacco use in the past 30 days (including e-cigarettes, cigarettes, and/or cigars), as well as a new variable `perceived_tobacco_use` equal to the maximum of the perceived cigarette and e-cigarette use. Then, create a new data frame `nyts_sub` that contains these two new columns as well as columns for sex, grades in the past year, psych distress, and family affluence. Finally, fit a logistic regression model with this new tobacco use variable as the outcome and all other selected variables as independent variables.

2. Perform stepwise selection on your model from Question 1 with `direction = "both"`, setting the upper scope of the model selection procedure to be a model including all two-way interactions and the lower scope to be a model including only an intercept. To specify all possible interactions, you can use the formula `"tobacco_use ~ .^2"`. Use the `tidy()` function to display the exponentiated estimated coefficients for the resulting model along with a confidence interval.

3. According to your model from Question 2, what is the estimated probability of tobacco use for a girl with mostly Cs, moderate psych distress, and a perceived tobacco use of 0.5? Use the `predict()` function to answer this question.

4. Construct a ROC curve for the model from Question 2 and find the AUC as well as the threshold that maximizes sensitivity and specificity.

15

Model Selection

In Chapter 13 and Chapter 14, we included one simple method for model selection, stepwise selection. This chapter expands upon our model selection tools in R by focusing on regularized regression. The two packages we cover are **glmnet** (Friedman, Tibshirani, and Hastie 2010) and **L0Learn** (Hazimeh, Mazumder, and Nonet 2023). These two packages focus on different types of model regularization.

```
library(HDSinRdata)
library(tidyverse)
library(glmnet)
library(L0Learn)
```

To demonstrate these packages, we use the same motivating example as in Chapter 13. Recall, that the NHANESsample dataset contains lead, blood pressure, BMI, smoking status, alcohol use, and demographic variables from NHANES 1999-2018. Our focus is looking at the association between blood lead levels and systolic blood pressure. We first create a single systolic blood pressure by averaging across all measurements. We also transform lead with a log transformation before dropping variables we want to exclude from our analysis.

```
# load in data
data(NHANESsample)

# transform SBP and lead
NHANESsample$SBP <-
  rowMeans(NHANESsample[c("SBP1", "SBP2", "SBP3", "SBP4")],
                     na.rm=TRUE)
NHANESsample$LEAD <- log(NHANESsample$LEAD)

# remove variables not to include in the model
nhanes <- NHANESsample %>%
  select(-c(ID, HYP, LEAD_QUANTILE, DBP1, DBP2, DBP3, DBP4,
            SBP1, SBP2, SBP3, SBP4, YEAR)) %>%
```

```
  na.omit()

# convert to factors
nhanes$SEX <- factor(nhanes$SEX)
nhanes$RACE <- factor(nhanes$RACE)
nhanes$EDUCATION <- factor(nhanes$EDUCATION)
nhanes$BMI_CAT <- factor(nhanes$BMI_CAT)
nhanes$ALC <- factor(nhanes$ALC)
```

15.1   Regularized Regression

Suppose we have a numeric data matrix $X \in \mathbb{R}^{n \times p}$ and outcome vector $y \in \mathbb{R}^n$. We let x_i denote the vector representing the ith row of X. This corresponds to the ith observation. When we refer to regularized regression, we are referring to solving the following optimization problem that minimizes the average loss plus a penalty term.

$$\min_{(\beta_0,\beta)\in\mathbb{R}^{p+1}} \frac{1}{n} \sum_{i=1}^{n} l(y_i, \beta_0 + \beta^T x_i) + \text{Pen}(\beta) \tag{15.1}$$

The function $l(y_i, \beta_0 + \beta^T x_i)$ represents the loss function. For linear regression, this corresponds to the squared error $(y_i - \beta_0 - \beta^T x_i)^2$. For logistic regression, this loss corresponds to the logistic loss function.

The penalty terms we implement include the following:

- L0 Norm: $\|\beta\|_0 = \sum_{j=1}^{p} 1(\beta_j \neq 0)$, the number of non-zero coefficients,

- L1 Norm: $\|\beta\|_1 = \sum_{j=1}^{p} |\beta_j|$, the sum of absolute values of the coefficients, and

- Squared L2 Norm: $\|\beta\|_2^2 = \sum_{j=1}^{p} \beta_j^2$, the sum of squared coefficients.

15.2   Elastic Net

We first consider L1 and L2 regularization. In particular, consider the following penalty term, referred to as elastic net regularization,

$$\lambda \left[\alpha\|\beta\|_1 + (1-\alpha)\|\beta\|_2^2 \right],$$

where λ is a complexity parameter and α controls the balance between the two norms. A model with only L1 regularization ($\alpha = 1$) corresponds to lasso regression while a model with only L2 regularization ($\alpha = 0$) corresponds to ridge regression. Note that the penalty depends on the scale of X and we typically assume each column has been standardized.

The **glmnet** package implements elastic net regularization. It assumes our data are in the form described previously. Therefore, we first create our numeric data matrix x and output vector y. Some of our variables are categorical, so in order to create a numeric matrix we need to one-hot encode them. We can do so using the `model.matrix()` function which takes in a formula and a data frame and creates the corresponding design matrix including creating dummy variables from factor variables and implementing any transformations. Note that we drop the first generated column which corresponds to the intercept. The transformation to our outcome does not impact the result.

```
x <- model.matrix(log(SBP) ~ ., nhanes)[, -1]
head(x)
#>   AGE SEXFemale RACEOther Hispanic RACENon-Hispanic White
#> 1  77         0                 0                       1
#> 2  49         0                 0                       1
#> 3  37         0                 0                       1
#> 4  70         0                 0                       0
#> 5  81         0                 0                       1
#> 6  38         1                 0                       1
#>   RACENon-Hispanic Black RACEOther Race EDUCATIONHS
#> ↳ EDUCATIONMoreThanHS
#> 1                      0              0           0                   1
#> 2                      0              0           0                   1
#> 3                      0              0           0                   1
#> 4                      0              0           0                   0
#> 5                      0              0           0                   0
#> 6                      0              0           0                   1
#>   INCOME SMOKEQuitSmoke SMOKEStillSmoke  LEAD BMI_CAT25<BMI<30
#> 1   5.00              0               0 1.609                0
#> 2   5.00              1               0 0.470                1
#> 3   4.93              0               0 0.875                0
#> 4   1.07              1               0 0.470                1
#> 5   2.67              0               1 1.705                1
#> 6   4.52              0               1 0.405                1
#>   BMI_CATBMI>=30 ALCYes
#> 1              0      1
#> 2              0      1
#> 3              1      1
#> 4              0      1
```

```
#> 5                    0       1
#> 6                    0       1
```

Our outcome vector corresponds to log transformed systolic blood pressure.

```
y <- log(nhanes$SBP)
```

The `glmnet()` function fits an elastic net regression model. This requires us to specify our input matrix x and response variable y. Additionally, we can specify the assumed distribution for y using the `family` argument. In our subsequent example, we fit this model with $\alpha = 1$ and 25 different values of λ. By default, `glmnet()` sets α to 1 and creates a grid of 100 different values of `lambda`. It is also the default to standardize x, which we can turn off by specifying `standardize = FALSE` in our function call.

```
mod_lasso <- glmnet(x, y, family = "gaussian", alpha = 1,
                    nlambda = 25)
```

If we plot the resulting object, we can see the model coefficients for each resulting model by plotting how the coefficient for each variable changes with the value of λ. The `plot()` function by default plots these against the penalty term but we can also specify to plot against the λ values on the log scale. The `label` argument adds a label to each line, though these are often hard to read. The numbers at the top of the plot indicate how many non-zero coefficients were included in the model for different λ values. Read the documentation `?glmnet` to see the other possible inputs including the `penalty.factor` and `weights` arguments.

```
plot(mod_lasso, xvar = "lambda", label = TRUE)
```

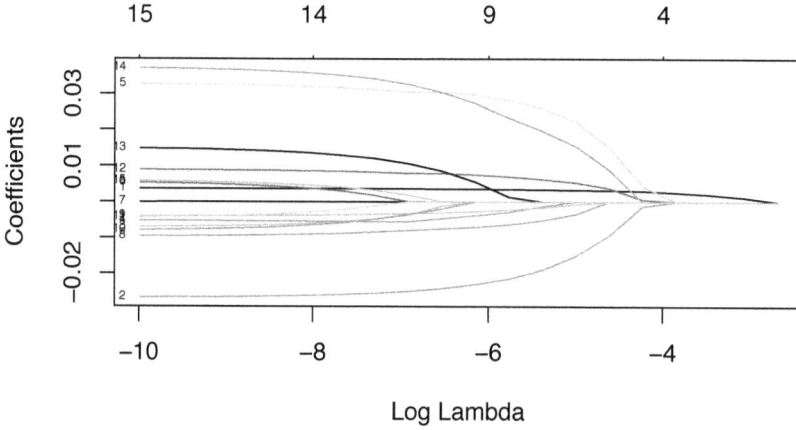

We can also print our results. This prints a matrix with the values of λ used.
For each λ value we can also see the number of non-zero coefficients (Df) and
the percent deviance explained (%dev).

```
print(mod_lasso)
#>
#> Call:  glmnet(x = x, y = y, family = "gaussian", alpha = 1, nlambda
  ↪ = 25)
#>
#>      Df %Dev Lambda
#> 1     0  0.0 0.0674
#> 2     1 11.6 0.0459
#> 3     1 17.0 0.0313
#> 4     1 19.5 0.0213
#> 5     4 21.0 0.0145
#> 6     5 23.1 0.0099
#> 7     7 24.3 0.0067
#> 8     8 24.9 0.0046
#> 9     9 25.2 0.0031
#> 10    9 25.4 0.0021
#> 11   12 25.6 0.0014
#> 12   13 25.6 0.0010
#> 13   14 25.7 0.0007
#> 14   14 25.7 0.0005
#> 15   14 25.7 0.0003
#> 16   14 25.7 0.0002
```

```
#> 17 14 25.7 0.0001
#> 18 14 25.7 0.0001
#> 19 15 25.7 0.0001
#> 20 15 25.7 0.0000
```

We can extract the model for a particular value of λ using the `coef()` function. The argument s specifies the value of λ. For the particular value of λ chosen in the following code, only age has a non-zero coefficient. Note that the `coef()` function returns the coefficients on the original scale.

```
coef(mod_lasso, s = 0.045920)
#> 16 x 1 sparse Matrix of class "dgCMatrix"
#>                           s1
#> (Intercept)           4.75241
#> AGE                   0.00121
#> SEXFemale                  .
#> RACEOther Hispanic         .
#> RACENon-Hispanic White .
#> RACENon-Hispanic Black .
#> RACEOther Race             .
#> EDUCATIONHS                .
#> EDUCATIONMoreThanHS        .
#> INCOME                     .
#> SMOKEQuitSmoke             .
#> SMOKEStillSmoke            .
#> LEAD                       .
#> BMI_CAT25<BMI<30           .
#> BMI_CATBMI>=30             .
#> ALCYes                     .
```

We can also use the `predict()` function to predict blood pressure for this particular model. In the function call, we have specified our value of λ as well as our data matrix x as the data to predict on.

```
pred_lasso <- predict(mod_lasso, s = 0.045920, newx = x)
```

This shows our observed model fit for a fairly high penalty term. In order to choose the best value of λ, we use 5-fold cross-validation. First, we randomly assign each observation to one of five folds using the `sample()` function. We can see that this splits the data into folds of roughly equal size.

```
set.seed(1)
foldid <- sample(1:5, size = nrow(x), replace = TRUE)
table(foldid)
#> foldid
#>    1    2    3    4    5
#> 6081 5967 6048 6188 6121
```

Next, we call the `cv.glmnet()` function which implements k-fold cross-validation across a grid of λ values. Similar to before, we specified x, y, and `alpha = 1`. This time, we also include the measure to use for cross-validation (mse indicates mean squared error) and provide the fold vector `foldid`. If you do not want to provide folds, you can instead use the `nfolds` argument to specify the number of folds desired and the `cv.glmnet()` function will create them. Plotting the returned object shows us the estimated mean squared error for different values of λ as well as error bars for each estimate. Similar to before, it also shows the number of non-zero coefficients at the top.

```
cv_lasso <- cv.glmnet(x, y, foldid = foldid, alpha = 1,
                      type.measure = "mse")
plot(cv_lasso)
```

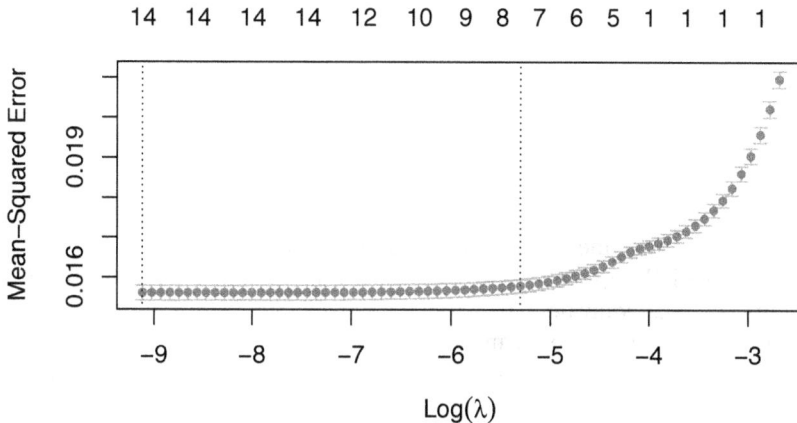

There are two vertical dashed lines included in the plot. These correspond to two values of λ that are stored in our object. The first is `lambda.min`. This corresponds to the λ value with the lowest estimated mean squared error. The other is `lambda.1se`. This corresponds to the largest λ value whose estimated mean squared error is within one standard error of the lowest value. As indicated in the plot, this corresponds to a model with fewer included coefficients and higher regularization.

We use the `lambda.min` value as our chosen λ value. To extract the coefficients corresponding to this λ value we again use the `coef()` function. However, this λ might not be one of the initial 25 used for our `mod_lasso` object. In this case, the `coef()` function uses linear interpolation to get the estimated coefficients. If we want to refit our model for this particular value of λ, we can instead specify the argument `exact = TRUE` and provide x and y.

```
lasso_coef <- coef(mod_lasso, s = cv_lasso$lambda.min,
                   exact = TRUE, x = x, y = y)
lasso_coef
#> 16 x 1 sparse Matrix of class "dgCMatrix"
#>                                s1
#> (Intercept)               4.63458
#> AGE                       0.00367
#> SEXFemale                -0.02652
#> RACEOther Hispanic       -0.00677
#> RACENon-Hispanic White   -0.00531
#> RACENon-Hispanic Black    0.03257
#> RACEOther Race            0.00493
#> EDUCATIONHS                   .
#> EDUCATIONMoreThanHS      -0.00942
#> INCOME                   -0.00396
#> SMOKEQuitSmoke           -0.00753
#> SMOKEStillSmoke          -0.00397
#> LEAD                      0.00880
#> BMI_CAT25<BMI<30          0.01452
#> BMI_CATBMI>=30            0.03688
#> ALCYes                    0.00547
```

We now repeat the same process for a model with $\alpha = 0$ and $\alpha = 0.5$. In this case, we call the `glmnet()` function with our chosen λ value to find the coefficients. This is equivalent to what we did for our lasso model. Last, we create a data frame with the estimated coefficients for each model. The `coef()` function returns a matrix, so this requires converting these to numeric vectors.

```
# cross-validation using same folds
cv_ridge <- cv.glmnet(x, y, foldid = foldid, alpha = 0,
                      type.measure = "mse")
cv_elastic <- cv.glmnet(x, y, foldid = foldid, alpha = 0.5,
                        type.measure = "mse")
```

```
# Refit model on full data with chosen lambda
mod_ridge <- glmnet(x, y, alpha = 0, lambda = cv_ridge$lambda.min)
mod_elastic <- glmnet(x, y, alpha = 0.5, lambda = cv_ridge$lambda.min)

# extract coefficients for a table
res_coef <- data.frame(name = c("Intercept", colnames(x)),
                       lasso = round(as.numeric(lasso_coef), 3),
                       ridge = round(as.numeric(coef(mod_ridge)), 3),
                       elastic = round(as.numeric(coef(mod_elastic)),
                                       3))
res_coef
#>                           name   lasso   ridge elastic
#> 1                    Intercept   4.635   4.646   4.650
#> 2                          AGE   0.004   0.003   0.003
#> 3                    SEXFemale  -0.027  -0.025  -0.020
#> 4          RACEOther Hispanic  -0.007  -0.007   0.000
#> 5    RACENon-Hispanic White   -0.005  -0.005  -0.002
#> 6    RACENon-Hispanic Black    0.033   0.031   0.027
#> 7              RACEOther Race    0.005   0.004   0.000
#> 8                 EDUCATIONHS    0.000   0.000   0.000
#> 9       EDUCATIONMoreThanHS   -0.009  -0.010  -0.006
#> 10                     INCOME  -0.004  -0.004  -0.002
#> 11           SMOKEQuitSmoke   -0.008  -0.006   0.000
#> 12          SMOKEStillSmoke   -0.004  -0.005   0.000
#> 13                       LEAD    0.009   0.011   0.008
#> 14        BMI_CAT25<BMI<30    0.015   0.014   0.000
#> 15          BMI_CATBMI>=30    0.037   0.035   0.022
#> 16                     ALCYes    0.005   0.004   0.000
```

The coefficients between the models are not so different. We can also compare
their mean squared errors, which are also similar. Since our lasso model was
fit on a grid of λ values, we again have to specify this value.

```
mean((nhanes$SBP - exp(predict(mod_lasso, newx = x,
                              s = cv_lasso$lambda.min)))^2)
#> [1] 268
mean((nhanes$SBP - exp(predict(mod_ridge, newx = x)))^2)
#> [1] 268
mean((nhanes$SBP - exp(predict(mod_elastic, newx = x)))^2)
#> [1] 270
```

15.3   Best Subset

The second package we introduce in this chapter is one that allows us to fit models with an L0 penalty term. The package **L0Learn** considers penalties of the following forms.

- L0 only: $\lambda||\beta||_0$
- L0L1: $\lambda||\beta||_0 + \gamma||\beta||_1$
- L0L2: $\lambda||\beta||_0 + \gamma||\beta||_2^2$

To fit a model with an L0 penalty term, we use the `L0Learn.fit()` function. Similar to `glmnet()`, we need to specify our input matrix `x` and response vector `y` as well as our penalty using the `penalty` argument. We can also specify a number of λ values to consider `nLambda` and specify the family through the loss function `loss`.

```
mod_l0 <- L0Learn.fit(x, y, penalty = "L0", loss = "SquaredError",
                      nLambda = 20)
```

Plotting the returned object also shows how the coefficients for each variable change with the penalty term, given by the support size or number of non-zero coefficients in this case. We can also print the returned object to see the different values of λ used and the corresponding number of included variables.

```
plot(mod_l0)
```

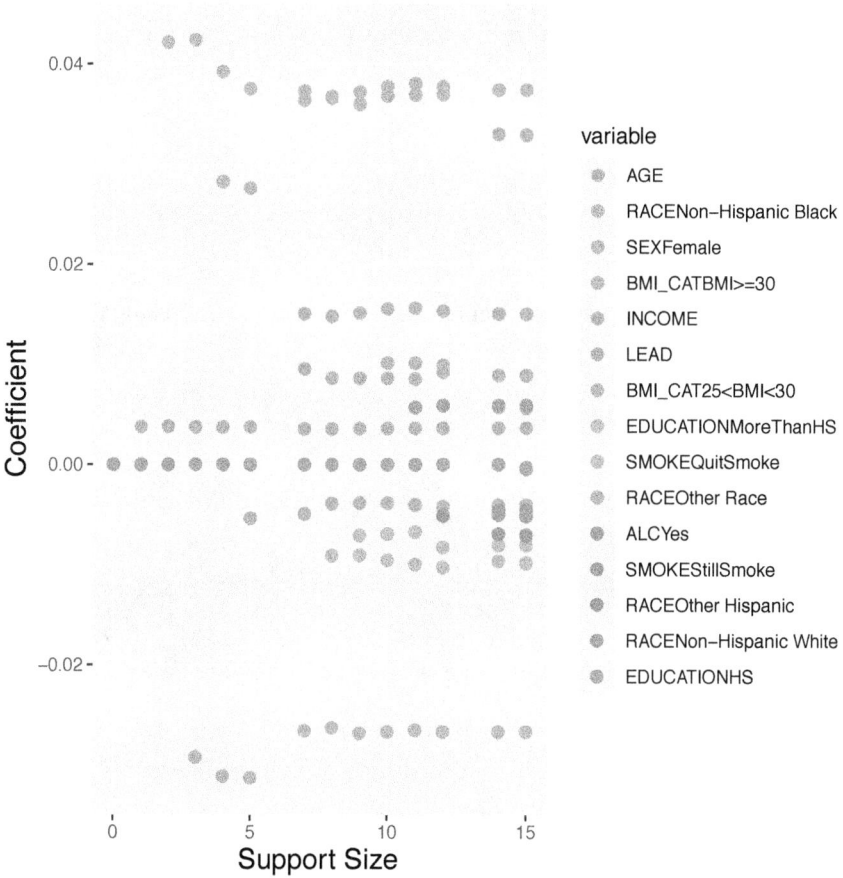

```
print(mod_l0)
#>      lambda gamma suppSize
#> 1  1.08e-01     0        0
#> 2  1.07e-01     0        1
#> 3  6.51e-03     0        2
#> 4  5.00e-03     0        3
#> 5  4.22e-03     0        4
#> 6  1.75e-03     0        5
#> 7  5.36e-04     0        7
#> 8  3.23e-04     0        8
#> 9  1.92e-04     0        9
#> 10 1.42e-04     0       10
#> 11 1.04e-04     0       11
#> 12 6.80e-05     0       12
```

```
#> 13 1.75e-05      0      14
#> 14 4.06e-07      0      15
#> 15 3.94e-07      0      15
#> 16 3.03e-08      0      15
#> 17 5.87e-09      0      15
#> 18 9.43e-10      0      15
#> 19 3.48e-10      0      15
#> 20 2.19e-10      0      15
```

To extract the model for a particular value, we can use the `coef()` function and specify the λ and γ values to use.

```
coef_l0 <- coef(mod_l0, lambda = 1.75475e-03, gamma = 0)
```

Unfortunately, this output doesn't include variable names so we add them manually.

```
rownames(coef_l0) <- c("Intercept", colnames(x))
coef_l0
#> 16 x 1 sparse Matrix of class "dgCMatrix"
#>
#> Intercept               4.63847
#> AGE                     0.00379
#> SEXFemale              -0.03130
#> RACEOther Hispanic      .
#> RACENon-Hispanic White  .
#> RACENon-Hispanic Black  0.03753
#> RACEOther Race          .
#> EDUCATIONHS             .
#> EDUCATIONMoreThanHS     .
#> INCOME                 -0.00535
#> SMOKEQuitSmoke          .
#> SMOKEStillSmoke         .
#> LEAD                    .
#> BMI_CAT25<BMI<30        .
#> BMI_CATBMI>=30          0.02760
#> ALLYes                  .
```

If instead we want to include a penalty with an L0 and L2 norm term, we can change our penalty argument to `penalty = L0L2` and specify a number of γ values to test.

```
mod_l0l2 <- L0Learn.fit(x, y, penalty = "L0L2",
                        loss = "SquaredError",
                        nLambda = 20, nGamma = 10)
```

The **L0Learn** package also includes a function to use cross-validation to choose these parameters. Unfortunately, it does not include an option to specify your own folds. Instead, we use the nFolds argument to specify to run 5-fold cross-validation. This function also allows us to specify a number of λ and γ values, or we can use the default number. Plotting the result shows the estimated mean squared error with error bars for each model and the corresponding support size.

```
cv_l0l2 = L0Learn.cvfit(x, y, loss = "SquaredError",
                        nFolds = 5, penalty = "L0L2")
plot(cv_l0l2)
```

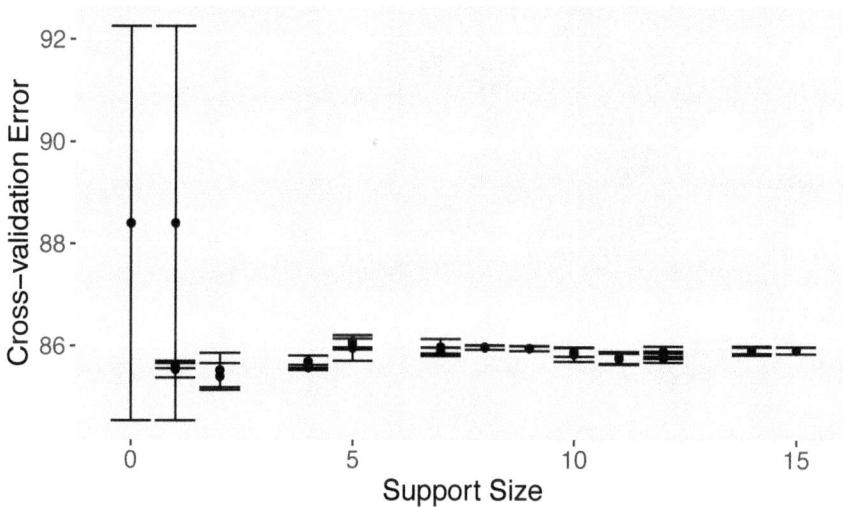

The returned results are stored in cvMeans. This is a list of matrices — one for each value of γ. To extract these into a more manageable form, we use the sapply() function to convert each matrix to a numeric vector and create a matrix of results. The columns of this matrix correspond to the 10 γ values used, and each column of this matrix corresponds to 100 λ values chosen for that particular value of γ. We use the which() function to find which one has the lowest estimated mean squared error.

```
cv_res <- sapply(cv_l0l2$cvMeans, as.numeric)
min_ind <- which(cv_res == min(cv_res), arr.ind = TRUE)
min_ind
#>      row col
#> [1,]  11  10
```

We can then extract out the corresponding γ and λ values through the `fit` object returned in our result.

```
gamma_min <- cv_l0l2$fit$gamma[[min_ind[2]]]
lambda_min <- cv_l0l2$fit$lambda[[min_ind[2]]][min_ind[1]]
```

We find the estimated coefficients for this model using the `coef()` function on the cross-validation object `cv_l0l2`.

```
cv_coef_l0 <- coef(cv_l0l2, gamma = gamma_min, lambda = lambda_min)
rownames(cv_coef_l0) <- c("Intercept", colnames(x))
cv_coef_l0
#> 16 x 1 sparse Matrix of class "dgCMatrix"
#>
#> Intercept               4.61671
#> AGE                     0.00382
#> SEXFemale               .
#> RACEOther Hispanic      .
#> RACENon-Hispanic White  .
#> RACENon-Hispanic Black  0.04216
#> RACEOther Race          .
#> EDUCATIONHS             .
#> EDUCATIONMoreThanHS     .
#> INCOME                  .
#> SMOKEQuitSmoke          .
#> SMOKEStillSmoke         .
#> LEAD                    .
#> BMI_CAT25<BMI<30        .
#> BMI_CATBMI>=30          .
#> ALCYes                  .
```

Last, we use the `predict()` function on `cv_l0l2` to evaluate our resulting model. To do so, we need to specify λ and γ as well as our data x. This model is much sparser than the ones in the previous section, but our mean squared error on our training data is a little higher.

```
pred_l0l2 <- predict(cv_l0l2, gamma = gamma_min,
                     lambda = lambda_min, newx = x)
mean((nhanes$SBP - exp(pred_l0l2))^2)
#> [1] 275
```

15.4 Exercises

For these exercises, we use the `nyts` data from Chapter 14. Our outcome of interest is whether or not someone uses any tobacco product.

1. Create a new variable `tobacco_use` representing any tobacco use in the past 30 days (including e-cigarettes, cigarettes, and/or cigars). Then, create a new data frame `nyts_sub` that contains this new column as well as columns for location, age, sex, race, whether someone identifies with the LGBT community, grades in the past year, perceived_cigarette use, perceived e-cigarette use, psych distress, and family affluence.

2. Create an outcome vector `y` corresponding to the column `tobacco_use` and a model matrix `x` containing all other covariates.

3. Fit a L1 (lasso), L2 (ridge), and L0 (best subset) penalized regression model using 5-fold cross-validation. Create a data frame with the corresponding coefficients for all models. Be sure to update the loss function to reflect our binary outcome.

4. Report the AUC and accuracy of these three models on the training data.

16

Case Study: Predicting Tuberculosis Risk

For this chapter, we use the `tb_diagnosis` dataset seen in Chapter 6 from the **HDSinRdata** package. These data contains information on 1,762 patients in rural South Africa and urban Uganda who presented at a health clinic with tuberculosis-related symptoms and who were tested for tuberculosis (TB) using Xpert MTB/RIF (Baik et al. 2020). Our goal is to conduct a similar regression analysis to Baik et al. (2020) and use these data to derive a risk model for screening patients for treatment while awaiting Xpert results. Unlike Baik et al. (2020), we do not restrict our analysis to simple integer risk score models.

```
library(tidyverse)
library(HDSinRdata)
library(gt)
library(gtsummary)
library(glmnet)
library(pROC)
```

Similar to Baik et al. (2020), we use the data from rural South Africa to derive our risk model and use the data from urban Uganda as a withheld validation set. Further, we divide the data from South Africa into a training and test set using a 70/30 split.

```
# data from package
data(tb_diagnosis)

# training data
tb_southafrica <- tb_diagnosis %>%
  filter(country == "South Africa") %>%
  select(-country) %>%
  na.omit()

# validation data
tb_uganda <- tb_diagnosis %>%
  filter(country == "Uganda") %>%
```

```
  select(-country) %>%
  na.omit()

# train/test split
train_index <- sample(1:nrow(tb_southafrica),
                      0.70*nrow(tb_southafrica),
                      replace = FALSE)

tb_train <- tb_southafrica[train_index,]
tb_test <- tb_southafrica[-train_index,]
```

The following table shows our data stratified by TB diagnosis. We observe that our data are well balanced between the two groups and that we see key differences in the distributions of our observed clinical and demographic variables. For example, those whose blood results confirmed TB generally had more observed symptoms and were more likely to have had symptoms for over two weeks.

```
tbl_summary(tb_southafrica, by = c(tb),
            label = list(age_group ~ "Age",
                         hiv_pos ~ "HIV Positive",
                         diabetes ~ "Diabetes",
                         ever_smoke ~ "Ever Smoked",
                         past_tb ~ "Past TB Diagnosis",
                         male ~ "Male",
                         hs_less ~ "< HS Education",
                         two_weeks_symp ~ "Symptoms for Two Weeks",
                         num_symptoms ~ "Number of TB Symptoms")) %>%
    modify_spanning_header(c("stat_1", "stat_2") ~
                           "**TB Diagnosis**") %>%
    as_gt()
```

	TB Diagnosis	
Characteristic	**0**, N = 705[1]	**1**, N = 702[1]
Age		
[55,99)	170 (24%)	102 (15%)
[15,25)	121 (17%)	85 (12%)
[25,35)	120 (17%)	166 (24%)
[35,45)	136 (19%)	202 (29%)
[45,55)	158 (22%)	147 (21%)
HIV Positive		
0	519 (74%)	331 (47%)

1	186 (26%)	371 (53%)
Diabetes		
0	683 (97%)	677 (96%)
1	22 (3.1%)	25 (3.6%)
Ever Smoked		
0	492 (70%)	419 (60%)
1	213 (30%)	283 (40%)
Past TB Diagnosis		
0	613 (87%)	574 (82%)
1	92 (13%)	128 (18%)
Male		
0	395 (56%)	275 (39%)
1	310 (44%)	427 (61%)
< HS Education		
0	73 (10%)	46 (6.6%)
1	632 (90%)	656 (93%)
Symptoms for Two Weeks		
0	258 (37%)	106 (15%)
1	447 (63%)	596 (85%)
Number of TB Symptoms		
1	427 (61%)	174 (25%)
2	181 (26%)	163 (23%)
3	67 (9.5%)	199 (28%)
4	30 (4.3%)	166 (24%)

[1]n (%)

16.1 Model Selection

Our goal is to predict TB diagnosis. We compare two risk models: a logistic regression model and a lasso logistic regression model. For both of these models, we fit our model on the training data. For the lasso model, we use 5-fold cross-validation to choose the penalty parameter. In the following code, we create a table with the estimated exponentiated coefficients.

```
# fit logistic model
mod_logistic <- glm(tb ~ ., data = tb_train, family = binomial)

# fit lasso model with CV
X_train <- model.matrix(tb~., data = tb_train)[, -1]
y_train <- tb_train[,1]
```

```
mod_lasso_cv <- cv.glmnet(X_train, y_train, alpha = 1,
                          family = "binomial", nfolds = 5)

# refit for given lambda
mod_lasso <- glmnet(X_train, y_train, alpha = 1, family = "binomial",
                    lambda = mod_lasso_cv$lambda.min)

# create data frame
coef_df <- data.frame(Logistic = signif(exp(coef(mod_logistic)), 3),
                      Lasso =
                          signif(exp(as.numeric(coef(mod_lasso))), 3))
coef_df
#>                        Logistic  Lasso
#> (Intercept)              0.0451 0.0671
#> age_group[15,25)         1.4300 1.1500
#> age_group[25,35)         2.8500 2.2600
#> age_group[35,45)         2.2400 1.8200
#> age_group[45,55)         1.5000 1.2300
#> hiv_pos1                 2.3800 2.3300
#> diabetes1                1.5100 1.2300
#> ever_smoke1              0.7410 0.8270
#> past_tb1                 1.3800 1.2900
#> male1                    2.5000 2.2300
#> hs_less1                 1.2100 1.1100
#> two_weeks_symp1          2.8500 2.6600
#> num_symptoms2            1.9900 1.8500
#> num_symptoms3            6.8900 6.1900
#> num_symptoms4            9.1400 8.1100
```

After fitting both models, we evaluate model performance on the withheld
test set using an ROC curve. The ROC curve shows similar discrimination for
both models. Therefore, we choose the lasso model for its potential sparsity
and parsimony.

```
par(mfrow = c(1,2))

# logistic regression model ROC
pred_test_logistic <- predict(mod_logistic, tb_test,
                              type = "response")
roc_test_logistic <- roc(predictor = pred_test_logistic,
                         response = tb_test$tb,
                         levels = c(0,1), direction = "<")
```

```
plot(roc_test_logistic, print.auc = TRUE)


# lasso model ROC
X_test <- model.matrix(tb~., data = tb_test)[,-1]
pred_test_lasso <- as.numeric(predict(mod_lasso, newx = X_test,
                                type = "response"))
roc_test_lasso <- roc(predictor = pred_test_lasso,
                  response = tb_test$tb,
                  levels = c(0,1), direction = "<")

plot(roc_test_lasso, print.auc = TRUE)
```

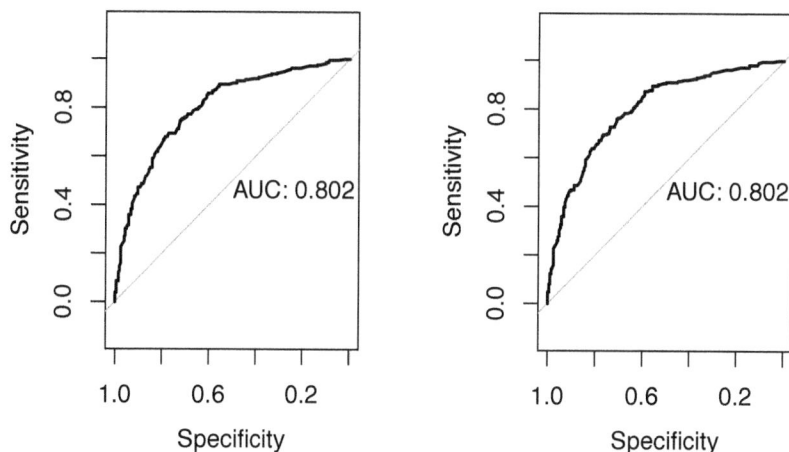

We refit the lasso model on the full data from South Africa and present the updated model in the subsequent code chunk.

```
# fit lasso model with CV
X_train_full <- model.matrix(tb~., data = tb_southafrica)[, -1]
y_train_full <- tb_southafrica[,1]
mod_cv_full <- cv.glmnet(X_train_full, y_train_full, alpha = 1,
                    family = "binomial", nfolds = 5)

# refit for given lambda
mod_full <- glmnet(X_train_full, y_train_full, alpha = 1,
                family = "binomial",
                lambda = mod_cv_full$lambda.min)
```

```
# create data frame
coef_df <- data.frame(
  Variable = c("Intercept", colnames(X_train_full)),
  Lasso = signif(exp(as.numeric(coef(mod_full))), 3))
coef_df
#>               Variable Lasso
#> 1            Intercept 0.102
#> 2    age_group[15,25) 1.000
#> 3    age_group[25,35) 1.830
#> 4    age_group[35,45) 1.350
#> 5    age_group[45,55) 1.000
#> 6             hiv_pos1 2.450
#> 7            diabetes1 1.380
#> 8          ever_smoke1 0.941
#> 9             past_tb1 1.090
#> 10              male1 2.050
#> 11            hs_less1 1.050
#> 12   two_weeks_symp1 2.290
#> 13      num_symptoms2 1.640
#> 14      num_symptoms3 4.970
#> 15      num_symptoms4 8.130
```

16.2 Evaluate Model on Validation Data

We then evaluate the lasso model on the withheld validation data. This data
comes from clinics in urban Uganda and contains only 387 observations. The
generated table shows that this population differs from our training population
including having a lower proportion of patients diagnosed with TB.

```
tbl_summary(tb_diagnosis, by = c(country),
            label = list(tb ~ "TB Diagnosis",
                         age_group ~ "Age",
                         hiv_pos ~ "HIV Positive",
                         diabetes ~ "Diabetes",
                         ever_smoke ~ "Ever Smoked",
                         past_tb ~ "Past TB Diagnosis",
                         male ~ "Male",
                         hs_less ~ "< HS Education",
```

```
                    two_weeks_symp ~ "Symptoms for Two Weeks",
                    num_symptoms ~ "Number of TB Symptoms")) %>%
    modify_spanning_header(c("stat_1", "stat_2") ~ "**Country**") %>%
    as_gt()
```

	Country	
Characteristic	**South Africa**, N = 1,407[1]	**Uganda**, N = 387[1]
TB Diagnosis		
0	705 (50%)	281 (73%)
1	702 (50%)	106 (27%)
Age		
[55,99)	272 (19%)	20 (5.2%)
[15,25)	206 (15%)	86 (22%)
[25,35)	286 (20%)	129 (33%)
[35,45)	338 (24%)	99 (26%)
[45,55)	305 (22%)	53 (14%)
HIV Positive		
0	850 (60%)	256 (66%)
1	557 (40%)	131 (34%)
Diabetes		
0	1,360 (97%)	383 (99%)
1	47 (3.3%)	4 (1.0%)
Ever Smoked		
0	911 (65%)	328 (85%)
1	496 (35%)	59 (15%)
Past TB Diagnosis		
0	1,187 (84%)	331 (86%)
1	220 (16%)	56 (14%)
Male		
0	670 (48%)	199 (51%)
1	737 (52%)	188 (49%)
< HS Education		
0	119 (8.5%)	30 (7.8%)
1	1,288 (92%)	357 (92%)
Symptoms for Two Weeks		
0	364 (26%)	63 (16%)
1	1,043 (74%)	324 (84%)
Number of TB Symptoms		
1	601 (43%)	156 (40%)
2	344 (24%)	128 (33%)
3	266 (19%)	68 (18%)
4	196 (14%)	35 (9.0%)

[1]n (%)

The ROC curve shows that the AUC on the validation data is lower than on the training data but still maintains meaningful discrimination.

```
# lasso validation roc
X_val <- model.matrix(tb~., data = tb_uganda)[, -1]
pred_val <- as.numeric(predict(mod_full, newx = X_val,
                                       type = "response"))
roc_val_lasso <- roc(predictor = pred_val,
                     response = tb_uganda$tb,
                     levels = c(0,1), direction = "<")

plot(roc_val_lasso, print.auc = TRUE)
```

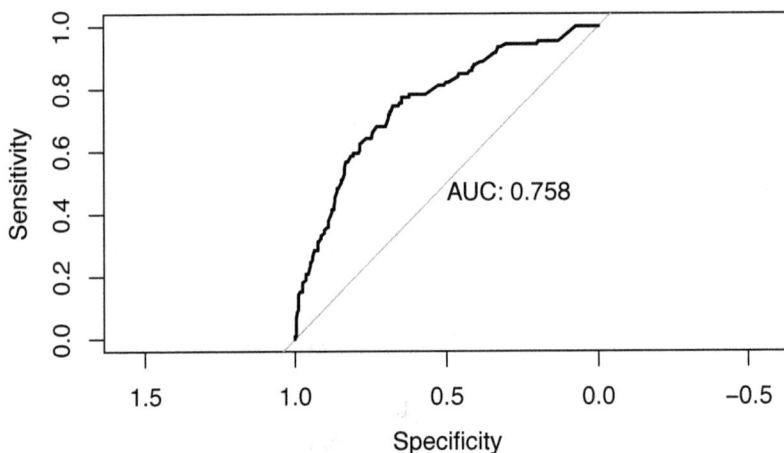

Part V

Writing Larger Programs

17

Logic and Loops

Now that we have seen a lot of the functionality of R, we can start to build up more structured code using programming structures. To start, we introduce *control flows*. Control flows are code blocks that determine a sequence of code to be run. The two types of control flows we introduce are if-else blocks and loops.

```
library(HDSinRdata)
library(tidyverse)
```

17.1   Logic and Conditional Expressions

You may recall that we introduced logical operators in Chapter 3. We used these operators through conditional expressions such as when we indexed a data frame or the `ifelse()` or `casewhen()` functions. For example, in the following code we have vectors of systolic and diastolic blood pressure measurements, and we write a logical operator to check if at least one of the systolic measurements is above 140 or if at least one of the diastolic measurements is above 90.

```
sbp_measurements <- c(131, 110, 125, 145, NA, 130)
dbp_measurements <- c(70, NA, 80)
any(sbp_measurements > 140, na.rm = TRUE) |
  any(dbp_measurements > 90, na.rm = TRUE)
#> [1] TRUE
```

Let's look at another example. Suppose these blood pressure measurements were taken consecutively but may have missing values. We want to create a single value to summarize the blood pressure for the patient. If we only have one blood pressure reading, then we use that value. However, if there is more than one blood pressure reading, then we drop the first observation and average the rest. We assume that not all values are NA. The following code uses an `ifelse()` function to do this by first checking if there is a single reading. If so, it takes the sum removing NA values to find that value. If not, we find all non-NA values and remove the first one before averaging.

```
sbp_measurements <- c(131, 110, 125, 145, NA, 130)
ifelse(sum(!is.na(sbp_measurements)) == 1,
       sum(sbp_measurements, na.rm = TRUE),
       mean(sbp_measurements[!is.na(sbp_measurements)][-1]))
#> [1] 128
```

We could also accomplish the same thing using a *control flow* called an *if-else statement*. An if-else statement follows the following structure. First, we have a conditional statement. If the conditional statement is true, then the code in the if statement, the code within the first set of curly braces, is run. If not, then the code in the else statement is run. In this way, the control flow controls how our code is executed.

```
if (conditional statement){
block of code if the statement is TRUE
} else{
block of code if the statement is FALSE
}
```

The next code chunk shows an example where the conditional statement is the same as previously. Note that since either the code in the if or else statement is run, the object `avg_val` is always defined.

```
sbp_measurements <- c(131, 110, 125, 145, NA, 130)
if(sum(!is.na(sbp_measurements)) == 1){
  avg_val <- sum(sbp_measurements, na.rm = TRUE)
} else{
  avg_val <- mean(sbp_measurements[!is.na(sbp_measurements)][-1])
}
avg_val
#> [1] 128
```

One of the things to notice is that an `if` statement can only take in a *single* Boolean. It cannot take in a vector of Boolean values like the `ifelse()` and `case_when()` functions can. In that way, the `ifelse()` function is useful because it can be applied to multiple instances, but it isn't as flexible if you want to run multiple lines of code depending on the logical statement since it doesn't allow you to include a code block.

Let's do another example of both an if-else statement and the `ifelse()` function to demonstrate this. In the following code, we use an if-else statement to determine if someone has hypertension. Note that here we have two lines of code that are run in each part: one line is printing the result and the other is storing a 0/1 value. Try changing the values of sbp and dbp.

```
sbp <- 130
dbp <- 80
if(sbp > 140 | dbp > 90){
  print("Hypertension")
  hyp <- 1
} else{
  print("No Hypertension")
  hyp <- 0
}
#> [1] "No Hypertension"
hyp
#> [1] 0
```

Now let's replicate this with the ifelse() function which allows us to take in paired vectors of blood pressure measurements and return a vector of 0/1 values for each observation. The difference here is that we cannot include a print statement since we are only allowed one return value.

```
sbp_measurements <- c(131, 110, 125, 145, 130)
dbp_measurements <- c(90, 75, 80, 90, 80)
hyp <- ifelse(sbp_measurements > 140 | dbp_measurements > 90, 1, 0)
hyp
#> [1] 0 0 0 1 0
```

Note that in the previous code we ignored NA values. In this case, changing sbp or dbp to NA causes an error in the if-else statement. This is because it does not understand which code block to run. The ifelse() can handle NA values and returns NA for observations with no TRUE/FALSE value. To accomplish this with the if-else statement, we can add in multiple conditions. In particular, we can add in more statements as follows. In this case, the first time we reach a true conditional statement, we run the code in that block. If no statements are true, then we run the last block of code. So we always run exactly one block of code.

```
if (conditional statement A){
block of code if the statement A is TRUE
} else if (conditional statement B){
block of code if the statement B is TRUE and statement A is FALSE
} else if (conditional statement C){
block of code if the statement C is TRUE and statement A and B are FALSE
```

```
} else{
block of code if statements A, B, and C are all FALSE
}
```

Let's use this with our hypertension example. In this case, we want to return NA if the answer is not known. Change the values so that you reach each code block. The order of the conditions matters because if the first statement is false, then we know at least one value is not NA. This also means that we would only check the fourth condition if the first three are false, which means that neither of the values can be NA.

```
sbp <- 130
dbp <- 80
if(is.na(sbp) & is.na(dbp)){
  # Both are NA
  hyp <- NA
} else if ((is.na(sbp) & dbp <= 90) | (is.na(dbp) & sbp <= 140)){
  # One is NA and the other is below the threshold
  hyp <- "Inconclusive"
} else if ((is.na(sbp) & dbp > 90) | (is.na(dbp) & sbp > 140)){
  # One is NA and the other is above the threshold
  hyp <- "Hypertension"
} else if (dbp > 90 | sbp > 140){
  # Neither are NA and at least one is above the threshold
  hyp <- "Hypertension"
} else{
  # Neither are NA and neither is above the threshold
  hyp <- "No Hypertension"
}
hyp
#> [1] "No Hypertension"
```

We can rearrange these conditions to have one less condition. In the following code chunk, we first check if both are NA. Then we check that at least one value is above the threshold. This statement uses the fact that both can't be NA since the first condition must be false. Next, in the third statement, if at least one value is NA, then that must mean the other is below the threshold, so the result is inconclusive.

```
sbp <- 130
dbp <- 80
if(is.na(sbp) & is.na(dbp)){
  # Both are NA
  hyp <- NA
```

```
} else if (sum(dbp > 90, sbp > 140, na.rm=TRUE) >= 1){
  # At least one is above the threshold - sum removes NA values
  hyp <- "Hypertension"
} else if (is.na(sbp) | is.na(dbp)){
  # Inconclusive
  hyp <- "Inconclusive"
} else{
  # Neither is NA and neither is above the threshold
  hyp <- "No Hypertension"
}
hyp
#> [1] "No Hypertension"
```

This can still seem like a lot of conditions to replicate what we did in a single line with an `ifelse()` function. In general, we prefer a simpler format. Consider the following code. In this case, we have two vectors x and y that we want to plot. First, we check whether these vectors are numeric. If not, we convert them to factors. Rather than returning a value as we do with an `ifelse()` function, we are changing our data depending on the type of x and y. Note that these statements do not contain an else statement. That is because we don't want to run any code when the condition is false. For these single-expression `if` statements, we technically don't need the curly braces for R to understand what code to run, but we consider it good practice to always wrap your code in curly braces when writing control flows.

```
# example x and y vectors
y <- factor(rbinom(100, 1, 0.3))
x <- rnorm(100, ifelse(y == 0, 0, 0.75))
# change x to factor(rbinom(100, 1, 0.3)) to observe

# convert x and y to factors if not numeric!
if (!is.numeric(x)){ x <- as.factor(x) }
if (!is.numeric(y)){ y <- as.factor(y) }

# find type of plot
if(is.factor(x) & is.factor(y)){
  # barplot
  p <- ggplot() + geom_bar(aes(x = x, fill = y), position = "dodge")
} else if (!is.factor(y) | !(is.factor(x))){
  # boxplot when one numeric, one factor
  p <- ggplot() + geom_boxplot(aes(x = x, y = y))
} else{
  # scatter plot when both numeric
```

```
  p <- ggplot() + geom_point(aes(x = x, y = y))
}
p
```

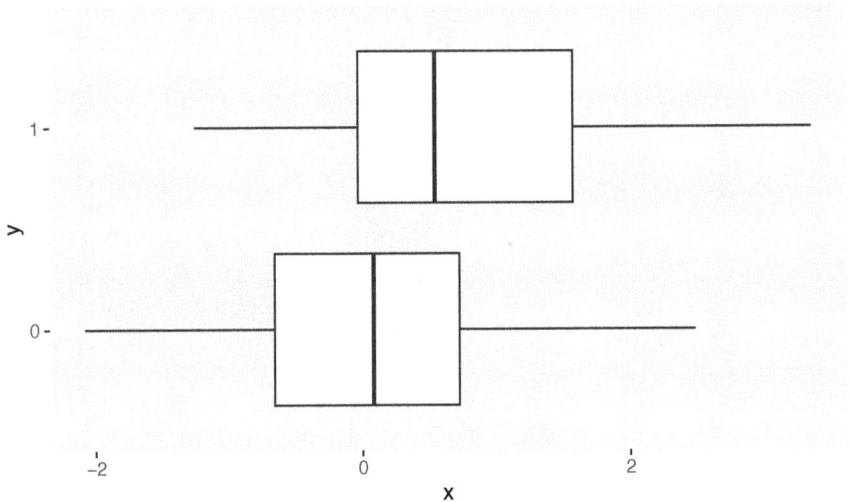

17.1.1 Practice Question

Use both an if-else statement and a `case_when()` function to find y as given
by the following function.

$$y = \begin{cases} 1 & x > 0 \\ 0 & x = 0 \\ 0.1 & x < 0 \end{cases}$$

```
# Insert your solution here:
x <- 2 # change x to different values to check your solution!
```

17.2 Loops

Another common control flow we use is loops. Loops capture code chunks we
want to run multiple times. For this example, we use the NHANESSample data
from the **HDSinRdata** package.

```
nhanes <- NHANESsample %>%
  select(c(RACE, SEX, SBP1, DBP1, HYP, LEAD)) %>%
  na.omit()
```

In the following code, we are fitting a simple linear regression model for systolic blood pressure with the single covariate of blood lead level for each race group and storing the associated coefficients and p-values. This code is repetitive, since we repeat the same steps for each group and the only element that is changing is the race group. This makes our code cluttered but also means we are prone to introducing errors. In fact, you can see that we have the wrong coefficient and p-value for the fourth model.

```
dat1 <- nhanes[nhanes$RACE == "Mexican American", ]
mod1 <- summary(lm(SBP1 ~ LEAD, data = dat1))
coef1 <- mod1$coefficients[2, 1]
pval1 <- mod1$coefficients[2, 4]

dat2 <- nhanes[nhanes$RACE == "Non-Hispanic White", ]
mod2 <- summary(lm(SBP1 ~ LEAD, data = dat2))
coef2 <- mod2$coefficients[2, 1]
pval2 <- mod2$coefficients[2, 4]

dat3 <- nhanes[nhanes$RACE == "Non-Hispanic Black", ]
mod3 <- summary(lm(SBP1 ~ LEAD, data = dat3))
coef3 <- mod3$coefficients[2, 1]
pval3 <- mod3$coefficients[2, 4]

dat4 <- nhanes[nhanes$RACE == "Other Hispanic", ]
mod4 <- summary(lm(SBP1 ~ LEAD, data = dat4))
coef4 <- mod3$coefficients[2, 1]
pval4 <- mod3$coefficients[2, 4]

dat5 <- nhanes[nhanes$RACE == "Other Race", ]
mod5 <- summary(lm(SBP1 ~ LEAD, data = dat5))
coef5 <- mod5$coefficients[2, 1]
pval5 <- mod5$coefficients[2, 4]

data.frame(
  group = c("Mexican American", "Non-Hispanic White",
            "Non-Hispanic Black", "Other Hispanic", "Other Race"),
  coefs = c(coef1, coef2, coef3, coef4, coef5),
  pvals = c(pval1, pval2, pval3, pval4, pval5))
#>                group coefs      pvals
```

```
#> 1    Mexican American 0.783  3.97e-11
#> 2 Non-Hispanic White 2.500  7.81e-138
#> 3 Non-Hispanic Black 2.005  1.83e-51
#> 4      Other Hispanic 2.005  1.83e-51
#> 5          Other Race 1.927  1.06e-11
```

We can rewrite this code slightly. In this case, we create an object i which represents the index of the group. This change means that the only thing that changes for each group is that we update the value of i. This is much less prone to errors, but still long.

```
# Initialize results data frame
race_values <- c("Mexican American", "Non-Hispanic White",
              "Non-Hispanic Black", "Other Hispanic", "Other Race")
df <- data.frame(
  group = race_values,
  coefs = 0,
  pvals = 0)

i <- 1
dat <- nhanes[nhanes$RACE == df$group[i], ]
mod <- summary(lm(SBP1 ~ LEAD, data = dat))
df$coef[i] <- mod$coefficients[2, 1]
df$pval[i] <- mod$coefficients[2, 4]

i <- 2
dat <- nhanes[nhanes$RACE == df$group[i], ]
mod <- summary(lm(SBP1 ~ LEAD, data = dat))
df$coef[i] <- mod$coefficients[2, 1]
df$pval[i] <- mod$coefficients[2, 4]

i <- 3
dat <- nhanes[nhanes$RACE == df$group[i], ]
mod <- summary(lm(SBP1 ~ LEAD, data = dat))
df$coef[i] <- mod$coefficients[2, 1]
df$pval[i] <- mod$coefficients[2, 4]

i <- 4
dat <- nhanes[nhanes$RACE == df$group[i], ]
mod <- summary(lm(SBP1 ~ LEAD, data = dat))
df$coef[i] <- mod$coefficients[2, 1]
df$pval[i] <- mod$coefficients[2, 4]
```

```
i <- 5
dat <- nhanes[nhanes$RACE == df$group[i], ]
mod <- summary(lm(SBP1 ~ LEAD, data = dat))
df$coef[i] <- mod$coefficients[2, 1]
df$pval[i] <- mod$coefficients[2, 4]

df
#>                   group coefs pvals  coef        pval
#> 1    Mexican American       0     0 0.783   3.97e-11
#> 2 Non-Hispanic White       0     0 2.500  7.81e-138
#> 3 Non-Hispanic Black       0     0 2.005   1.83e-51
#> 4      Other Hispanic       0     0 1.242   8.46e-09
#> 5          Other Race       0     0 1.927   1.06e-11
```

We now write this code as a *for loop*. A for loop contains two pieces. First, we
have an *iterator*. An iterator traverses an object that has a natural order. Most
of the time we traverse over vectors, but we could also have a list object. The
second piece is a code block. This code is run for each value of the iterator.

```
for (iterator_name in object){
code to run for each value of the iterator
}
```

Two simple for loops are given in the next code chunk. In the first loop, our
iterator goes through the vector 1:5, whereas in the second one our iterator
iterates through the vector of names. In the first loop, we traverse the numbers
1 to 5 and for each number we run the code that squares the number. In each
iteration, we name the current number we are on to be i. That means that
the first time through the loop i is equal to 1, the second time i has value 2,
etc. In the second loop, our iterator is also a vector, but this time it is names.
In this case, in each iteration the object name represents the current name we
are on as we traverse the vector of names. In particular, the first time through
the loop name is equal to "Alice", the second time name has value "Bob", and
so forth.

```
for (i in 1:5){
  print(sqrt(i))
}
#> [1] 1
#> [1] 1.41
#> [1] 1.73
#> [1] 2
#> [1] 2.24
```

```
names <- c("Alice", "Bob", "Carol")
for (name in names){
  print(paste("Hello,", name))
}
#> [1] "Hello, Alice"
#> [1] "Hello, Bob"
#> [1] "Hello, Carol"
```

Let's apply this to our example. First, we use a numeric iterator i that takes on values 1 to 5. This directly replicates our previous code in which the value of i changed for each race group. Our result matches our previous result.

```
df <- data.frame(group = race_values, coefs = 0, pvals = 0)

for (i in 1:5){
  dat <- nhanes[nhanes$RACE == df$group[i], ]
  mod <- summary(lm(SBP1 ~ LEAD, data = dat))
  df$coef[i] <- mod$coefficients[2, 1]
  df$pval[i] <- mod$coefficients[2, 4]
}
df
#>                  group coefs pvals  coef       pval
#> 1    Mexican American     0     0 0.783   3.97e-11
#> 2  Non-Hispanic White     0     0 2.500  7.81e-138
#> 3  Non-Hispanic Black     0     0 2.005   1.83e-51
#> 4       Other Hispanic     0     0 1.242   8.46e-09
#> 5          Other Race     0     0 1.927   1.06e-11
```

Let's show a different way we could write the same loop. This time we set our iterator to be the race group name. In this case, we update how we are storing the coefficients and p-values because we are not iterating over an index.

```
coefs <- c()
pvals <- c()

for (group in race_values){
  dat <- nhanes[nhanes$RACE == group, ]
  mod <- summary(lm(SBP1 ~ LEAD, data = dat))
  coefs <- c(coefs, mod$coefficients[2, 1])
  pvals <- c(pvals, mod$coefficients[2, 4])
}
```

```
data.frame(group = race_values, coefs = coefs, pvals = pvals)
#>                  group coefs      pvals
#> 1    Mexican American 0.783   3.97e-11
#> 2 Non-Hispanic White 2.500  7.81e-138
#> 3 Non-Hispanic Black 2.005   1.83e-51
#> 4      Other Hispanic 1.242   8.46e-09
#> 5          Other Race 1.927   1.06e-11
```

Another type of loop is a *while loop*. A while loop does not have an iterator. Instead, a while loop checks a condition. If the condition is true, the loop runs the code in the code block. If the condition is false, it stops and breaks out of the loop. That is, the code is run until the condition is no longer met.

```
while (condition){
code to run each iteration
}
```

The following code gives an example of a simple while loop. In this case, the loop keeps dividing x by 2 until it is below a certain value of 3. In this case, x starts above 3, so the condition starts off being true, and we would divide x by 2 to get 50. Since 50 is still greater than 3, the code block is run again, etc. Once x reaches a value of 1.5625, the condition no longer holds and the code stops. Note that if the condition was x > -1, it would hold indefinitely, creating what is called an infinite loop.

```
x <- 100
while(x > 3){
  x <- x/2
}
x
#> [1] 1.56
```

Let's do another example with a bigger code block. The following code creates a Poisson process of arrivals where in each iteration we generate the next arrival time by drawing from an exponential distribution. Once we reach the end of the time interval (i.e., the current time is greater than 10) we stop. If we re-run this chunk of code, we might get a different length vector.

```
arrivals <- c()
time <- 0
next_arrival <- rexp(1, rate = 3)

# Find the time of all arrivals in the time period [0,10]
```

```
while(time+next_arrival <= 10){
  # Update list of arrivals and current time
  arrivals <- c(arrivals, next_arrival)
  time <- time + next_arrival

  # Generate the next arrival
  next_arrival <- rexp(1, rate = 3)
}
```

Given that we have two types of loops, how do you know which to use? You should use a for loop when you know how many times you go through the loop and/or if there is a clear object to iterate through. On the other hand, while loops are useful if you don't know how many times you go through the loop and you want to iterate through the loop *until* something happens. Within a for loop, you can also break out early using the break operator. This stops the loop similar to a while loop but is sometimes less succinct. The following code loops through the blood pressure measurements we defined earlier to find if any of the observations meet the criteria for hypertension.

```
# Start with assumption that the result is FALSE
res <- FALSE
for (i in 1:length(sbp_measurements)){

  # If above threshold, update the result and stop the loop
  if (sbp_measurements[i] > 140 | dbp_measurements[i] < 90){
    res <- TRUE
    break
  }
}
```

17.2.1   Practice Question

Use a loop to find the smallest integer number x such that $2.3^x \geq 100$. The answer should be 6.

```
# Insert your solution here:
```

17.3 Avoiding Control Flows with Functions

We just introduced logic and loops, and now I'm going to tell you to avoid them when you can. Control flows are very useful programming structures, but sometimes the same thing can be done without them. For example, we can find whether there is at least one observation that has hypertension using a single line of code.

```
any(sbp_measurements > 140 | dbp_measurements > 90)
#> [1] TRUE
```

Another example we saw previously was using an `ifelse()` or `case_when()` function instead of an if-else statement. These two functions are *vectorized functions*. That means that the function is evaluated on a vector of values rather than having to loop through each value separately. Vectorized functions return a vector or results of the same size as your input. That means that if you needed to do a computation on every element of a vector, you could either loop through all the elements and call that function *or* you can take advantage of the vectorized structure and call the function on the whole vector. This is generally cleaner and more efficient. The `any()` function is not a vectorized function since it returns a single TRUE/FALSE value, but it also helps to make our code cleaner.

Another tool that can help with brevity in this manner is the family of *apply functions*. These are loop-hiding functions. In Chapter 3, we saw the `apply(X, MARGIN, FUN)` function. This function called the function `FUN` on either the rows (`MARGIN = 1`) or columns (`MARGIN = 2`) of `X`, which is data frame or matrix `X`. In the next code chunk, we generate a random matrix `X` and compute the column means using a loop and using the `apply()` function. We can see that the version with the `apply()` function is simpler.

```
X <- matrix(rnorm(100), nrow = 20, ncol = 5)

# Apply mean function
apply(X, 2, mean)
#> [1]  0.0768 -0.1682 -0.4058  0.0328 -0.1283

# Loop through columns
means <- rep(0, ncol(X))
for (i in 1:ncol(X)){
  means[i] <- mean(X[, i])
}
```

17 Logic and Loops

```
means
#> [1]  0.0768 -0.1682 -0.4058  0.0328 -0.1283
```

Another loop-hiding function is `lapply(X, FUN)`. This function applies the function X to each element of X. In this case, X functions like an iterator, and FUN is a function representing what we want to do in each iteration. The result is returned as a list of the function output for each value of X. We use this function in the regression context we saw earlier. Here, X is our vector of groups, and we have written a custom function to be able to call that code on each group. We learn how to write our own functions in Chapter 18.

```
find_lm_results <- function(group){
    # Runs simple linear regression and returns coefficient and p-value
    dat <- nhanes[nhanes$RACE == group, ]
    mod <- summary(lm(SBP1 ~ LEAD, data = dat))
    return(mod$coefficients[2, c(1, 4)])
}
```

```
lapply(race_values, find_lm_results)
#> [[1]]
#> Estimate Pr(>|t|)
#> 7.83e-01 3.97e-11
#>
#> [[2]]
#>   Estimate  Pr(>|t|)
#>   2.50e+00 7.81e-138
#>
#> [[3]]
#> Estimate Pr(>|t|)
#> 2.01e+00 1.83e-51
#>
#> [[4]]
#> Estimate Pr(>|t|)
#> 1.24e+00 8.46e-09
#>
#> [[5]]
#> Estimate Pr(>|t|)
#> 1.93e+00 1.06e-11
```

Another useful function is `sapply(X, FUN)`. This function operates similarly to `lapply()`. However, it then tries to simplify the output to be either a vector or matrix. You can remember the difference by remembering the l in `lapply()` stands for list, and the s in `sapply()` stands for simplify.

```
sapply(race_values, find_lm_results)
#>              Mexican American Non-Hispanic White Non-Hispanic Black
#> Estimate            7.83e-01             2.50e+00             2.01e+00
#> Pr(>|t|)            3.97e-11             7.81e-138            1.83e-51
#>           Other Hispanic Other Race
#> Estimate        1.24e+00   1.93e+00
#> Pr(>|t|)        8.46e-09   1.06e-11
```

The last loop-hiding function we introduce is `replicate(n, expr)`. This runs
the code expression `expr` n times and returns the results. By default, this
simplifies the output similar to `sapply()`. If you set `simplify=FALSE`, it returns
a list. The following code generates a random matrix and computes the column
means six times.

```
replicate(6, colMeans(matrix(rnorm(100), ncol = 5)))
#>            [,1]    [,2]    [,3]     [,4]     [,5]     [,6]
#> [1,]   0.30815   0.278  0.4122 -0.1929   0.1030   0.0692
#> [2,]   0.21620   0.225 -0.2344 -0.0579 -0.0966   0.1656
#> [3,]   0.00271  -0.147  0.0628  0.1923   0.3118   0.0875
#> [4,]  -0.04880   0.239  0.1706 -0.0846   0.1923 -0.1693
#> [5,]   0.31253   0.183 -0.4122  0.5335   0.1544 -0.3784
```

17.4 Exercises

For these exercises, we use the `pain` data from the **HDSinRdata** package.
You can use the help operator `?pain` to learn more about the source of these
data and to read its column descriptions.

1. Create a new column `PAT_RACE_SIMP` that represents a patient's race
   using three categories: White, Black, or Other. First, do this using
   the `case_when()` function. Then, use a loop and if-else statement to
   accomplish the same thing.

2. For each category of your new column `PAT_RACE_SIMP`, subset the
   data to that group and find the five body regions with the highest proportion of patients with pain. Your solution should use two
   nested loops. Then, rewrite your code without using a loop.

3. The following code sorts a numeric vector x but is missing comments

to explain the steps. Read through the code and add your own comments to explain how this works.

```
x <- c(1,3,0,3,2,6,4)

n <- length(x)
for (i in 1:(n-1)){

  next_ind <- i
  for (j in (i+1):n){
    if (x[j] < x[next_ind]){
      next_ind <- j
    }
  }

  temp <- x[i]
  x[i] <- x[next_ind]
  x[next_ind] <- temp
}

x
#> [1] 0 1 2 3 3 4 6
```

4. Write code using a loop that generates a series of Bernoulli random variables with probability of success of 0.5 until at least $r < -6$ successes occur. What distribution does this correspond to?

18

Functions

Functions are an important part of creating reproducible research and clean code. So far we have been using many useful functions from base R and available packages by learning how to specify the inputs and use the output. We now shift to writing our own functions. To start, we need to understand the arguments and return values of functions as well as the scope of objects used or created within functions. We also talk about how to document, test, and debug your functions so that we can ensure they are correct and easy to use. We use the **testthat** package to create simple tests for our functions.

```
library(testthat)
library(tidyverse)
```

One type of function we have already written is an *anonymous function*. These are functions that are not saved or given a name. These functions typically exist if we want to input a function argument to another function but we don't want to save that function for future use. For example, in the following code, we use the apply() function on a data frame to find the proportion of observations that are NA for each column. Note that since the function is so short, it is easy enough to define within the apply() function call by just including the code for what is returned. For functions with more than one line, you would not want to use an anonymous function and would need to define the function.

```
df <- data.frame(x1 = c(NA, 1, 1, 0),
                 x2 = c(0, 1, 0, 0),
                 x3 = c(0, 0, NA, NA))
apply(df, 2, function(x) sum(is.na(x)) / length(x))
#>   x1   x2   x3
#> 0.25 0.00 0.50
```

18.1   Components of a Function

To start storing functions, we need to give them a name and define their input (arguments) and output (return values). To do so, we assign a function name to a function object as shown in the following code. This example function has two arguments `arg1` and `arg2` and returns `output`.

```
function_name <- function(arg1, arg2){
  code to compute output from arguments
  return(output)
}
```

Take a look at the following simple function. The name of this function is `say_hello`, and there is no input (arguments) or output (return values) associated with this function. Instead, it just prints out a hello statement.

```
say_hello <- function(){
  print("Hello!")
}
```

Running the previous code creates an object called `say_hello` of the class `function`. We can run this function by calling it using empty parentheses (since there are no input arguments).

```
class(say_hello)
#> [1] "function"
```

```
say_hello()
#> [1] "Hello!"
```

We can add to this function by instead adding our first argument called `name` which is a string and then printing "Hello, [name]!". In the next code chunk, we use the `paste0()` function which concatenates the string arguments into a single string.

```
say_hello <- function(name){
  print(paste0("Hello, ", name, "!"))
}
say_hello("Weici")
#> [1] "Hello, Weici!"
```

18.1.1 Arguments

Arguments are inputs passed to functions so that they can complete the desired computation. We can also have default values for these arguments. In this case, those arguments do not have to be specified when calling the function. For example, `rnorm(10)` uses the default value for the mean to understand which distribution we want to use. In the following function, we find the Euclidean distance from a given (x,y,z) coordinate and the origin (0,0,0) with a default value of zero for all values.

```
dist_to_origin <- function(x = 0,y = 0,z = 0){
  return(((x - 0)^2 + (y - 0)^2 + (z - 0)^2)^(0.5))
}
```

If we call this function with no arguments, it uses all the default values.

```
dist_to_origin()
#> [1] 0
```

However, if we call the function with one argument, the function assumes this first argument is x. Similarly, it assumes the second value is y and the third value is z. If we want to give the arguments without worrying about the order, we can specify them using their names (see the last line in the following code chunk).

```
dist_to_origin(1)
#> [1] 1
dist_to_origin(1, 2)
#> [1] 2.24
dist_to_origin(1, 2, 3)
#> [1] 3.74
dist_to_origin(y = 2, z = 3)
#> [1] 3.61
```

Besides passing in numeric values, strings, data frames, lists, or vectors, we can also pass other types of objects in as arguments to a function. For example, we can take another function in as an argument. In the next example, we create two functions. The first function calculates the Euclidean distance between two points. The second one computes the distance from a given point to the origin. Note that this updated function to find the distance to the origin is more flexible and written in a cleaner manner. First, it allows us to input a point of any length. Second, it allows us to specify the distance function used. This also demonstrates calling a function within another function.

Try out calling `euclidean_dist()` and `dist_to_origin()` on different values.

```
euclidean_dist <- function(pt1, pt2){
  # Finds the Euclidean distance from pt1 to pt2
  return(sqrt(sum((pt1- pt2)^2)))
}

dist_to_origin <- function(pt1, dist_func = euclidean_dist){
  # Finds the distance from pt1 to the origin
  origin <- rep(0, length(pt1))
  return(dist_func(pt1, origin))
}

dist_to_origin(c(1,1))
#> [1] 1.41
```

18.1.2   Practice Question

Write a function that calculates the Manhattan distance between two points
`pt1` and `pt2`, where the Manhattan distance is the sum of absolute differences
between points across all the dimensions. To check your solution, you should
check that the distance between points `pt1 <- c(1,-1,1.5)` and `pt2 <- c(0.5,
2.5, -1)` is 6.5.

```
# Insert your solution here:
```

Another type of argument to a function can be a formula. If you have used
linear regression in R, you have seen this in practice. In the following code,
we fit a simple linear model where we specify a model formula y~x as the first
argument. We are also using default arguments for `rnorm()` on the first two
lines.

```
x <- rnorm(mean = 3, n = 100)
y <- x + rnorm(sd = 0.2, n = 100)

lm(y ~ x)
#>
#> Call:
#> lm(formula = y ~ x)
#>
#> Coefficients:
```

```
#> (Intercept)                  x
#>      0.0671          0.9946
```

18.1.3 Return Values

If we read the documentation for lm() by calling ?lm, we can see that there
are a lot of arguments that have default values. The other thing to note about
the lm documentation is that there are multiple values returned. In fact, the
type of object returned is a list containing all the different things we want to
know about the results such as the coefficients.

```
simp_model <- lm(y ~ x)
simp_model$coefficients
#> (Intercept)                  x
#>      0.0671          0.9946
```

Since R only allows you to return one object, packaging the return values into a
list is a useful way to return multiple outputs from a function. In the following
example, we create a function coin_flips() that takes in a probability prob
and a number of iterations n (with default value 10) and simulates n coin flips
where the coin has a probability of prob of landing on heads. The function
returns the percentage of trials that were heads and the results of the coin flips.
We can access each of these returned values by using the names percent_heads
and results.

```
coin_flips <- function(prob, n = 10){
  # Flips a coin with probability prob of heads for n trials

  results <- rbinom(n = n, size = 1, prob = prob)
  return(list(percent_heads = sum(results)/n, results = results))
}
trial <- coin_flips(0.6)
trial$percent_heads
#> [1] 0.5
trial$results
#>  [1] 0 0 0 1 1 1 0 1 0 1
```

One important thing to know about R and return values: if you don't specify
a return statement but assign the output of our function to an object, it
will assign the value to the last computed object by default. In the following
code, the value returned is 3. Avoid unexpected behavior by always using the
return() function.

```
ex_return <- function(){
  x <- 2
  y <- 3
}
result <- ex_return()
result
#> [1] 3
```

18.1.4 Scope of Objects

When working within functions and calling functions, we want to remember
the scope of our objects. *Global objects* are objects defined outside of functions.
These values can also be accessed outside or inside functions. For example, the
object y is defined outside of a function and so is a global object, meaning we
can use its value inside the function.

```
y <- "Cassandra"

ex_scope <- function(){
  return(paste("Hey,", y))
}

ex_scope()
#> [1] "Hey, Cassandra"
```

If we change the value of a global object within a function however, it does
not update the value outside of the function. In the subsequent code chunk,
we add 1 to y inside the function, but it does not change the value of y after
the function is done. Every time we run a function, R creates a new sub-
environment inside, which can access the values of global objects but also
creates its own *local objects*. In this case, the function creates its own object
y, which is a local object that is a copy of the original object.

As another example, the function also creates a local object called z which
ceases to exist after we run the function. If we try to print z on the last line,
we would get an error that z is not found. All objects created inside functions
only exist in that sub-environment and are erased when we are no longer in
the function. Therefore, we want to make sure we return any values we want
to store.

```
y <- 5
```

```
ex_local <- function(x){
  y <- y + 1
  z <- x * y
  return(y + z)
}
```

```
ex_local(2)
#> [1] 18
y
#> [1] 5
```

To update global objects within a function, you can use the <<- operator (global assignment operator). This looks for an object in the global environment and updates its value (or creates an object with this value if none is found). For example, the following function updates the value of the global objects y. As a general practice, we should be careful using global objects within a function, and it often is safer to use input arguments and return values instead.

```
y <- 5
```

```
ex_update_global <- function(x){
  y <<- y + 1
  return(y + x)
}
```

```
ex_update_global(2)
#> [1] 8
y
#> [1] 6
```

18.1.5 Functions within Functions and Returning Functions

Sometimes we see functions written inside other functions. Writing functions within functions can be useful to separate out some part of the code or to give that function access to the local environment objects. In the following example, the inner function has access to the value of x even though we have not passed it as an argument. The downside of this structure is that the function add_x() does not exist outside the function, so we cannot call it in other code.

```
add_x_seq <- function(x){
  # Adds x to 1:10 and returns
  add_x <- function(y){
      return(y + x)
  }

  return(add_x(1:10))
}

add_x_seq(3)
#>  [1]   4   5   6   7   8   9 10 11 12 13
#add_x(3) # would return an error
```

If we want to use the created function, we can return it. In the updated example, we return an anonymous function. By doing so, we create a unique function for each x value.

```
add_x <- function(x){
  # Returns a function to add x to any value
  return(function(y) y + x)
}

add2 <- add_x(2)
add2(1:10)
#>  [1]   3   4   5   6   7   8   9 10 11 12

add10 <- add_x(10)
add10(1:10)
#>  [1]  11 12 13 14 15 16 17 18 19 20
```

18.2 Documenting Functions

The functions we wrote had minimal comments or documentation. When creating functions, we should document them including any information about the format of the input and output. We do so using comments that precede the function and start with #'. This style of function documentation is called *roxygen*. The following code chunk shows an example for our Euclidean distance function. You can see we provided information about the two arguments and the return value. The roxygen style is the style used for published R packages.

```
#' Euclidean distance
#'
#' @description Calculates the Euclidean distance between two points
#'
#' @param pt1 numeric vector
#' @param pt2 numeric vector
#' @return the Euclidean distance from pt1 to pt2
euclidean_dist <- function(pt1, pt2){
  return((sum((pt1 - pt2)^2))^0.5)
}
```

Each comment should start with a pound sign and backtick. The first block of lines is the introduction, and the first line of the comment block is reserved for the title. This is the first information we want the user to know about the function and should be a single line. For all other information besides the title, we use certain tags.

- @description This tag should be placed first and is a place where you can briefly put more information about the function beyond the title. You can also add more details with the @details tag.

- @param This tag comes before each input argument's description. For each argument, we want to include the name and type, but we might also include information on how that argument is used.

- @return This tag documents the returned object and specifies the type. If we are returning a list, then we might include information about each object in the list.

18.2.1 Practice Question

Write the documentation for the following coin flip function.

```
#' Insert your solution here:
coin_flips <- function(prob, n = 10){
  results <- rbinom(n = n, size = 1, prob = prob)
  return(list(percent_heads = sum(results)/n, results = results))
}
```

18.3 Debugging and Testing

As we write more complex code and functions, we want to learn how to test our code. When it comes to testing code, a good mantra is "test early and test often". So avoid writing too much code before running and checking that the results match what you expect. Here are some simple principles that are applicable to debugging in any setting.

- Start simple and build up in steps.
- Check your syntax by checking that all parentheses (), brackets [], and curly braces {} match where you expect.
- Check that object names are correct and you don't have any accidental typos or that you are accidentally using the same name for different objects.
- Restart your R session and re-run all code.
- Check if you use the same object name for different objects.
- Localize your error by printing out the values of objects at each stage or use break points in R.
- Modify your code one piece at a time and check all test values again to avoid introducing new errors.

For example, suppose we want to write a function that finds any pairs of numeric columns with a Pearson correlation with absolute value above a certain threshold. We want our code to be structured so that it makes sense, is flexible to our needs, and avoids unnecessary work. To start building up this function, we need to first think about the inputs and outputs we want. This is called a *top-down approach*. Sketching out the overall steps your code needs to complete before writing any of them can help to improve your structure and avoid having to rewrite large pieces.

In this case, our input to this function is a data frame which could contain a mixture of numeric and categorical columns and a threshold correlation value with a default value of 0.6. We want to return a data frame with the pairs and their correlation. This gives us a template for our documentation.

```
#' Find pairs of columns with strong correlation
#'
#' @description Finds all pairs of numeric columns with strong Pearson
#' correlation and returns the pairs in a data frame
#'
#' @param df data frame
#' @param threshold positive numeric threshold value to define a
#' strong correlation as one with absolute value above the threshold
#' @return data frame with one row for each pair of columns
#' with high correlation containing the names of the columns
```

```
#' and the corresponding correlation
high_cor <- function(df, threshold = 0.6){
  return()
}
```

Next, to start simple, we want to create some artificial data we can use to test our function. We use the `mvnrorm()` function from the **MASS** package (Venables and Ripley 2002) to control the correlation between our columns and add in a categorical column that should be ignored by our function.

```
set.seed(4)
cor_mat <- matrix(c(1, 0.9, 0.4, 0,
                    0.9, 1, 0.3, 0,
                    0.4, 0.3, 1.0, 0,
                    0, 0, 0, 1.0), nrow = 4)
m <- round(MASS::mvrnorm(100, c(0,0,0,0), Sigma = cor_mat), 3)
test_df <- as.data.frame(m)
test_df$V5 <- sample(c("A", "B", "C"), 100, replace = TRUE)
high_cor(test_df)
#> NULL
```

We can use the `cor()` function to find the Pearson correlation.

```
cor(test_df[,-5])
#>         V1       V2      V3      V4
#> V1  1.0000   0.9006   0.324 -0.0797
#> V2  0.9006   1.0000   0.291 -0.0702
#> V3  0.3241   0.2912   1.000 -0.2306
#> V4 -0.0797  -0.0702  -0.231  1.0000
```

Great, now let's roughly sketch out the steps we need to complete.

1. Subset the data to only numeric columns.
2. Find the correlation of all pairs of columns.
3. Check if a pair has a strong correlation.
4. If so, add it to our results.

Let's start with step 1. Before putting code into our function, we are going to test our steps on our example data. To do so, we use the `select_if()` function from the **dplyr** package.

```
df_numeric <- select_if(test_df, is.numeric)
head(df_numeric)
#>        V1      V2      V3      V4
#> 1 -0.656   0.417   1.188   0.685
#> 2  0.117  -0.336  -1.611  -0.115
#> 3  1.229   0.617   0.241  -0.356
#> 4  0.478   0.121   1.176  -0.106
#> 5  1.546   1.914   0.366   0.045
#> 6  0.416   0.110   1.630  -1.726
```

This worked. Next we need to find the strong correlations. Now, we can use the correlation function to find the correlations. We then want to iterate through all pairs to check if the absolute value of the correlation is above our threshold. We use a loop for this. In our first attempt, we create a nested for loop where i is the index of one column and j is the index of the second column in the pair. We can see we must have some mistakes because we are getting pairs where i and j are equal to each other, and we are also getting zeros. Note how we are using print statements. This helps us to identify that we need to add parentheses for the first for loop, and we need to update j to start at i+1.

```
cor_mat <- cor(df_numeric)
for (i in 1:nrow(cor_mat) - 1){
  for (j in (i:nrow(cor_mat))){
    print(paste(i, j))
  }
}
#> [1] "0 0"
#> [1] "0 1"
#> [1] "0 2"
#> [1] "0 3"
#> [1] "0 4"
#> [1] "1 1"
#> [1] "1 2"
#> [1] "1 3"
#> [1] "1 4"
#> [1] "2 2"
#> [1] "2 3"
#> [1] "2 4"
#> [1] "3 3"
#> [1] "3 4"
```

Let's try again. This time we create a variable n which is the number of columns.

```
cor_mat <- cor(df_numeric)
n <- nrow(cor_mat)
for (i in 1:(n-1)){
  for (j in ((i+1):n)){
    print(paste(i, j))
  }
}
#> [1] "1 2"
#> [1] "1 3"
#> [1] "1 4"
#> [1] "2 3"
#> [1] "2 4"
#> [1] "3 4"
```

Next, we need to add an if statement to check whether there is a correlation above the given threshold. In this case, to check if our code is working correctly, we use a print statement for only those that meet the condition.

```
n <- nrow(cor_mat)
for (i in 1:(n-1)){
  for (j in ((i+1):n)){
    if(abs(cor_mat[i,j]) > 0.6){
      print(paste(i, j))
    }
  }
}
#> [1] "1 2"
```

We have sketched out our code more thoroughly, so we have a good idea of how we want to compute our result. We now move to writing our function. Importantly, we need to make sure that we use our input arguments now rather than our test values. In the subsequent version, we also add in a results data frame that we use to keep track of our results, and we add an additional argument for how to deal with NA values in calculating the correlations. The output matches what we expect for our test data frame.

```
#' Find pairs of columns with strong correlation
#'
#' @description Finds all pairs of numeric columns with strong Pearson
#' correlation and returns the pairs in a data frame
#'
#' @param df data frame
```

```
#' @param threshold positive numeric threshold value to define a
#' strong correlation as one with absolute value above the threshold
#' @param use an optional character string giving a method for
#' computing correlations in the presence of missing values.
#' This must be (an abbreviation of) one of the strings "everything",
#' "all.obs", "complete.obs", "na.or.complete", or
#' "pairwise.complete.obs".
#' @return data frame with one row for each pair of columns
#' with high correlation containing the names of the columns
#' and the corresponding correlation
high_cor <- function(df, threshold = 0.6, use = "everything"){

  # create result data frame
  res <- data.frame(name1 = vector("character"),
                    name2 = vector("character"),
                    cor = vector("numeric"))

  # subset to numeric columns
  df_numeric <- select_if(df, is.numeric)

  # find correlations and variable names
  cor_mat <- cor(df_numeric, use = use)

  # go through pairs to find those with high correlations
  n <- nrow(cor_mat)
  for (i in 1:(n-1)){
    for (j in ((i+1):n)){
      if(abs(cor_mat[i,j]) > threshold){
        res <- add_row(res,
                       name1 = colnames(cor_mat)[i],
                       name2 = colnames(cor_mat)[j],
                       cor = cor_mat[i,j])
      }
    }
  }
  return(res)
}
high_cor(test_df)
#>   name1 name2   cor
#> 1    V1    V2 0.901
```

We can prevent unexpected behavior of our functions by using stop() functions to limit a function to be run on certain types of arguments. This is helpful
if other people will use your function or if you might forget any assumptions

you built into the function. The `stop()` function stops the execution of the current expression and returns a message. In the following example, we check to make sure that the point given is a numeric vector. Further, we check to see whether the vector has length 0 and return 0 if it does.

```
#' Distance to the origin
#'
#' @description Calculates the distance from a single numeric vector
#' to the origin
#'
#' @param pt1 numeric vector
#' @param dist_fun function to compute the distance with, default is
#' Euclidean distance
#' @return the distance from pt1 to origin in the same dimension
dist_to_origin <- function(pt1, dist_func = euclidean_dist){

  # check format of input
  if(!(is.vector(pt1) & is.numeric(pt1))){
    stop("pt1 must be a numeric vector")
  }
  if(length(pt1) == 0){
    return(0)
  }

  # calculate the distance
  origin <- rep(0, length(pt1))
  return(dist_func(pt1, origin))
}
```

18.3.1 Unit Tests

We know our function `high_cor()` works on a single example. To thoroughly test our functions, we want to run them on several different input values. These types of tests are called *unit tests*. We try to vary these test values to cover a wide range of possibilities. For example, for a numeric argument, test positive and negative input values. For a vector input, test an empty vector, a vector of length 1, and a vector with multiple values. If you discover an error, we need to go back to debugging mode to resolve it.

To test our function, we use the **testthat** package (Wickham 2011). This includes several functions that can check our expectations. For example, there is the `expect_equal(object, expected)` function which checks whether object matches `expected` up to a given numeric tolerance. If we want to only check the values of our objects but not the attributes, we can set the argument `ignore_attr = FALSE`. Other functions from this package are expect_error(object) which can be used to test that an error message was returned and expect_true(object) which can be used to test whether a condition is met.

```
testthat::expect_equal(paste0("A","B"), "AB")
testthat::expect_true(mean(c(1,2,3)) > 1)
```

In the following code chunk, we demonstrate some tests for the `dist_to_origin()` function. Our tests here focus on the format of the vector. We should test each function separately, so we would write a separate batch of tests for the Euclidean distance function.

```
# check error message for character vector
expect_error(dist_to_origin(c("A")),
                     "pt1 must be a numeric vector")

# check error message for not a vector
expect_error(dist_to_origin(matrix(0)),
                     "pt1 must be a numeric vector")

# check for empty numeric vector
testthat::expect_equal(dist_to_origin(vector("numeric")), 0)

# check length 1 vector
testthat::expect_equal(dist_to_origin(c(2)), 2)

# check length 3 vector
testthat::expect_equal(dist_to_origin(c(2,8.5,3)), 9.233093,
                     tolerance = 0.0001)
```

18.3.2   Practice Question

Following are a series of tests for the function `high_cor()` with different data frame sizes and types of columns. Unfortunately, not all of the tests are working. Use your debugging skills to fix the function to pass the tests and write at least one additional test.

```
# mixed data frame - should return a data frame with three columns
expect_equal(high_cor(test_df),
             data.frame(name1 = "V1", name2 = "V2",
                     cor = 0.9011631), tolerance = 0.001)
```

```
# change threshold - lower, should have three pairs
expect_equal(high_cor(test_df, 0.2)$cor,
            c(0.9011631, 0.31765407, 0.30748633),
            tolerance = 0.001)

# change threshold - higher, should be empty
expect_equal(high_cor(test_df, 0.95)$cor, vector("numeric"),
            tolerance = 0.001)

# single numeric column - should return an empty data frame
expect_equal(high_cor(test_df[,4:5])$cor, vector("numeric"))

# single row - should return an empty data frame
expect_equal(high_cor(test_df[1,])$cor, numeric())
```

18.4 Exercises

For each question, be sure to document your function(s) using roxygen style documentation.

1. Standardizing a variable means subtracting the mean and then dividing through by the standard deviation. Create a function called `standardize_me()` that takes a numeric vector as an argument, and returns the standardized version of the vector. Write at least three unit tests to check that the result is correct.

2. Suppose we have two binary vectors x and y each of length n. Let m_1 be the number of indices where x or y has a 1 and m_2 be the number of indices where both x and y equal 1. For example, if x <- (1,1,0) and y <- c(0,1,0) then $m_1 = 2$ and $m_2 = 1$. The Jaccard distance is defined as $1 - m_2/m_1$ and measures the dissimilarity between two binary vectors. Write a function `jaccard_dist()` that takes in two binary vectors and returns the Jaccard distance between the two.

3. For this question we use a subset of the `pain` data from the **HDSinRdata** package. Recall, that this data contains binary variables representing where people experienced pain. Write a function that takes in a data frame with all binary columns and returns a matrix with the Jaccard distance between all observations. That is, if D is the returned matrix, then D[i,j] is the Jaccard distance between

observation i and observation j. Apply your function to the pain
data and plot the distribution of these distances.

```
library(HDSinRdata)
#> Warning: package 'HDSinRdata' was built under R version
 ↳  4.4.1
pain_sub <- pain[1:500,]
```

4. The function in the following code chunk is supposed to take in a
   positive integer and calculate how many positive integer divisors it
   has (other than 1 and itself). However, the function is not getting
   the right results. Debug the function. Then, think about ways you
   could improve this function by changing the structure, documentation, and adding argument checks.

```
total <- 0
divisors <- function(x){
  for(i in 1:x){
    if (i %% x){
      total <- total + 1
      i <- i + 1
    }
  }
  return(total)
  }

divisors(2)
#> [1] 1
divisors(6)
#> [1] 5
```

5. In this problem, you create our own summary table. To start, create
   a function that takes in a data frame and returns a summary table
   that reports the mean and standard deviation for all continuous variables and the count and percentage for all categorical variables. An
   example is given in Figure 18.1. Call your function on the NHANES
   dataset with the columns selected in the subsequent code to match
   what is shown in the figure.

```
nhanes_df <- NHANESsample %>%
  select(c(AGE, SEX, LEAD, HYP, SMOKE))
```

Variable	Level	Summary Statistic
AGE	-	49.178 (17.776)
SEX	Male	16468 (52.7%)
	Female	14797 (47.3%)
LEAD	-	1.805 (1.813)
HYP	-	0.553 (0.497)
SMOKE	NeverSmoke	15087 (48.3%)
	QuitSmoke	8861 (28.3%)
	StillSmoke	7317 (23.4%)

Figure 18.1: Example Summary Table.

19

Case Study: Designing a Simulation Study

Simulation studies are an ideal setting for utilizing functions. When conducting a simulation study, we often need to generate data, run statistical methods, and collect results, and we replicate this for a large number of simulations. Functions will ensure that we can write cleaner and reproducible code. In this case study, we will write the code for a simulation study that is based on the analysis by Hastie, Tibshirani, and Tibshirani (2020), which compared different methods for sparse regression. For our purposes, we will focus on the comparison between lasso and ridge regression, introduced in Chapter 15.

Our goal is to understand the predictive power of the two models for different data settings. We will generate our training and test data using the following data generating mechanism which relies on the number of observations n, the number of predictors p, the sparsity $s \leq p$, predictor correlation level ρ, and ν signal-to-noise ratio.

1. We define a vector of coefficients $\beta \in \mathbb{R}^p$ which has its first s components equal to 1 and the rest equal to 0. Note that our model will not have an intercept.

2. We draw the rows of the predictor matrix $X \in \mathbb{R}^{n \times p}$ from a multivariate normal distribution $N_p(0, \Sigma)$, where $\Sigma \in \mathbb{R}^{p \times p}$ has entry (i, j) equal to $\$\rho\{|i - j|\}$.

3. We draw the outcome $y \in \mathbb{R}^n$ from a normal distribution $N(X\beta, \sigma^2 I)$, where $\sigma^2 = \frac{\beta\Sigma\beta}{\nu}$. This ensures that the data has signal-to-noise ratio, defined as $\text{Var}(x^T\beta)/\text{Var}(\sigma^2)$, equal to ν.

After generating our data, we will use 5-fold cross-validation to fit a lasso or ridge regression model on the training data to get estimated coefficients $\hat{\beta}$. Last, we will predict on the withheld test set. The evaluation metrics we are interested in are the time to fit the model (in seconds), the relative test error

$$\text{RTE} = \frac{(\hat{\beta} - \beta)^T \Sigma (\hat{\beta} - \beta) + \sigma^2}{\sigma^2},$$

and the proportion of variance explained

$$PVE = 1 - \frac{(\hat{\beta} - \beta)^T \Sigma (\hat{\beta} - \beta) + \sigma^2}{\beta^T \Sigma \beta + \sigma^2}.$$

In Hastie, Tibshirani, and Tibshirani (2020), they vary all five parameters n, p, s, ρ, and ν to observe how the data generation impacts these metrics.

19.1   Outlining Our Approach

Before coding our method, let's recap the steps we will need to perform for a single simulation and practice top-down programming. In a single simulation, we need to generate our training and test data, fit our models, and store the results in a way that we can use later. There are two potential sketches of how we can program this code shown in Figure 19.1. Take a look at the differences. In the first, we are storing the data we generate and have a separate function for each method. In the second, we have a function that calculates our end metrics for an inputted model, and we have a function that runs through the different methods. A benefit of the first approach is that it will be more flexible; if we think of another method we want to compare, we would be easily able to add it without having to re-run any other code. A benefit of the second approach is that we are ensuring that the results stored for each method are the same. Of course, you could also do a hybrid between the two and use a metrics function in the first approach.

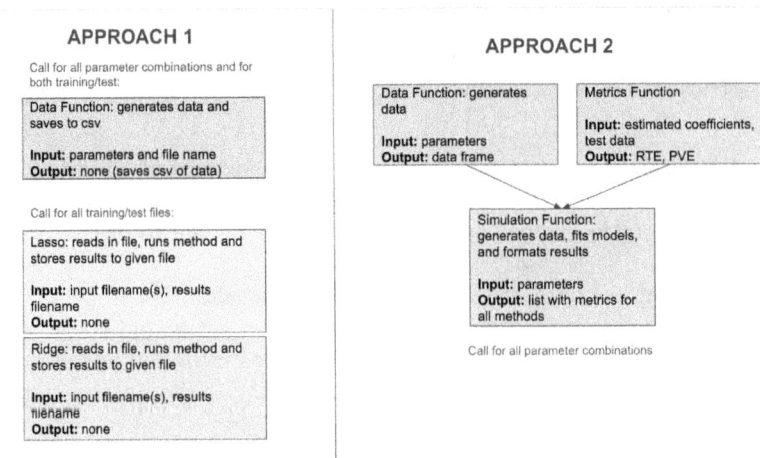

Figure 19.1: Example Approaches to Sketching out Functions.

Let's take a closer look at the second approach. For our metrics function, we have missed some inputs we will need. In particular, in order to calculate our end metrics, we will need to know the true coefficients β, the covariance matrix Σ, and the level of noise σ. Therefore, rather than returning a data frame, we will return a list that will contain X, y, and these values. For the first approach, this would require saving this information in a text file. Comparing between our two options, we will implement the second approach that does not store data. Another thing we can notice in our current sketch is that we likely want to store the results as a csv file, so rather than returning a list, we should return a vector that will correspond to a row in this file. Our final sketch is shown in Figure 19.2.

FINAL APPROACH

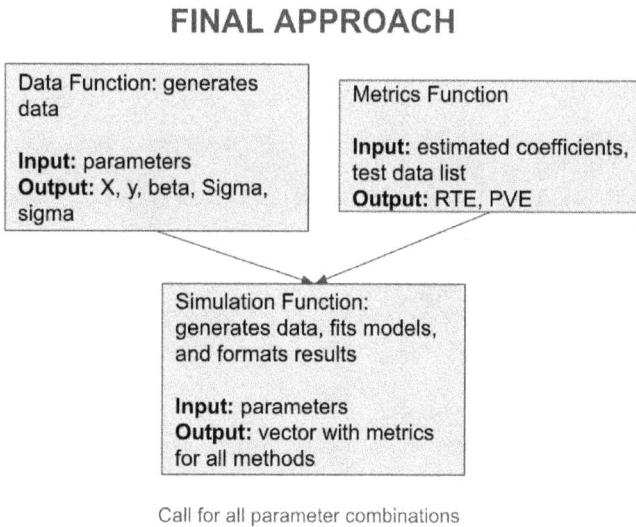

Figure 19.2: Updated Function Sketch.

19.2 Coding Our Simulation Study

We first load in the packages we will use. We will use the **MASS** package for the mvrnorm() function, which generates data from a multivariate normal distribution, we will use the **glmnet** package to implement our lasso and ridge models, and we will use the **tidyverse** and **patchwork** packages for summarizing and plotting the results.

```
library(MASS)
library(tidyverse)
library(patchwork)
library(glmnet)
```

We start by writing our function to generate our data. Our input here will be the parameters n, p, s, ρ, and ν and our output will be a list.

```
#' Simulate data
#'
#' @param n Number of observations
#' @param p Number of variables
#' @param s Sparsity level (number of non-zero coefficients)
#' @param snr Signal-to-noise ratio
#' @param rho Predictor correlation level
#' @return List containing simulated covariate matrix `X`,
#' outcome vector `y`, true coefficient vector `beta`,
#' covariate matrix `Sigma`, and variance of y `sigma`
simulate_data <- function(n, p, s, snr, rho) {

  # Generate covariance matrix
  cov_mat = matrix(0, nrow = p, ncol = p)
  for (row in 1:p) {
    for (col in 1:p) {
      cov_mat[row, col] = rho^(abs(row-col))
    }
  }

  # Generate X
  x <- mvrnorm(n=n, mu=rep(0,p), Sigma = cov_mat)

  # Generate beta values
  b <- rep(0, p)
  b[1:s] <- 1

  # find values
  mu <- x %*% b
  intercept <- -mean(mu)

  # Calculate variance
  var <- as.numeric((t(b) %*% cov_mat %*% b)/snr)

  # Generate y values
```

```
y <- mvrnorm(mu = mu, Sigma = var*diag(n))

    return(list(X = x, y = y, beta = b, Sigma = cov_mat, sigma = var))
}
```

Next, we will write a function for our model metrics. The only input we need from our model is the estimated coefficients. Otherwise, all of the information comes from the data we generate with the function we just wrote. We will utilize this list format to extract the values needed for our formulas.

```
#' Return model metrics
#'
#' @param coef_est Vector with estimated coefficients
#' @param test_data Withheld test set (`simulate_data()` output)
#' @return Vector with relative test error (RTE) and proportion
#' of variance explained (PVE).
get_metrics <- function(coef_est, test_data) {

  # Extract out values needed
  coef_true <- test_data$beta
  Sigma <- test_data$Sigma
  var_y <- test_data$sigma

  # Calculate relative test error
  RTE <- (t(coef_est - coef_true) %*% Sigma %*%
            (coef_est - coef_true) + var_y) /
          var_y

  # Calculate PVE
  # Proportion of variance explained
  PVE <- 1 - (t(coef_est - coef_true) %*% Sigma %*%
              (coef_est - coef_true) + var_y) /
    (var_y + t(coef_true %*% Sigma %*% coef_true))


  return(c(RTE = RTE, PVE = PVE))
}
```

Next, we will write a function that takes in the given parameters, fits the two models, and outputs the evaluation metrics. In this case, we will let the parameters be a named vector that contains all the components needed for the data simulation. We will also include an optional argument to set the random seed. In the code below, we find the time it takes to fit each model using `Sys.time()`. This function finds the current system time. Therefore, we can find the difference between them using the `difftime()` function. We also make sure to format the lasso and ridge results in the same manner.

```
#' Model selection simulation
#'
#' @param params named vector containing all parameters needed for
#' data generation (rho, snr, n, p, s)
#' @param seed (optional) random seed to set before setting folds,
#' by default not used
#' @return Vector with parameter values, results
model_selection <- function(params, seed = NULL) {

  # Extract out parameters
  n <- params['n']
  p <- params['p']
  s <- params['s']
  snr <- params['snr']
  rho <- params['rho']

  # Generate training and test data
  train <- simulate_data(n, p, s, snr, rho)
  test <- simulate_data(n, p, s, snr, rho)

  # Set folds, if needed
  if (!is.null(seed)){
    set.seed(seed)
  }
  k <- 5
  folds <- sample(1:k, nrow(train$X), replace=TRUE)

  # Lasso model
  start_lasso <- Sys.time()
  lasso_cv <- cv.glmnet(train$X, train$y, nfolds = k, foldid = folds,
                        alpha = 1, family = "gaussian",
                      intercept=FALSE)
  lasso_mod <- glmnet(train$X, train$y, lambda = lasso_cv$lambda.min,
                      alpha = 1, family = "gaussian", intercept=FALSE)
  end_lasso < Sys.time()

  # Get lasso results
  lasso_time <- as.numeric(difftime(end_lasso, start_lasso,
                                    units = "secs"))
  lasso_results <- c(lasso_time,
```

```
                    get_metrics(coef(lasso_mod)[-1], test))
  names(lasso_results) <- c("lasso_sec", "lasso_RTE", "lasso_PVE")

  # Ridge model
  start_ridge <- Sys.time()
  ridge_cv <- cv.glmnet(train$X, train$y, nfolds = k, foldid = folds,
                        alpha = 0, family = "gaussian",
                        intercept=FALSE)
  ridge_mod <- glmnet(train$X, train$y, lambda = ridge_cv$lambda.min,
                      alpha = 0, family = "gaussian", intercept=FALSE)
  end_ridge <- Sys.time()

  # Get ridge results
  ridge_time <- as.numeric(difftime(end_ridge, start_ridge,
                                    units = "secs"))
  ridge_results <- c(ridge_time,
                    get_metrics(coef(ridge_mod)[-1], test))
  names(ridge_results) <- c("ridge_sec", "ridge_RTE", "ridge_PVE")

  # Full results
  res <- c(n, p, s, snr, rho, lasso_results, ridge_results)

  return(res)
}
```

19.3 Results

Now it's time to run our simulation! We first need to find the combinations of parameters we want to use in our simulation design. In our case, we will set $n = 500$, $\rho = 0.35$, and $s = 10$. We will vary $p \in \{50, 100\}$ and the signal-to-noise ratio $\nu \in \{0.1, 0.5, 1.5\}$. We also want to run each possible combination of parameters ten times so that we can average across the results. We use the expand.grid() function to create a matrix that contains a row for each simulation.

```
# Set up parameter grid
rho_grid <- c(0.35)
snr_grid <- c(0.1, 0.5, 1.5)
n_grid <- c(500)
```

```
p_grid <- c(50, 100)
s_grid = c(10)
iter_grid <- 1:5
param_grid <- expand.grid(rho = rho_grid, snr = snr_grid, n = n_grid,
                          p = p_grid, s = s_grid, iter = iter_grid)

# convert to numeric
param_grid <- as.matrix(param_grid)
head(param_grid)
#>        rho snr   n   p  s iter
#> [1,] 0.35 0.1 500  50 10    1
#> [2,] 0.35 0.5 500  50 10    1
#> [3,] 0.35 1.5 500  50 10    1
#> [4,] 0.35 0.1 500 100 10    1
#> [5,] 0.35 0.5 500 100 10    1
#> [6,] 0.35 1.5 500 100 10    1
```

Recall that our main function took in a named vector that contained all needed parameters. This allows us to use an `apply()` function to run our simulation. In order to summarize by method, we pivot the results to a longer form with a column for method.

```
# Run experiments
results <- apply(param_grid, 1, model_selection) %>% t()

# Convert to long data frame
results <- as.data.frame(results) %>%
  pivot_longer(cols = starts_with(c("lasso", "ridge")),
               names_to = c("method", ".value"), names_sep="_")
```

Finally, we summarize our results. For example, we can create a table with the average time for each method grouped by the data dimensions. We observe that ridge regression was slower on average than lasso.

```
avg_time <- results %>%
  group_by(method, n, p) %>%
  summarize(avg_seconds = round(mean(sec),3)) %>%
  ungroup()
avg_time
#> # A tibble: 4 x 4
#>   method     n     p avg_seconds
#>   <chr>  <dbl> <dbl>       <dbl>
```

```
#> 1 lasso     500     50       0.019
#> 2 lasso     500    100       0.03
#> 3 ridge     500     50       0.022
#> 4 ridge     500    100       0.045
```

We can also create summary plots of our evaluation metrics similar to Hastie, Tibshirani, and Tibshirani (2020). To do so, we create one last function that will create a plot of the relative test error and percentage of variance explained across different signal-to-noise ratios. This allows us to regenerate this plot for different parameter settings.

```
#' Generate RTE and PVE plots for a given set of parameters
#'
#' @param results Data frame with simulation results
#' @param n_input Number of observations
#' @param p_input Number of variables
#' @param s_input Sparsity level
#' @return ggplot object
generate_plot <- function(results, n_input, p_input, s_input) {

  setting <- results %>%
    filter(n == n_input, p == p_input, s == s_input) %>%
    group_by(method, snr) %>%
    summarize(mean_RTE = mean(RTE, na.rm = TRUE),
              sd_RTE = sd(RTE, na.rm = TRUE),
              mean_PVE = mean(PVE, na.rm = TRUE),
              sd_PVE = sd(PVE, na.rm = TRUE))

  rte_plot <- ggplot(setting) +
    geom_point(aes(x = snr, y = mean_RTE, color = method)) +
    geom_errorbar(aes(x = snr, ymin = mean_RTE - sd_RTE,
                      ymax = mean_RTE + sd_RTE, color = method),
                  alpha = 0.8, width = 0.2) +
    geom_line(aes(x = snr, y = mean_RTE, color = method)) +
    theme_bw() +
    theme(legend.position = "bottom") +
    labs(x = "SNR", y = "RTE", color = "")


  pve_plot <- ggplot(setting) +
    geom_point(aes(x = snr, y = mean_PVE, color = method)) +
    geom_errorbar(aes(x = snr, ymin = mean_PVE - sd_PVE,
                      ymax = mean_PVE + sd_PVE, color = method),
```

```
                     alpha = 0.8, width = 0.2) +
    geom_line(aes(x = snr, y = mean_PVE, color = method)) +
    theme_bw() +
    theme(legend.position = "bottom") +
    labs(x = "SNR", y = "PVE", color = "")

  full_plot <- rte_plot + pve_plot

  return(full_plot)
}
generate_plot(results, 500, 50, 10)
```

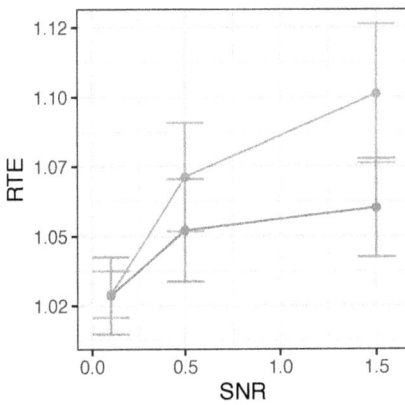 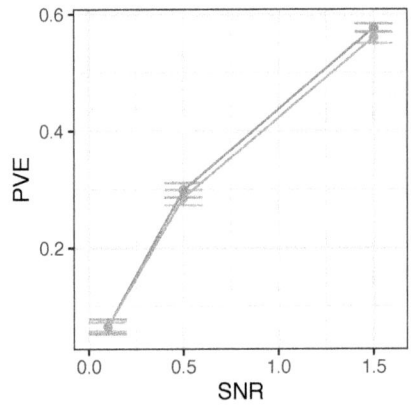

```
generate_plot(results, 500, 100, 10)
```

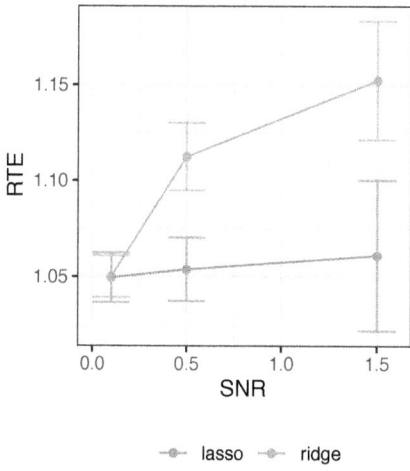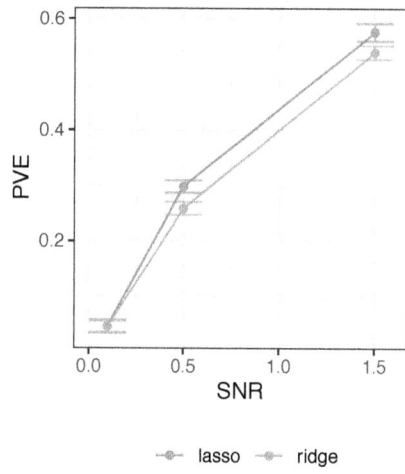

20

Writing Efficient Code

When we talk about efficient code, we are talking about computational efficiency or writing code that is fast to execute. For this topic, we need to peek under the hood to consider how R is implementing our code in order to understand what can slow down our code. We use the **microbenchmark** package (Mersmann 2023) to time our code execution. For demonstration, we use a subset of the `pain` dataset from the **HDSinRdata** package.

```r
library(microbenchmark)
library(HDSinRdata)
library(tidyverse)

data(pain)
pain <- pain %>%
  select(-c(BMI, GH_MENTAL_SCORE, GH_PHYSICAL_SCORE,
                  PROMIS_PAIN_BEHAVIOR)) %>%
  na.omit()
```

The function `Sys.time()` returns the current system time. This allows us to find the net time required to execute a chunk of code. For example, the following code finds how long it takes to loop through the data to find the number of people who had an improvement in pain.

```r
start_time <- Sys.time()
num <- 0
for (i in 1:nrow(pain)){
  if (pain$PAIN_INTENSITY_AVERAGE[i] <=
      pain$PAIN_INTENSITY_AVERAGE.FOLLOW_UP[i]){
    num <- num + 1
  }
}
end_time <- Sys.time()
end_time - start_time
#> Time difference of 0.0198 secs
```

Using `Sys.time()` is a simple approach to time our code. The function `microbenchmark()` from the **microbenchmark** package allows us to replicate an expression multiple times to get an average execution time. We can pass multiple expressions to this function and specify a unit of measurement and number of times to replicate each expression.

```
microbenchmark(first expression, second expression, units ="ms",
  times = 10)
```

For example, we time the same expression as previously using this package. This time we get some summary statistics in milliseconds. We used the default 100 times to replicate this expression.

```
microbenchmark( pain_inc = {
  num <- 0
  for (i in 1:nrow(pain)){
    if (pain$PAIN_INTENSITY_AVERAGE[i] <=
        pain$PAIN_INTENSITY_AVERAGE.FOLLOW_UP[i]){
      num <- num + 1
    }
  }
}, unit = "ms")
#> Warning in microbenchmark(pain_inc = {: less accurate nanosecond
↳ times
#> to avoid potential integer overflows
#> Unit: milliseconds
#>      expr  min   lq mean median   uq  max neval
#>  pain_inc 16.1 16.5 18.3   17.8 18.4 65.3   100
```

20.1   Use Fast and Vectorized Functions

R is known as a slower programming language. In part, R sacrifices computation time to make it more welcoming to new programmers. However, not all of R is actually written in R. Many functions that are in base R are actually written in C or Fortran. These functions are significantly faster than if we wrote them ourselves. When possible, we should use base R functions rather than writing our own. Let's take a look at the difference in time when we write our own summation function compared to using the `sum()` function.

```
my_sum <- function(x){
  out <- 0
```

```
  for (i in 1:length(x)){
    out <- out + x[i]
  }
  return(out)
}


x <- 1:100000
microbenchmark(sum_function = my_sum(x),
               builtin_sum = sum(x),
               unit = "ms")
#> Unit: milliseconds
#>          expr      min       lq     mean   median       uq    max neval
#>  sum_function 2.182020 2.2e+00 2.298618 2.252089 2.292556 3.61021
#>  100
#>   builtin_sum 0.000041 8.2e-05 0.000474 0.000082 0.000246 0.00459
#>  100
```

This also simplifies our code to a single line. Looking back at our first example, we can also simplify our code. We did not need to loop through our data. Instead, we should use a vectorized approach that checks for pain improvement across all observations and then sum up the TRUE/FALSE values.

```
microbenchmark({
  vector_pain = sum(pain$PAIN_INTENSITY_AVERAGE <=
                      pain$PAIN_INTENSITY_AVERAGE.FOLLOW_UP)
}, unit = "ms")
#> Unit: milliseconds
#>
#> expr
#> {      vector_pain = sum(pain$PAIN_INTENSITY_AVERAGE <=
#> pain$PAIN_INTENSITY_AVERAGE.FOLLOW_UP) }
#>    min     lq    mean median     uq    max neval
#> 0.0155 0.0156 0.0168 0.0157 0.0159 0.0459    100
```

This is much faster. Loops are notoriously slow in R so you often hear the advice to avoid loops. Using apply functions like `apply()` and `sapply()` are loop-hiding functions. Using these functions instead of an explicit loop doesn't improve the efficiency of our code except that by using these functions we often simplify our code as a byproduct of rewriting our code.

The true functions that can improve efficiency over loops are *vectorized* functions, which can be evaluated on a vector of values. Vectorizing our code means that we are thinking about a vector approach rather than computing something for each element of the vector and looping through these values. A vectorized function returns output that is the same dimensions as the input and operates on these elements in an efficient manner.

The following code chunk shows a simple example of comparing taking the square root of each individual element or calling the `sqrt()` function, which is a vectorized function. Vectorized functions still have to operate on each element, but that loop is often written in C or Fortran rather than R making it significantly faster, so this is a special case where we can utilize the speed of some functions.

```
microbenchmark(loop_sqrt = {
  for (i in 1:length(x)){
    x[i] <- sqrt(x[i])
  }
  }, sqrt = sqrt(x), unit = "ms")
#> Unit: milliseconds
#>       expr   min   lq  mean median    uq   max neval
#> loop_sqrt 4.427 4.55 4.946  4.659 4.978 11.98   100
#>      sqrt 0.099 0.14 0.159  0.151 0.165  0.41   100
```

20.1.1 Practice Question

First, read the documentation of the function `tapply()`. This is another function in the apply function library that was not covered in Chapter 17. Rewrite the following code without using a loop using the `tapply()` function. Would you expect this approach to be faster? Why or why not?

```
mean_pain <- c()
pat_races <- unique(pain$PAT_RACE)

for (r in pat_races){
  mean_pain[r] <- mean(pain$PAIN_INTENSITY_AVERAGE[pain$PAT_RACE ==
  ↪ r])
}
```

20.2 Avoid Copies and Duplicates

Another aspect of our programs that can slow down our operations is any time we need to create a large object. Look at the following code. First, we create a matrix m. We then create a matrix n that is equal to m. Last, we update n by taking the logarithm of all elements plus one, differentiating it from m. R creates copies upon modification. This means that when we initialize n we have not actually created a second matrix in memory. Instead, we have two names for the same matrix. On the third line, we want to update n, so we need to actually create a second matrix that is different from m.

```
m <- matrix(rpois(100000, 6), ncol=1000)
n <- m
n <- log(n + 1)
```

This is different from the subsequent code which updates m itself. In this case, R can modify the matrix in place by going through each element and updating its value rather than creating a new matrix. As the size of our data grows, creating copies can be expensive. Imagine, m being a large genetic dataset with RNA-sequencing data. First, this object may take up a lot of memory, so creating a copy may mean we could run out of memory. Second, copying over all this information is expensive.

```
m <- log(m + 1)
```

Let's consider another case. In the following code, we have two functions that both find the proportion of people within 1, 2, and >2 standard deviations from the mean for one of the PROMIS instrument variables. When we input pain as an argument to the first function, we do not create a copy of it since we haven't modified the data frame. However, once we create a new column, this means that we have to copy the full data frame. The second function instead takes in a single column, requiring us to copy only this information. The difference in execution time shows an edge to the second method, but the difference is small. This indicates that actually computing this new column and finding the proportions takes more time than the duplication.

```
code_promis1 <- function(df){
  # create new column with categories
  df$PAIN_PHYSICAL_FUNCTION_CUT <- case_when(
    abs(df$PROMIS_PHYSICAL_FUNCTION-50) <= 10 ~ "<= 1SD",
    abs(df$PROMIS_PHYSICAL_FUNCTION-50) <= 20 ~ "<= 2 SD",
    TRUE ~ "> 2SD")

  # get proportions
  res <- prop.table(table(df$PAIN_PHYSICAL_FUNCTION_CUT))
  return(res)
}
```

```
code_promis2 <- function(v){
  # create new column with categories
  v <- case_when(
    abs(v-50) <= 10 ~ "<= 1SD",
    abs(v-50) <= 20 ~ "<= 2 SD",
    TRUE ~ "> 2SD")

  # get proportions
  res <- prop.table(table(v))
  return(res)
}


microbenchmark(code_promis1(pain),
               code_promis2(pain$PROMIS_PHYSICAL_FUNCTION),
               unit = "ms")
#> Unit: milliseconds
#>                                           expr   min    lq  mean median
#>                             code_promis1(pain) 0.644 0.693 0.813  0.715
#>   code_promis2(pain$PROMIS_PHYSICAL_FUNCTION) 0.619 0.665 0.770
#> ↳ 0.685
#>     uq  max neval
#>  0.756 3.77   100
#>  0.708 3.93   100
```

Another time when we create copies of objects is when we modify their size. Functions like `cbind()`, `rbind()`, and `c()` create a new object that needs to copy over information to create one vector, matrix, or data frame. If we know the size of the final vector, matrix, or data frame, we can pre-allocate that space and fill in values. This means that the computer won't have to repeatedly find more space. For example, take a look at the two ways to simulate a random walk in one dimension in the following code chunk. In the first method, the length of the vector v changes on each iteration of the loop, whereas in the second v always has length n.

```
rw1 <- function(n){
  v <- c(0)
  for (i in 2:n){
    v[i] <- v[i-1] + rbinom(1, 1, 0.5)
  }
  return(v)
}
```

```
rw2 <- function(n){
  v <- rep(0, n)
  for (i in 2:n){
    v[i] <- v[i-1] + rbinom(1, 1, 0.5)
  }
}


microbenchmark(rw1(10000), rw2(10000), unit="ms")
#> Unit: milliseconds
#>         expr  min   lq mean median   uq   max neval
#>   rw1(10000) 5.10 5.25 5.84   5.36 5.92 10.64   100
#>   rw2(10000) 4.27 4.35 4.68   4.39 4.58  9.32   100
```

This also works for data frames or matrices. In the following code chunk, we generate a random matrix in three ways. The first creates the matrix with a single line, the second initializes an empty matrix and then fills in each row, and the last dynamically updates the size of the matrix on each iteration.

```
random_mat1 <- function(n){
  m <- matrix(sample(1:3, n^2, replace = TRUE), nrow = n)
  return(m)
}


random_mat2 <- function(n){
  m <- matrix(nrow = n, ncol = n)
  for (i in 1:n){
    m[i,] <- sample(1:3, n, replace = TRUE)
  }
}


random_mat3 <- function(n){
  m <- NULL
  for (i in 1:n){
    m <- rbind(m, sample(1:3, n, replace = TRUE))
  }
  return(m)
}


microbenchmark(random_mat1(100),
               random_mat2(100),
               random_mat3(100),
               unit = "ms")
#> Unit: milliseconds
```

```
#>                expr    min    lq  mean median    uq  max neval
#>   random_mat1(100) 0.226 0.244 0.265  0.249 0.256 1.59   100
#>   random_mat2(100) 0.494 0.508 0.544  0.521 0.536 2.52   100
#>   random_mat3(100) 1.075 1.163 1.384  1.189 1.233 5.01   100
```

This demonstrates that if you need to update the values of a vector, matrix, or data frame, try to do as much reassignment at once. For example, changing the whole column at a time is better than changing the individual values. This avoids additional copies.

20.2.1   Practice Question

The following code fits a linear model for each racial group and records the coefficient. Rewrite this code so that we pre-allocate the results vector and use the **microbenchmark** to compare the efficiency between the two approaches.

```
coefs <- c()
pat_races <- unique(pain$PAT_RACE)
for (r in pat_races){
  df <- pain[pain$PAT_RACE == r, ]
  if (nrow(df) > 3){
    new_coef <- lm(PROMIS_DEPRESSION ~ PROMIS_ANXIETY,
                 data = df)$coefficients[2]
    coefs <- c(coefs, new_coef)
  }
}
```

20.3   Parallel Programming

Another approach to make our code more efficient is using parallel processing. When we run loops in R, only one iteration is run at a time. For example, the following code runs a random walk 100 times in serial. Parallel processing allows us to execute multiple calls to this function at the same time. This is done by running these processes on separate cores, or processors, on your machine. For example, if we had six cores available, we would be able to run 1/6 of the replications on each processor and reduce our overall computation time. The **parallel** package (R Core Team 2024) contains functions to implement parallel processing on different operating systems. Unfortunately, this functionality is often not supported within RStudio and is not covered in this book. We recommend using the mclapply() function from the **parallel** package to implement parallel processing using forking. This does not work on Windows but is much simpler to implement. For parallel processing on Windows, we recommend looking into the socket approach using the parLapply() function in the **parallel** package.

```
replicate(100, rw1(1000))
```

20.4 Exercises

1. The following code chunk includes four attempts to create a new column LOWER_BACK to the pain data. Note that the second and third attempts are vectorized, whereas the first and fourth are not. Time each approach and order the approaches from fastest to slowest.

```r
# Attempt 1: loop
pain$LOWER_BACK <- vector(mode="logical", length=nrow(pain))
for (i in 1:nrow(pain)) { # for every row
  if ((pain$X218[i] == 1) | (pain$X219[i] == 1)) {
    pain$LOWER_BACK[i] <- TRUE
  } else {
    pain$LOWER_BACK[i] <- FALSE
  }
}

# Attempt 2: logic
pain$LOWER_BACK <- ((pain$X218[i] == 1) |
                    (pain$X219[i] == 1))

# Attempt 3: which
pain$LOWER_BACK <- FALSE
true_ind <- which((pain$X218[i] == 1) | (pain$X219[i] == 1))
pain$LOWER_BACK[true_ind] <- TRUE

# Attempt 4: apply
back_pain <- function(x){
  if((x['X218'] == 1) | (x['X219'] == 1)){
    return(TRUE)
  }
```

```
    return(FALSE)
  }
pain$BACK_PAIN <- apply(pain, 1, back_pain)
```

2. Examine the following code and determine what is being computed. Then, rewrite the code to make it more efficient. Use the **microbenchmark** package to compare the execution time, and explain why your approach is more efficient.

```
n <- 100000
x1 <- rnorm(n, 10, 1)
x2 <- rbinom(n, 1, 0.2)
y <- numeric(0)

for (i in 1:n){
  if (x2[i] == 1){
    y[i] <- rnorm(1,2 *x1[i], 0.7)
  } else{
    y[i] <- rnorm(1, 1+3*x1[i], 0.2)
  }
}
df <- data.frame(x1 = x1, x2 = x2, y = y)
```

3. Suppose we want to find the five most frequently reported pain regions by racial group. Code your solution (a) using at least one loop and (b) pivoting the data on the body region columns and then using **dplyr** functions to summarize. Compare the efficiency of both approaches.

Part VI

Extra Topics

21

Expanding Your R Skills

Throughout this book, we have covered some popular packages as well as many of the specific functions from these packages. However, it would be impossible to cover all of the packages, functions, and options that are available in R. In this chapter, we talk about how to use new packages, interpret error messages, debugging, and overall good programming practices to help you take your R programming to the next level.

21.1 Reading Documentation for New Packages

As you start to apply the tools from this book to your own work or in new settings, you may need to install and use new packages or encounter some unexpected errors. Practicing reading package documentation and responding to error messages helps you expand your R skills beyond the topics covered here. We demonstrate these skills using the **stringr** package (Wickham 2022), which is a package that is part of the **tidyverse** and has several functions for dealing with text data.

```
library(tidyverse)
library(HDSinRdata)
```

Every published package has a CRAN website. This website contains a reference manual that contains the documentation for the functions and data available in the package. Most often, the website also includes useful vignettes that give examples of how to use the functions in the package. The site also tells you what the requirements for using the package are, who the authors of the package are, and when the package was last updated. For example, take a look at the CRAN site for **stringr**[1] and read the vignette "Introduction to String R"[2].

We use the **stringr** package to demonstrate cleaning up text related to a

---

[1] https://cran.r-project.org/web/packages/stringr/index.html
[2] https://cran.r-project.org/web/packages/stringr/vignettes/stringr.html

PubMed search query for a systematic review. An example search query is given in the following code chunk and is taken from Gue et al. (2021). Our first goal is to extract the actual search query from the text along with all the terms used in the query. We can assume that the search query is either fully contained in parentheses or is a sequence of parenthetical phrases connected with AND or OR. Our goal is to extract the search query as well as all the individual search terms used in the query, but we have to get there in a series of steps.

```
sample_str <- " A systematic search will be performed in PubMed,
Embase, and the Cochrane Library, using the following search query:
('out-of-hospital cardiac arrest' OR 'OHCA') AND ('MIRACLE 2' OR
'OHCA' OR 'CAHP' OR 'C-GRAPH' OR 'SOFA' OR 'APACHE' OR 'SAPS' OR
'SWAP' OR 'TTM')."
```

The first thing we want to do with the text is clean up the white space by removing any trailing, leading, or repeated spaces. In our example, the string starts with a trailing space and there are also multiple spaces right before the search query. Searching for "white space" in the **stringr** reference manual, we find the `str_trim()` and `str_squish()` functions. Read the documentation for these two functions. You should find that `str_squish()` is the function we are looking for and that it takes a single argument.

```
sample_str <- str_squish(sample_str)
sample_str
#> [1] "A systematic search will be performed in PubMed, Embase, and
↳  the Cochrane Library, using the following search query:
↳  ('out-of-hospital cardiac arrest' OR 'OHCA') AND ('MIRACLE 2' OR
↳  'OHCA' OR 'CAHP' OR 'C-GRAPH' OR 'SOFA' OR 'APACHE' OR 'SAPS' OR
↳  'SWAP' OR 'TTM')."
```

21.2 Trying Simple Examples

The premise of testing a function on a single string is a good example of starting with a simple case. Rather than applying your function to your full dataset right away, you want to first make sure that you understand how it works on a simple example and on which you can anticipate what the outcome should look like. Our next task is to split the text into words and store this as a character vector. Read the documentation to determine why we use the `str_split_1()` function. We then double-check that the returned result is indeed a vector and print the result.

```
sample_str_words <- str_split_1(sample_str, " ")
class(sample_str_words)
#> [1] "character"
sample_str_words
#>  [1] "A"                "systematic"       "search"
#>  [4] "will"             "be"               "performed"
#>  [7] "in"               "PubMed,"          "Embase,"
#> [10] "and"              "the"              "Cochrane"
#> [13] "Library,"         "using"            "the"
#> [16] "following"        "search"           "query:"
#> [19] "('out-of-hospital" "cardiac"          "arrest'"
#> [22] "OR"               "'OHCA')"          "AND"
#> [25] "('MIRACLE"        "2'"               "OR"
#> [28] "'OHCA'"           "OR"               "'CAHP'"
#> [31] "OR"               "'C-GRAPH'"        "OR"
#> [34] "'SOFA'"           "OR"               "'APACHE'"
#> [37] "OR"               "'SAPS'"           "OR"
#> [40] "'SWAP'"           "OR"               "'TTM')."
```

We now want to identify words in this vector that have starting and/or end parentheses. The function `grepl()` takes in a character vector x and a pattern to search for. It returns a logical vector for whether or not each element of x has a match for that pattern.

```
grepl(sample_str_words, ")")
#> Warning in grepl(sample_str_words, ")"): argument 'pattern' has
#>   length
#> > 1 and only the first element will be used
#> [1] FALSE
```

That didn't match what we expected. We expected to have multiple TRUE/FALSE values outputted, one for each word. Let's read the documentation again.

21.3   Deciphering Error Messages and Warnings

The previous warning message gives us a good clue for what went wrong. It says that the inputted pattern has length >1. However, the pattern we gave it is a single character. In fact, we specified the arguments in the wrong order. Let's try again. This time we specify x and `pattern`.

```
grepl(x = sample_str_words, pattern = ")")
#>  [1] FALSE FALSE FALSE FALSE FALSE FALSE FALSE FALSE FALSE FALSE
#>  ↳ FALSE
#> [12] FALSE FALSE FALSE FALSE FALSE FALSE FALSE FALSE FALSE FALSE
#>  ↳ FALSE
#> [23]  TRUE FALSE FALSE FALSE FALSE FALSE FALSE FALSE FALSE FALSE
#>  ↳ FALSE
#> [34] FALSE FALSE FALSE FALSE FALSE FALSE FALSE FALSE  TRUE
```

That fixed it. However, it won't work if we change that to an opening parenthesis. Try it out for yourself to see this. The error message says that it is looking for an end parenthesis. In this case, the documentation does not help us. Let's try searching "stringr find start parentheses" using an online search engine. Our search results indicate that we may need to use backslashes to tell R to read the parentheses literally rather than as a special character used in a regular expression (a technique often referred to as "escaping" a character). Investigating the reason for an error, including using online material, is an important skill for a programmer to have.

```
grepl(x = sample_str_words, pattern = "\\(")
#>  [1] FALSE FALSE FALSE FALSE FALSE FALSE FALSE FALSE FALSE FALSE
#>  ↳ FALSE
#> [12] FALSE FALSE FALSE FALSE FALSE FALSE FALSE  TRUE FALSE FALSE
#>  ↳ FALSE
#> [23] FALSE FALSE  TRUE FALSE FALSE FALSE FALSE FALSE FALSE FALSE
#>  ↳ FALSE
#> [34] FALSE FALSE FALSE FALSE FALSE FALSE FALSE FALSE FALSE
```

When a function doesn't return what we expect it to, it is a good idea to first test whether the arguments we gave it match what we expect, then re-read the documentation, and then look for other resources for help. For example, we could check that `sample_str_words` is indeed a character vector, then re-read the **stringr** documentation, and then search our problem.

21.3.1 Debugging Code

The following code is supposed to extract the search query from the text as well as find the individual search terms used in the query. However, the code is incorrect. You can try out two test strings given to see why the code output is wrong. Practice reading through the code to understand what it is trying to do. The comments are there to help explain the steps, but you may also want to print the output to figure out what it is doing.

```
sample_strA <- " A systematic search will be performed in PubMed,
Embase, and the Cochrane Library, using the following search query:
('out-of-hospital cardiac arrest' OR 'OHCA') AND ('MIRACLE 2' OR
'OHCA' OR 'CAHP' OR 'C-GRAPH' OR 'SOFA' OR 'APACHE' OR 'SAPS' OR
'SWAP' OR 'TTM')."

sample_strB <- "Searches will be conducted in MEDLINE via PubMed, Web
of Science, Scopus and Embase. The following search strategy will be
used:(child OR infant OR preschool child OR preschool children OR
preschooler OR pre-school child OR pre-school children OR pre school
child OR pre school children OR pre-schooler OR pre schooler OR
children OR adolescent OR adolescents)AND(attention deficit disorder
with hyperactivity OR ADHD OR attention deficit disorder OR ADD OR
hyperkinetic disorder OR minimal brain disorder) Submitted "


sample_str <- sample_strB

# separate parentheses, remove extra white space, and split into words
sample_str <- str_replace(sample_str, "\\)", " \\) ")
sample_str <- str_replace(sample_str, "\\(", " \\( ")
sample_str <- str_squish(sample_str)
sample_str_words <- str_split_1(sample_str, " ")

# find indices with parentheses
end_ps <- grepl(x = sample_str_words, pattern = "\\)")
start_ps <- grepl(x = sample_str_words, pattern = "\\(")

# find words between first and last parentheses
search_query <- sample_str_words[which(end_ps)[1]:which(start_ps)[1]]
search_query <- paste(search_query, collapse=" ")
search_query
#> [1] ") adolescents OR adolescent OR children OR schooler pre OR
 ↳   pre-schooler OR children school pre OR child school pre OR
 ↳   children pre-school OR child pre-school OR preschooler OR children
 ↳   preschool OR child preschool OR infant OR child ("

# find search terms
search_terms <- str_replace_all(search_query, "\\)", "")
search_terms <- str_replace_all(search_query, "\\(", "")
sample_terms <- str_squish(search_query)
```

```
search_terms <- str_split_1(search_terms, " AND | OR ")
search_terms
#>  [1] ") adolescents"      "adolescent"        "children"
#>  [4] "schooler pre"       "pre-schooler"       "children school
 ↳ pre"
#>  [7] "child school pre"   "children pre-school" "child pre-school"
 ↳
#> [10] "preschooler"        "children preschool" "child preschool"
 ↳
#> [13] "infant"             "child "
```

21.4   General Programming Tips

As you write more complex code and functions, we want to focus on practicing good programming principles. This helps when you need to share or update your code or when you inevitably run into errors or unexpected behavior. Following are some general programming tips and how they relate to communication and debugging.

1. **Consistent Naming.** Use consistent and informative names for your objects and functions. For example, you can see that within this text we have only used lowercase letters, underscores (_), and occasionally numbers in our names. These names should also be informative and unique. This makes it easier to check for typos or duplicate names when debugging. When debugging, check that you haven't used the same name for different objects or different names for the same object. You can do this by using the ls() function to find all current objects or by checking your environment pane.

```
# Recommended
ages <- c(65, 33, 27, 88)
age_mean <- mean(ages)

# Not recommended
x <- c(65, 33, 27, 88)
x1 <- mean(ages)
```

2. **Make Your Code Readable.** Readable code requires several elements of communication. As with writing an essay, we need to break our code into digestible and structured pieces. First, code should be broken into blocks, using white space to separate steps, and should use correct levels of indentation (one extra level of indentation for each new loop, if/else statement, or function). This means that closing curly braces should be on their own line indicating the end of the block. This makes it easy to check that all parentheses (), brackets [], and curly braces {} match. Additionally, you should use line breaks to avoid going over 80 characters on a single line of code. RStudio has an option to re-format or re-indent your code under the Code tab.

Besides the structure of your code, writing helpful comments and function documentation is key for making your code readable. A good rule of thumb is to write comments for yourself a year from now; you might remember the project goal, but you won't remember what x represents. You likely do not need a comment for every line of code but you might need comments to explain the overall goal of a code block or to clarify lines that aren't self-explanatory.

In the following code, we have not used indentation. This makes it hard to see the structure of the code such as what lines of code are in the loop or if statement. The function does not have any roxygen documentation. However, we have added too many comments. The comments here are repetitive with the code. Last, we named the function `unique()`, which is already a function in R.

```
# Not recommended
unique <- function(x){
y <- c() # results
if (length(x) == 0){ # check length 0
return(NULL)} # return NULL
for(i in length(x)){  # loop through x
if(!(x[i] %in% y)){  # check if x[i] in y
y <- c(y, x[i]) }} # add x[i] to y
return(y) # return y
}
```

We rewrite the function addressing these comments. The end result is much easier to read.

```
#' Find unique elements of a vector
#'
#' @param x vector
#' @return new vector with duplicates removed
own_unique <- function(x){

  # check for empty vector
  if (length(x) == 0){
    return(NULL)
  }

  # otherwise y will be unique values
  y <- c()

  for(i in 1:length(x)){
    # if value of x is not in y, we add it
    if(!(x[i] %in% y)){
      y <- c(y, x[i])
    }
  }

  return(y)
}
```

3. **Don't Repeat Yourself.** Repeating code increases the likelihood of errors. Additionally, it makes it hard to update our code later on. When we find ourselves repeating code, we should use a function. If you find yourself repeating constants, you should define these values as an object. The subsequent code uses a single line of code to convert categorical variables to factors and stores a vector of which columns are categorical.

```
dry_df <- data.frame(age = ages,
                     tb = c(1, 0, 0, 0),
                     heart_rate = c(60, 82, 76, 72),
                     gender = c("Female", "Male", "Nonbinary",
                                "Female"))

# convert factor variables
cat_vars <- c("tb", "gender")
dry_df[cat_vars] <- lapply(dry_df[cat_vars], factor)
```

4. **Practice Reading Documentation.** Whenever you are using a new function, you should read the documentation first. When debugging, you should check that the input arguments to a function match what is expected and check the examples. Reading these examples also helps when writing your own documentation so you can better understand how to communicate to your audience.

5. **Start Simple, Build Up.** If we write a large amount of code at once and then it fails to work, it's hard to understand what went wrong. Instead, we should build up our code or functions in small steps and check it after each step. When it comes to testing code, a good mantra is *test early and test often*. So, try to avoid writing too much code before running and checking that the results match what you expect. If you do end up writing a big chunk of code, you can localize your error by checking the values of objects at different points.

6. **Get Comfortable Asking for Help.** In software engineering, it's a known tip to have a rubber ducky (or other adorable object) at your desk to talk through your code. Having to verbalize and explain your approach can be really helpful for debugging. R's error messages can sometimes hint at what the error might stem from, but they are not always direct. Searching for error messages you don't understand might give you a better understanding of the problem.

21.5 Exercises

These exercises focus on reading function documentation and debugging.

1. Suppose we want to replace the words "Thank you" in the following string with the word "Thanks". Why does the following code fail? How can we correct it?

```
string <- "Congratulations on finishing the book!
Thank you for reading it."
str_sub(string, c(35, 42)) <- "Thanks"
string
#> [1] "Congratulations on finishing the bThanks"
#> [2] "Congratulations on finishing the book! \nTThanks"
```

2. The subsequent code uses the NHANESsample data from the **HDSin-**

Rdata package. The goal of the code is to plot the worst diastolic blood pressure reading against the worst systolic blood pressure reading for each patient, colored by hypertension status. However, the code currently generates an error message. What is wrong with the code? There are four errors for you to identify and fix.

```
data(NHANESsample)

nhanes_df <- NHANESsample %>%
  mutate(worst_DBP = max(DBP1, DBP2, DBP3, DBP4),
     worst_SBP = max(SBP1, SBP2, SBP3, SBP4))

ggplot() %>%
  geom_point(data = nhanes_df,
               aes(x = worst_SBP, y = worst_DBP),
               color = HYP)
```

3. The following code uses the `breastcancer` data from the **HDSin-Rdata** package. The goal is to create a logistic regression model for whether or not the diagnosis is benign or malignant and then to create a calibration plot for the model, following the code from Chapter 14. Debug and fix the code. Hint: there are three separate errors.

```
data(breastcancer)

model <- glm(diagnosis ~ smoothness_worst + symmetry_mean +
          texture_se + radius_mean,
        data = breastcancer, family = binomial)

pred_probs <- predict(model)

num_cuts <- 10
calib_data <-  data.frame(prob = pred_probs,
               bin = cut(pred_probs, breaks = num_cuts),
               class = mod_start$y)

calib_data <- calib_data %>%
       group_by(bin) %>%
       summarize(observed = sum(class)/n(),
             expected = sum(prob)/n(),
             se = sqrt(observed * (1 - observed) / n())))
```

```
calib_data

ggplot(calib_data) +
  geom_abline(intercept = 0, slope = 1, color = "red") +
  geom_errorbar(aes(x = expected, ymin = observed - 1.96 *
  ↪ se,
                  ymax = observed + 1.96 * se),
            color = "black", width = .01)+
  geom_point(aes(x = expected, y = observed)) +
  labs(x="Expected Proportion", y="Observed Proportion") +
  theme_minimal()
```

22

Writing Reports in Quarto

This chapter introduces you to Quarto, which is a document format that combines Markdown text with code. Writing in Quarto helps you write reproducible code and create polished reports to present your analyses. Quarto is similar to R Markdown but is compatible with other programming languages and incorporates some new features that make it easier to write nice reports. If you already use R Markdown, it's easy to transition to Quarto.

```
library(tidyverse)
library(HDSinRdata)
library(kableExtra)
library(gt)

data(NHANESsample)
```

22.1 Starting a Quarto File

To create a Quarto file, you need to have RStudio installed as an application. For more recent versions of RStudio, Quarto is already installed. If you have an older version, you can install Quarto[1]. We also recommend the **kableExtra** package (Zhu 2021) for formatting your tables.

Now that you have these packages downloaded, opening a new Quarto file is very similar to opening a new R file, which was covered in Chapter 1. Just like opening a new R file, you'll want to go to File -> New File, but instead of selecting 'R Script', you'll now select 'Quarto Document...'. This should bring up a window that looks like Figure 22.1.

First, enter a title of your choosing for your report and type your name in the Author field (note that you can always change these later) and then click on OK. You should also choose which type of file you would like to generate, a PDF, HTML, or WORD document. This opens an Quarto file that has

---

[1]https://quarto.org/docs/get-started/

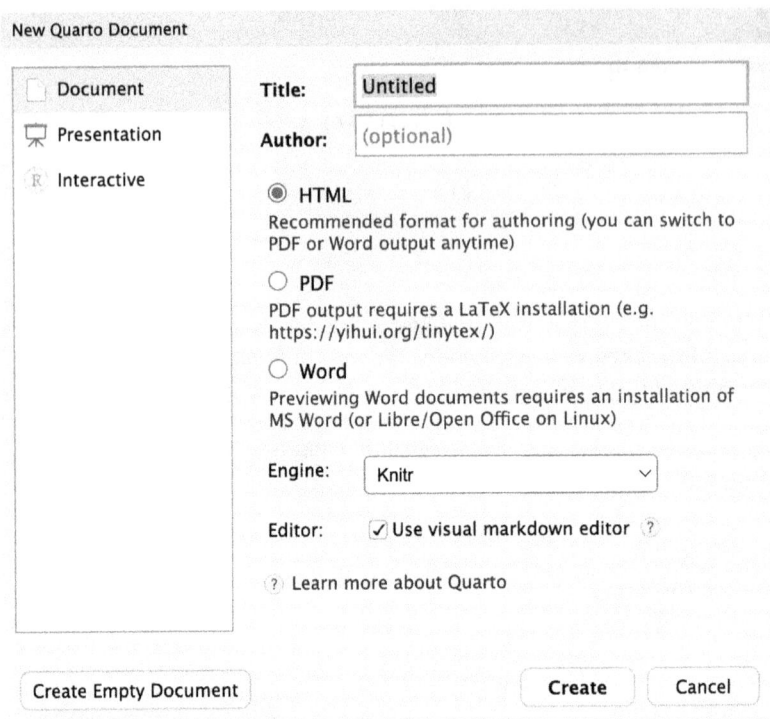

Figure 22.1: Creating a New R Quarto Document.

the extension .qmd. Make sure to save this file with a suitable name in your desired location on your computer by selecting File -> Save, and then you're ready to start writing your report! Your file should now look like Figure 22.2.

At the top of this pane is a toggle between source and visual mode. In visual mode, we can see that we have a text toolbar including options to bold text or add a list. If we switch to source mode, our text reveals the underlying Markdown in Figure 22.3 and the toolbar disappears. This chapter focuses on teaching you to edit in source mode, but you can always switch to visual mode if you prefer.

We write all of the text and code that we would like to include in your report in this .qmd file, and then produce a nicely formatted report from this file by 'rendering' the file. We can either render to HTML, PDF, or WORD by clicking on the Render button ⇨ Render from the toolbar at the top of the page. To update our format from PDF, we change the text in the top block to format: html or format: word.

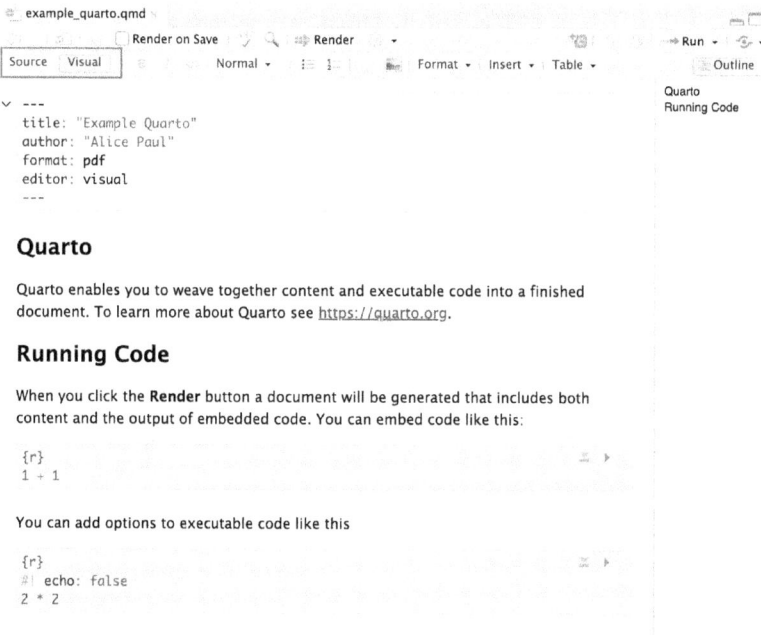

Figure 22.2: A New Quarto Document.

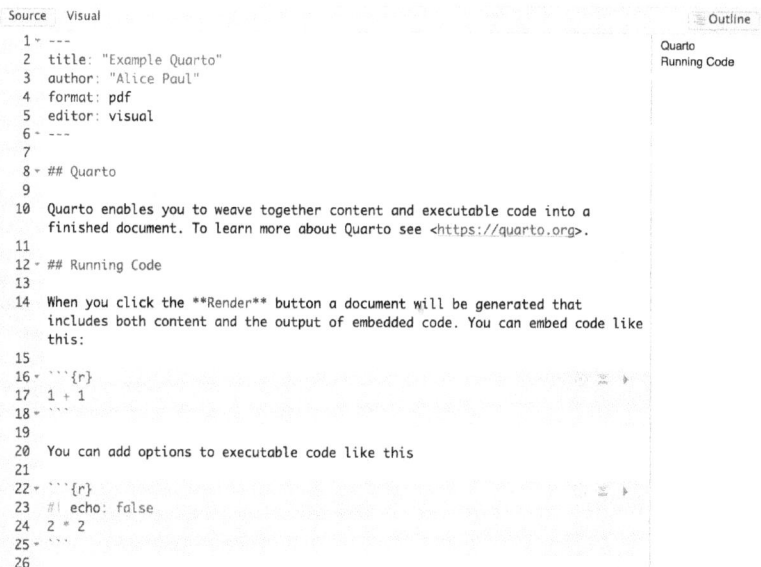

Figure 22.3: Source Mode.

22.1.1 Adding Code Chunks

Each of the darker gray rectangles is called a code chunk. All of the code used to generate your report goes in these chunks, and all of your text writing goes outside of them. Each code chunk starts with ```` ```{r} ```` and ends with ```` ``` ````. To create a chunk, you can

- click on this green "add chunk" symbol 🟢 ▾ in the toolbar at the top of the page,
- type ```` ```{r} ```` and ```` ``` ````, or
- use the keyboard shortcut **Ctrl + Alt + I** (**Cmd + Option + I** on Macs).

To run the code in a chunk, you can either use the keyboard shortcut **Ctrl + Enter** (**Cmd + Return** on Mac), or you can use one of the following buttons at the top right of the chunks: ⬇ runs all chunks above the current chunk, and ▶ runs the current chunk.

22.1.2 Customizing Chunks

You can specify whether you want to include the code and/or its various output in your final report by adding the following commands, preceded by `#|`, at the top of the code chunk:

- `include: false` makes it so that neither code nor its output appears in your report.
- `echo: false` makes it so that the output of the code but not the code itself appears in your report.
- `message: false`, `warning: false`, and `error: false` make it so that messages, warnings, and errors (respectively) that are generated from the code in the chunk won't appear in your report.

Here we can also specify a label for our code chunk. For example, if we wanted to include a chunk that displayed our code but did not execute it, we could include the following.

```{r}
#| label: example-chunk
#| echo: true
#| eval: false

x <- c(1,2,3)
```

To apply the same options to all chunks in the document at once, you can add them to the first chunk at the very top of your Quarto that has the label `label: setup` using the `knitr::opts_chunk$set()` function. These are called the global settings. For example, using the following code for your first code chunk ensures that none of the errors, warnings, or messages from any of the code chunks appear in your final report. It is also good practice to load all the packages you are using for your report within this first code chunk using the `library()` function. For example, we load the **tidyverse** and **HDSinRdata** packages.

```{r}
#| label: setup
#| include: false
knitr::opts_chunk$set(echo = TRUE, warning = FALSE,
 error = FALSE, echo = FALSE)
library(tidyverse)
library(HDSinRdata)
```

If you want to display the code for your report in a code appendix, you can easily do this by creating an empty code chunk at the end of your .qmd file that looks like the following. This finds all other chunks and displays the code.

```{r ref.label = knitr::all_labels()}
#| echo: true
#| eval: false
```

22.2 Formatting Text in Markdown

To add text to your report, you can simply type directly into the Quarto file, between the code chunks. This code is formatted using Markdown, which allows us to specify how to format and display the text when it is knit. For example, adding a single asterisk * on either side of some text italicizes it, while adding a double asterisk ** on either side of text makes it bold. To indicate code, you can use backticks `.

```
regular text regular text
```

```
*italicized text* italicized text
```

```
**bold text** bold text
```

```
`code text` code text
```

To create headers and sections, you can add the # symbol in front of your text. Adding more of these symbols makes the headers smaller, which is useful for making sub-headers (see Figure 22.4).

```
# Header
```

```
## Smaller Header
```

```
### Even Smaller Header
```

Header

Smaller Header

Even Smaller Header

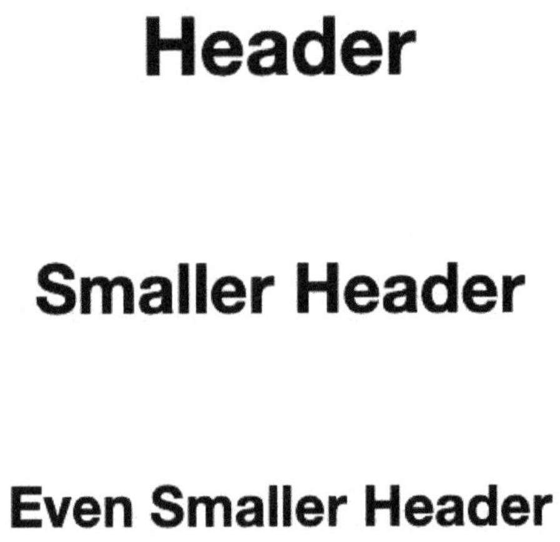

Figure 22.4: Example Header Sizes.

You can also add links [text](www.example.com) and images ![alt text](#fig-label image.png). In the latter example, fig-label becomes the label of the image we can use to cross-reference it, while image.png is the image file name (see Figure 22.5).

Example link.[2]

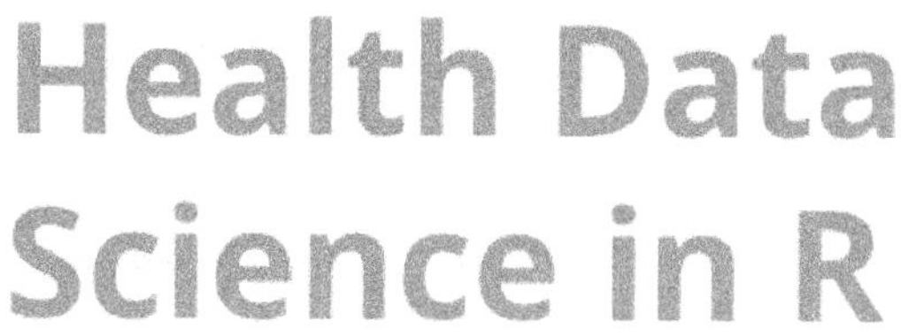

Health Data Science in R

Figure 22.5: Example Image.

The Markdown Guide[3] has a great cheat sheet[4] as well as more resources for formatting Markdown text.

You can also have inline R code by using single backticks around your code `{r} max(c(1,2,3))`. The code must start with r to be run when knit. This allows you to reference variables in your text. For example, we could display the variance of a column in our data without having to copy the value over `{r} round(var(cars$speed),2)`.

22.3 Formatting Figures and Tables

Often, you'll want to include figures generated by your code in your report, and you can customize these figures by changing the chunk options for the chunks that produce them. To change the size of a figure, you can add in the chunk option fig-width: 3 with your desired size in inches. To add a nice caption to a figure in your report, you can add fig-cap : 'Your Desired Caption.' option. To name a figure, you want to start your label with fig- such as fig-myfigure.

By default, the figures generated by your code chunks are allowed to 'float' in Quarto. This means that the figures might move away from where they were coded or referenced in the final report. To prevent this behavior, you can

---

[2]https://alicepaul.github.io/health-data-science-using-r/
[3]https://www.markdownguide.org/
[4]https://www.markdownguide.org/cheat-sheet/

customize the chunk that contains the code to produce the figure by adding `fig-pos : 'H'` to that chunk's options. If you want to prevent floating for all figures, add `fig-pos : 'H'` to the first code chunk in the file (the one that starts with the `knitr::opts_chunk$set()` function). Figure 22.6 shows the resulting figure.

```{r}
#| label: fig-myfigure
#| fig-width: 3
#| fig-pos: "H"
#| fig-cap: "Blood Lead Level by Education"

data(NHANESsample)
ggplot(subset(NHANESsample, !is.na(EDUCATION))) +
geom_boxplot(aes(x = EDUCATION, y = log(LEAD)), fill = 'lightblue') +
theme_bw() +
labs(y = "Log Blood Lead Level") +
scale_x_discrete("Education")
```

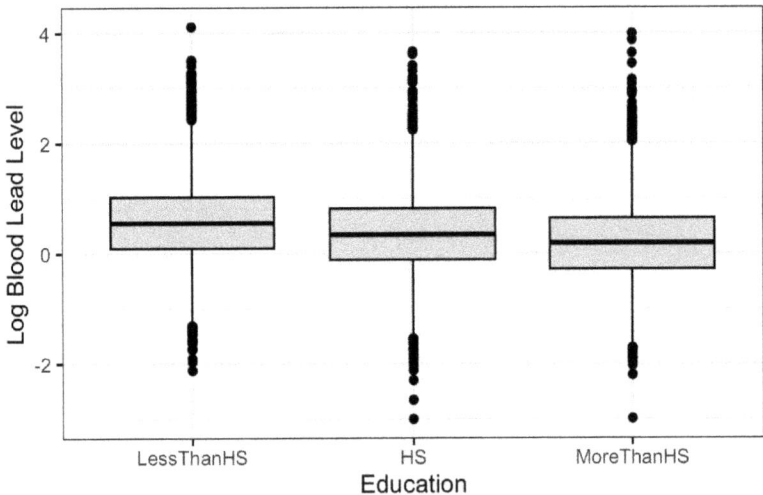

Figure 22.6: Blood Level by Education.

If you want to make data frames, matrices, or tables from your raw R output more polished and aesthetically pleasing, you can use the **gt** and **kableExtra** packages. Be sure to load the package you are using to the code chunk at the top of your Quarto file that contains all of your libraries.

Table 22.1

```
NHANESsample %>%
  select(AGE, SEX, EDUCATION, INCOME, LEAD) %>%
  head()
#>    AGE    SEX  EDUCATION INCOME LEAD
#> 1   77   Male MoreThanHS   5.00  5.0
#> 2   49   Male MoreThanHS   5.00  1.6
#> 3   37   Male MoreThanHS   4.93  2.4
#> 4   70   Male LessThanHS   1.07  1.6
#> 5   81   Male LessThanHS   2.67  5.5
#> 6   38 Female MoreThanHS   4.52  1.5
```

To demonstrate the abilities of these packages, let's suppose that we wanted to display the head of the first few columns of the NHANESsample data from the **HDSinRdata** package. The following code produces the corresponding output in the knitted pdf report. You can see in Table 22.1 that it essentially just copies the raw output from R, which is rather messy.

We use the kable() and kable_styling() functions from the **kableExtra** package to produce a more nicely formatted table. The kable() function generates a table from a data frame. The kable() function allows you to specify some display options for your table. For example, you can add a caption to your table using the caption argument, and you can change the names of the columns in the table using the col.names argument. The kable_styling() has additional options available. Similar to the fig-pos = H command described for figures in the previous section, adding "HOLD_position" to the kable_styling() function prevents the table from floating on the report; adding "scale_down" scales the table so that it fits in the margins of the paper. The updated code and output are shown in the following code chunk and Table 22.2. See the documentation for the kable() and kable_styling() functions for more options available.

```
NHANESsample %>%
  select(AGE, SEX, EDUCATION, INCOME, LEAD) %>%
  head() %>%
  kable(col.names = c("Age", "Sex", "Education Level",
                      "Poverty Income Ratio", "Lead Level")) %>%
  kable_styling(latex_options = c("scale_down", "HOLD_position"))
```

Table 22.2: Head of the NHANES Sample Dataset

Age	Sex	Education Level	Poverty Income Ratio	Lead Level
77	Male	MoreThanHS	5.00	5.0
49	Male	MoreThanHS	5.00	1.6
37	Male	MoreThanHS	4.93	2.4
70	Male	LessThanHS	1.07	1.6
81	Male	LessThanHS	2.67	5.5
38	Female	MoreThanHS	4.52	1.5

In the previous code chunk, we saw that `kable()` produces a much nicer table in the knitted pdf that is more suitable for a data analysis report. In Chapter 4, we also introduced the **gt** package. This package is an alternative package to **kableExtra** that allows you to format each part of the table and includes options for formatting the columns, adding footers or subtitles, or grouping your table. See the package introduction[5] for more details about this package. An example `gt` table is given in the following code and output. Note that for tables, we want to start our label with `tbl-` and can include a caption using the `tbl-cap` option. The resulting table from the code chunk below is shown in Figure 22.7.

```{r}
#| label: tbl-gt-ex
#| tbl-cap: "Head of the NHANES Sample Data"

NHANESsample %>%
select(AGE, SEX, EDUCATION, INCOME, LEAD) %>%
head() %>%
gt() %>%
tab_header(title = "Head of the NHANES Sample Data") %>%
cols_label(AGE ~ "Age",
    SEX ~ "Sex",
    EDUCATION ~ "Education Level",
    INCOME ~ "Poverty Income Ratio",
    LEAD ~ "Lead Level")
```

22.3.1 Using References

Quarto automatically adds figure and table numbers to the figures and tables in your report. By using the label options, we can also reference our figures

---

[5]https://gt.rstudio.com/articles/intro-creating-gt-tables.html

Head of the NHANES Sample Dataset				
Age	Sex	Education Level	Poverty Income Ratio	Lead Level
77	Male	MoreThanHS	5.00	5.0
49	Male	MoreThanHS	5.00	1.6
37	Male	MoreThanHS	4.93	2.4
70	Male	LessThanHS	1.07	1.6
81	Male	LessThanHS	2.67	5.5
38	Female	MoreThanHS	4.52	1.5

Figure 22.7: Head of the NHANES Sample Data.

easily by using their names: `@fig-figname` or `@tab-tablename`. The knitted pdf substitutes the appropriate figure or table number into your text. Additionally, we can reference sections by adding in labels to the section header. For example, we added the tag `#sec-awesome` for the section in the following text and can now reference it using `@sec-awesome`.

`## Awesome Stuff {#sec-awesome}`

22.4 Adding in Equations

Another useful option in Markdown is to add in mathematical equations. If you want to insert math equations, you can do so by writing LaTeX expressions. To write a math equation inline, you put a single dollar sign $ on either side of your equation, and to write a math equation on its own line, you put a double dollar sign $$ on either side of the equation, like so:

Here's an equation that is inline with the text: `$5x^2 + 9x^3$` produces $5x^2 + 9x^3$. On the other hand, here's an equation that is on its own line: `$$5x^2 + 9x^3$$` produces

$$5x^2 + 9x^3$$

Here is some other LaTeX notation that you should know in order to write common equations: * To create a fraction, type `\frac{numerator}{denominator}`. For example, `\frac{2}{3}` produces $\frac{2}{3}$. * To create a subscript, type `_`. For example, x_{2} produces x_2. * To create a superscript, type ^. For example, x^{2} produces x^2.

If you want to learn more about how to write in LaTeX, Art of Problem Solving[6] provides a great reference for LaTeX symbols, and Overleaf[7] provides a helpful introduction to LaTeX in general.

22.5 Exercises

The exercise for this chapter is to recreate this example pdf[8] created from an Quarto file. You will need to use the NHANESsample data from the **HDSinR-data** package.

---

[6]https://artofproblemsolving.com/wiki/index.php/LaTeX:Symbols
[7]https://www.overleaf.com/learn/latex/Tutorials#Learn_LaTeX_in_30_minutes
[8]https://github.com/alicepaul/health-data-science-using-r/blob/main/book/refs/example_quarto.pdf

References

Alter, Benedict J, Nathan P Anderson, Andrea G Gillman, Qing Yin, Jong-Hyeon Jeong, and Ajay D Wasan. 2021. "Hierarchical Clustering by Patient-Reported Pain Distribution Alone Identifies Distinct Chronic Pain Subgroups Differing by Pain Intensity, Quality, and Clinical Outcomes." *PLoS One* 16 (8): e0254862.

Baik, Yeonsoo, Hannah M Rickman, Colleen F Hanrahan, Lesego Mmolawa, Peter J Kitonsa, Tsundzukana Sewelana, Annet Nalutaaya, et al. 2020. "A Clinical Score for Identifying Active Tuberculosis While Awaiting Microbiological Results: Development and Validation of a Multivariable Prediction Model in Sub-Saharan Africa." *PLoS Medicine* 17 (11): e1003420.

Centers for Disease Control and Prevention (CDC). 1999-2018. "National Health and Nutrition Examination Survey Data (NHANES)." U.S. Department of Health and Human Services. http://www.cdc.gov/nchs/nhanes.htm.

———. 2021. "National Youth Tobacco Survey (NYTS)." U.S. Department of Health and Human Services. https://www.cdc.gov/tobacco/data_statistics/surveys/nyts/index.htm.

Di Lorenzo, Paolo. 2024. *Usmap: US Maps Including Alaska and Hawaii.* https://CRAN.R-project.org/package=usmap.

Fox, John, Sanford Weisberg, and Brad Price. 2023. *car: Companion to Applied Regression.* https://CRAN.R-project.org/package=car.

Friedman, Jerome, Robert Tibshirani, and Trevor Hastie. 2010. "Regularization Paths for Generalized Linear Models via Coordinate Descent." *Journal of Statistical Software* 33 (1): 1–22. https://doi.org/10.18637/jss.v033.i01.

Gue, Ying X., Krishma Adatia, Rahim Kanji, Tatjana Potpara, Gregory Y. H. Lip, and Diana A. Gorog. 2021. "Out-of-Hospital Cardiac Arrest: A Systematic Review of Current Risk Scores to Predict Survival." *American Heart Journal* 234: 31–41. https://doi.org/10.1016/j.ahj.2020.12.011.

Guidotti, Emanuele. 2022. "A Worldwide Epidemiological Database for COVID-19 at Fine-Grained Spatial Resolution." *Scientific Data* 9 (1): 112. https://doi.org/10.1038/s41597-022-01245-1.

Guidotti, Emanuele, and David Ardia. 2020. "COVID-19 Data Hub." *Journal of Open Source Software* 5 (51): 2376. https://doi.org/10.21105/joss.02376.

Hastie, Trevor, Robert Tibshirani, and Ryan Tibshirani. 2020. "Best Subset, Forward Stepwise or Lasso? Analysis and Recommendations Based on Extensive Comparisons." *Statistical Science* 35 (4).

Hazimeh, Hussein, Rahul Mazumder, and Tim Nonet. 2023. *L0Learn: Fast Algorithms for Best Subset Selection.* https://CRAN.R-project.org/pack age=L0Learn.

Hothorn, Torsten, Achim Zeileis, Richard W. Farebrother, and Clint Cummins. 2022. *lmtest: Testing Linear Regression Models.* https://CRAN.R-project. org/package=lmtest.

Huang, Ziyao. 2022. "Association Between Blood Lead Level with High Blood Pressure in US (NHANES 1999–2018)." *Frontiers in Public Health* 10: 836357.

Iannone, Richard, Joe Cheng, Barret Schloerke, Ellis Hughes, Alexandra Lauer, and JooYoung Seo. 2023. *gt: Easily Create Presentation-Ready Display Tables.* https://CRAN.R-project.org/package=gt.

Kortsmit, Katherine. 2023. "Abortion Surveillance—United States, 2021." *MMWR. Surveillance Summaries* 72.

Mersmann, Olaf. 2023. *Microbenchmark: Accurate Timing Functions.* https: //CRAN.R-project.org/package=microbenchmark.

Müller, Kirill. 2023. *Hms: Pretty Time of Day.* https://CRAN.R-project.org/ package=hms.

Neuwirth, Erich. 2022. *RColorBrewer: ColorBrewer Palettes.* https://CRAN .R-project.org/package=RColorBrewer.

Park-Lee, Eunice, Andrea S Gentzke, Chunfeng Ren, Maria Cooper, Michael D Sawdey, S Sean Hu, and Karen A Cullen. 2023. "Impact of Survey Setting on Current Tobacco Product Use: National Youth Tobacco Survey, 2021." *Journal of Adolescent Health* 72 (3): 365–74.

Pedersen, Thomas Lin. 2022. *patchwork: The Composer of Plots.* https://CR AN.R-project.org/package=patchwork.

R Core Team. 2024. *R: A Language and Environment for Statistical Computing.* Vienna, Austria: R Foundation for Statistical Computing. https: //www.R-project.org/.

Raifman, Julia, Kristen Nocka, David Jones, Jacob Bor, Sarah Lipson, Jonathan Jay, Megan Cole, et al. 2022. "COVID-19 US State Policy Database." Inter-university Consortium for Political; Social Research. http s://doi.org/10.3886/E119446V143.

Robin, Xavier, Natacha Turck, Alexandre Hainard, Natalia Tiberti, Frédérique Lisacek, Jean-Charles Sanchez, and Markus Müller. 2023. *pROC: Display and Analyze ROC Curves.* http://expasy.org/tools/pROC/.

Robinson, David, Alex Hayes, and Simon Couch. 2023. *broom: Convert Statistical Objects into Tidy Tibbles.* https://CRAN.R-project.org/package= broom.

Roser, Max, and Hannah Ritchie. 2013. "Maternal Mortality." https://ourw orldindata.org/maternal-mortality.

Schloerke, Barret, Di Cook, Joseph Larmarange, Francois Briatte, Moritz Marbach, Edwin Thoen, Amos Elberg, and Jason Crowley. 2021. *GGally: Extension to ggplot2.* https://CRAN.R-project.org/package=GGally.

Sjoberg, Daniel D., Joseph Larmarange, Michael Curry, Jessica Lavery,

Karissa Whiting, and Emily C. Zabor. 2023. *gtsummary: Presentation-Ready Data Summary and Analytic Result Tables.* https://CRAN.R-project.org/package=gtsummary.

Spinu, Vitalie, Garrett Grolemund, and Hadley Wickham. 2023. *lubridate: Make Dealing with Dates a Little Easier.* https://CRAN.R-project.org/package=lubridate.

Texas Health & Human Services Commission. 2016-2021. "Induced Terminations of Pregnancy." Texas Department of State Health Services. https://www.hhs.texas.gov/about/records-statistics/data-statistics/itop-statistics.

Venables, W. N., and B. D. Ripley. 2002. *Modern Applied Statistics with S.* Fourth Edition. New York: Springer. https://www.stats.ox.ac.uk/pub/MASS4/.

Warren, Michael S, and Samuel W Skillman. 2020. "Mobility Changes in Response to COVID-19." *arXiv Preprint arXiv:2003.14228.*

Wickham, Hadley. 2011. "Testthat: Get Started with Testing." *The R Journal* 3: 5–10. https://journal.r-project.org/archive/2011-1/RJournal_2011-1_Wickham.pdf.

———. 2016. *Ggplot2: Elegant Graphics for Data Analysis.* Springer-Verlag New York. https://ggplot2.tidyverse.org.

———. 2022. *stringr: Simple, Consistent Wrappers for Common String Operations.* https://CRAN.R-project.org/package=stringr.

———. 2023. *tidyverse: Easily Install and Load the Tidyverse.* https://CRAN.R-project.org/package=tidyverse.

Wickham, Hadley, and Jennifer Bryan. 2023. *readxl: Read Excel Files.* https://CRAN.R-project.org/package=readxl.

Wickham, Hadley, Romain François, Lionel Henry, Kirill Müller, and Davis Vaughan. 2023. *dplyr: A Grammar of Data Manipulation.* https://CRAN.R-project.org/package=dplyr.

Wickham, Hadley, Jim Hester, and Jennifer Bryan. 2023. *readr: Read Rectangular Text Data.* https://CRAN.R-project.org/package=readr.

Wickham, Hadley, Evan Miller, and Danny Smith. 2023. *haven: Import and Export 'SPSS', 'Stata' and 'SAS' Files.* https://CRAN.R-project.org/package=haven.

Wickham, Hadley, Davis Vaughan, and Maximilian Girlich. 2023. *tidyr: Tidy Messy Data.* https://CRAN.R-project.org/package=tidyr.

Yoshida, Kazuki, and Alexander Bartel. 2022. *Tableone: Create 'Table 1' to Describe Baseline Characteristics with or Without Propensity Score Weights.* https://CRAN.R-project.org/package=tableone.

Zhu, Hao. 2021. *kableExtra: Construct Complex Table with Kable and Pipe Syntax.* https://CRAN.R-project.org/package=kableExtra.

Index

For Product Safety Concerns and Information please contact our EU
representative GPSR@taylorandfrancis.com
Taylor & Francis Verlag GmbH, Kaufingerstraße 24, 80331 München, Germany

www.ingramcontent.com/pod-product-compliance
Lightning Source LLC
Chambersburg PA
CBHW060758220326
41598CB00022B/2483

9 7 8 1 0 3 2 7 2 9 9 3 0